# Metabolic Dysfunction-Associated Steatotic Liver Disease

Nahum Méndez-Sánchez • Xingshun Qi
Editors

# Metabolic Dysfunction-Associated Steatotic Liver Disease

## Prevalence, research insights and the future directions

Springer

*Editors*
Nahum Méndez-Sánchez
Faculty of Medicine
National Autonomous University
of Mexico
Mexico City, Mexico

Liver Research Unit
Medica Sur Clinic and Foundation
Mexico City, Mexico

Xingshun Qi
Department of Gastroenterology
General Hospital of Nor Theater
Command
Shenyang, China

ISBN 978-981-97-9521-5 ISBN 978-981-97-9519-2 (eBook)
https://doi.org/10.1007/978-981-97-9519-2



This Springer imprint is published by the registered company Springer Nature Singapore Pte Ltd.
The registered company address is: 152 Beach Road, #21-01/04 Gateway East, Singapore 189721, Singapore

# Preface

Welcome to the comprehensive exploration of metabolic dysfunction-associated steatotic liver disease (MASLD). In recent years, this condition has emerged as a significant health challenge worldwide, reflecting the alarming rise in metabolic disorders and their intricate relationship with liver health.

MASLD represent a paradigm shift in our understanding of liver disease, highlighting the multifaceted interplay between metabolic dysfunction, inflammation, and hepatic steatosis. As the global prevalence of obesity, diabetes, and other metabolic syndromes continues to surge, so does the incidence of this liver condition. This underscores the urgent need for a deeper understanding and effective management strategies to combat their impact on public health.

This book is the result of a collective effort to unravel the complexities surrounding MASLD. It offers an in-depth examination of their epidemiology, pathophysiology, clinical manifestations, diagnosis, and management strategies. Through the collaboration of esteemed experts in hepatology and allied disciplines, we aim to provide a multidisciplinary perspective that empowers healthcare professionals to tackle these conditions effectively.

The evolution of terminology from non-alcoholic fatty liver disease (NAFLD) to MASLD underscores a more nuanced understanding of this disease. By embracing these changes, we acknowledge the multifactorial nature of MASLD, characterized by intricate interactions between metabolic dysfunction, inflammation, and fibrosis.

In this book, readers will find a synthesis of cutting-edge research findings alongside practical insights drawn from clinical experience. From fundamental mechanisms to the latest diagnostic modalities and therapeutic interventions, our aim is to empower clinicians, researchers, and students with the knowledge and tools needed to confront the challenges posed by MASLD.

We extend our deepest gratitude to the contributors whose expertise and dedication have enriched this project. Their commitment to advancing the field of hepatology and improving patient care is truly commendable.

To healthcare professionals, researchers, and students, we offer this book as a valuable resource for understanding MASLD. May it serve as a catalyst for ongoing advancements in unraveling the complexities of these diseases, improving their management, and ultimately contributing to their prevention.

Mexico City, Mexico Nahum Méndez-Sánchez
Shenyang, China Xingshun Qi

# Contents

# Introduction of MASLD

# 1

Nahum Méndez-Sánchez, Mariana M. Ramírez-Mejía,
and Mohammed Eslam

## 1.1 Introduction

The historical trajectory of non-alcoholic fatty liver disease (NAFLD) reflects the evolving understanding of this disorder. Coined in 1980, the term NAFLD initially described a steatotic liver disease (SLD) unrelated to excessive alcohol consumption, delimiting a specific cluster of patients at that time [1]. In the current landscape of liver diseases, NAFLD has emerged as the predominant cause of chronic liver disease (CLD), affecting one third of global population [2]. Through the years, numerous investigations and clinical observations have deepened our understanding of NAFLD, revealing its complex pathogenesis, broad clinical spectrum and associated complications, making the term NAFLD outdated, not encompassing the complexity and multifaceted nature of the disease [3, 4].

N. Méndez-Sánchez (✉) · M. M. Ramírez-Mejía
Faculty of Medicine, National Autonomous University of Mexico, Mexico City, Mexico

Liver Research Unit, Medica Sur Clinic and Foundation, Mexico City, Mexico
e-mail: nmendez@medicasur.org.mx

M. Eslam
Storr Liver Centre, Westmead Institute for Medical Research, Westmead Hospital and University of Sydney, Westmead, NSW, Australia
e-mail: mohammed.eslam@sydney.edu.au

In recent years, a major paradigm shift has led to the introduction of the term metabolic dysfunction-associated fatty liver disease (MAFLD), which aims to more comprehensively understand and classify SLD [5–7]. This conceptual change emerged from the collective reflections of an international group of experts during a consensus conference held in 2020 [7]. Recognizing the need for a unified terminology that encompasses the various metabolic factors and associated liver disorders commonly observed in patients with NAFLD, MAFLD emerged as a more inclusive and contemporary term.

On this basis, the term metabolic dysfunction-associated steatotic liver disease (MASLD) was introduced in 2023. MASLD not only recognizes the metabolic aspect of SLD, but also aims to remove the stigma associated with this condition and recognizes the overlap between MASLD and alcoholic liver disease (ALD) under the term MetALD [8]. The introduction of MASLD and MAFLD marks a transformative phase, as it provides a clearer and more inclusive framework for the diagnosis, research, and clinical management of this increasingly prevalent liver disorder. This terminological evolution marks a substantive breakthrough in the field of liver disease, laying the foundation for future strides in diagnosis and treatment [9].



N. Méndez-Sánchez, X. Qi (eds.), *Metabolic Dysfunction-Associated Steatotic Liver Disease*,
https://doi.org/10.1007/978-981-97-9519-2_1

## 1.2 Historical Perspective: From NAFLD to MASLD

### 1.2.1 Evolution of Terminology

The initial descriptions of SLD and the evolution of its nomenclature reflect the dynamic nature of medical terminology. In the nineteenth century, Thomas Adisson, a prominent physician, made the pioneering observation of liver histologic changes associated with SLD, particularly in individuals with a history of excessive alcohol consumption [10].

Subsequently, pathologists worldwide documented similar histological changes, primarily associated with excessive food consumption and sedentary lifestyle. These changes were characterized by liver fat accumulation, perilobular fibrosis and cirrhosis [11]. As the understanding of the disorder progressed, it became evident that SLD was not exclusive to those with a history of alcohol abuse. Instead, it was observed in individuals who exhibited metabolic dysregulations associated with obesity and diabetes [12, 13]. In 1980, Ludwig et al. introduced for the first time the term nonalcoholic steatohepatitis (NASH). This term was associated with histological alterations such as lobular hepatitis, focal necrosis, inflammatory infiltrate and Mallory bodies in liver biopsies of patients who denied excessive alcohol consumption [14]. Later in 1986, Schaffner and Thaler introduced the term NAFLD to describe a milder form of liver steatosis. Concurrently, systemic metabolic alterations were observed in patients exhibiting these histological features, including obesity, hyperlipidemia, hyperglycemia, hyperinsulinemia, and hypertension [10]. The evolution of terminology from historical descriptions to the introduction of NAFLD reflects the ongoing refinement in understanding and categorizing SLD.

### 1.2.2 The Transition to MASLD

In the twenty-first century, the growing concern about NAFLD prompted worldwide discussions on the necessity to rename this pathology. The main catalyst for this debate was the recognition that NAFLD did not adequately reflect the complex pathophysiology of the disease. Its focus revolved primarily around the exclusion of possible causes before a diagnosis was established, which contributed to the perception of misrepresentation [3, 15]. In response to this recognition, a landmark shift was made in 2020 with the introduction of the term MAFLD.

This conceptualization emerged from an international consensus among experts, which underscored the crucial role of metabolic dysfunction in the development and progression of the disease [5–7]. As a key component of this evolution, diagnostic criteria for MAFLD were introduced (Sect. 1.3.3), which provided a more nuanced and comprehensive approach to identifying affected individuals. By integrating metabolic parameters into the diagnostic criteria, the medical community recognized the systemic nature of MAFLD, acknowledging that the condition extends beyond localized liver manifestations [16–18]. This conceptual shift from NAFLD to MAFLD was a catalyst for a broader reevaluation of our understanding of liver diseases in the context of metabolic health. It prompted a reexamination of the relationship between metabolic dysregulation and liver disorders [9, 19, 20].

The momentum gained with the adoption of MAFLD paved the way for another significant advance in 2023: the introduction of MASLD. Driven by international liver societies, MASLD shared similar diagnostic criteria to those previously proposed for MAFLD (Sect. 1.3.3). Noteworthy in the introduction of MASLD is the acknowledgment that even moderate alcohol consumption can contribute to the development of this condition. This recognition added a layer of complexity to the understanding of SLD [8].

## 1.3 Understanding MASLD

### 1.3.1 Generalities and Definition

Liver steatosis, also known as hepatic steatosis, refers to the abnormal accumulation of fat in hepatocytes. This condition is characterized by the presence of intrahepatic fat of at least 5% of liver weight, which can interfere with normal liver function [21, 22]. Fat accumulation in hepatocytes can lead to a series of metabolic and inflammatory changes, which mark the onset of the spectrum of MASLD [23–25]. Beyond the quantitative definition of hepatic steatosis, MASLD encompasses a broader understanding of liver diseases associated with metabolic dysregulation. This change in nomenclature recognizes that hepatic steatosis is not isolated, but often coexists with systemic metabolic abnormalities, such as obesity, insulin resistance (IR), dyslipidemia, and hypertension [26–28].

### 1.3.2 Clinical Spectrum

The clinical spectrum of MASLD is very wide, ranging from patients with low or normal body mass index (BMI) who are metabolically dysfunctional to metabolically dysfunctional overweight/obese patients [29, 30].

In the initial stage, individuals with MASLD may present with simple steatosis without significant inflammation. This stage is usually asymptomatic and may be discovered incidentally during routine imaging studies or investigations for unrelated health problems. Early detection at this stage offers the opportunity to intervene to prevent disease progression [31–33]. As the disease progresses, a subset of individuals may develop metabolic steatohepatitis (MASH), characterized by inflammation and hepatocellular injury. MASH is a more aggressive form of MASLD and carries a higher risk of progression to advanced liver disease, such as fibrosis and cirrhosis [30, 34, 35]. Progression of MASH can lead to the development of liver fibrosis, in which there is an abnormal accumulation of scar tissue in the liver. Advanced fibrosis can progress to cirrhosis, characterized by widespread liver scarring and impaired liver function. In these stages, the risk of complications increases, such as portal hypertension, ascites and hepatocellular carcinoma (HCC) [36, 37].

### 1.3.3 Diagnostic Criteria

The shift in diagnostic criteria from NAFLD to MAFLD and MASLD is a major advance in the understanding of liver disorders. While NAFLD diagnosis historically relied on the exclusion of significant alcohol consumption and other causes of liver steatosis [38]. MASLD take a more inclusive approach, recognizing the intricate connection between metabolic health and liver pathology. A notable aspect of the MASLD diagnostic criteria is the inclusion of metabolic risk factors as integral components. These risk factors go beyond traditional considerations of alcohol consumption and include conditions such as obesity, IR, dyslipidemia, and hypertension [7, 8] (Tables 1.1 and 1.2). The MAFLD and MASLD criteria provide a more inclusive framework, recognizing that liver steatosis can occur in individuals with variable metabolic risk profiles. These criteria address the limitations of the previous exclusionary approach and encompass a broader population susceptible to metabolically associated liver disease [39, 40]. Furthermore, within the MASLD definition, a distinctive subclassification is introduced, termed MetALD. This category combines the presence of metabolic risk factors with high alcohol intake, with defined weekly limits (140–350 g for females and 210–420 g for males). The recognition of MetALD underlines the complexity of liver disorders, acknowledging scenarios where metabolic factors and alcohol intake may interact to influence liver health [8].

**Table 1.1** Diagnostic criteria for metabolic dysfunction-associated fatty liver disease (MAFLD)

| | Overweight or obesity | Lean/normal weight | Diabetes mellitus |
|---|---|---|---|
| Hepatic steatosis | **Evidence of hepatic steatosis in adults**<br>(by imaging techniques, histological techniques or serum biomarkers) | | |
| Metabolic factor | Overweight or obesity<br>(BMI >25 kg/m$^2$ in Caucasians and >23 kg/m$^2$ in Asians) | Lean/normal weight<br>(BMI <25 kg/m$^2$ in Caucasians and <23 kg/m$^2$ in Asians)<br>**Plus at least 2 metabolic risk abnormalities:**<br>Waist circumference ≥102/88 cm in Caucasian men and women (or ≥90/80 cm in Asian men and women).<br>Blood pressure ≥130/85 mmHg or drug treatment.<br>Plasma triglycerides ≥150 mg/dL or drug treatment.<br>Plasma HDL-cholesterol ≤40 mg/dL for men and <50 mg/for women or drug treatment.<br>Prediabetes (fasting glucose levels 100–125 mg/dL or HbA1c 5.7–6.4% or 2-hour post-load glucose levels 140–199 mg/dL).<br>Homeostasis model assessment-insulin resistance score ≥2.5.<br>Plasma hs-C reactive protein level >2 mg/L. | **Diabetes mellitus**<br>(according to widely accepted international criteria) |

**Table 1.2** Diagnostic criteria for metabolic dysfunction-associated steatotic liver disease (MASLD)

| | |
|---|---|
| Hepatic steatosis | **Evidence of hepatic steatosis in adults**<br>(By imaging techniques or histological techniques) |
| Metabolic factor | **At least 1 of the 5 cardiometabolic criteria**<br>BMI ≥25 kg/m$^2$ (≥23 kg/m$^2$ Asia) or waist circumference 94/80 cm in men and women or ethnicity adjusted.<br>Fasting serum glucose ≥5.6 mmol/L (100 mg/dL) or 2-h post-load glucose levels ≥7.8 mmol/L (≥140 mg/dL) or HbA1c ≥5.7% (39 mmol/L) or type 2 diabetes or treatment for type 2 diabetes.<br>Blood pressure >130/85 mmHg or specific antihypertensive drug treatment.<br>Plasma triglycerides ≥1.70 mmol/L (150 mg/dL) or lipid lowering treatment.<br>Plasma HDL-cholesterol ≤1.0 mmol/L (40 mg/dL) in men and <1.3 mmol/L (50 mg/dL) in women or lipid lowering treatment. |

## 1.4 Conclusion

The evolution of liver disease terminology from NAFLD to MASLD signifies a transformative phase in our understanding of metabolic-associated liver disorders. This journey has been shaped by historical observations, clinical insights, and international consensus, reflecting the dynamic nature of medical terminology. The introduction of MAFLD in 2020 and MASLD in 2023 represents a pivotal shift toward a more inclusive and contemporary framework for diagnosing and managing liver diseases. MASLD not only acknowledges the diverse metabolic risk factors contributing to liver pathology but also incorporates a broader spectrum of affected individuals. This paradigm shift holds the potential for future advances in diagnosis, research and treatment, offering more precise and effective strategies for navigating the complexities of metabolic liver disorders.

## References


1. Schaffner F, Thaler H. Nonalcoholic fatty liver disease. Prog Liver Dis. 1986;8:283–98.
2. Younossi ZM, Golabi P, Paik JM, Henry A, Van Dongen C, Henry L. The global epidemiology of nonalcoholic fatty liver disease (NAFLD) and nonalcoholic steatohepatitis (NASH): a systematic review. Hepatology. 2023;77(4):1335–47.
3. Loria P, Lonardo A, Carulli N. Should nonalcoholic fatty liver disease be renamed? Dig Dis. 2005;23(1):72–82.
4. Demirtas CO, Yilmaz Y. Metabolic-associated Fatty Liver Disease: time to integrate ground-breaking new terminology to our clinical practice? Hepatol Forum. 2020;1(3):79–81.
5. Eslam M, Alkhouri N, Vajro P, Baumann U, Weiss R, Socha P, et al. Defining paediatric metabolic (dysfunction)-associated fatty liver disease: an international expert consensus statement. Lancet Gastroenterol Hepatol. 2021;6(10):864–73.
6. Eslam M, El-Serag HB, Francque S, Sarin SK, Wei L, Bugianesi E, George J. Metabolic (dysfunction)-associated fatty liver disease in individuals of normal weight. Nat Rev Gastroenterol Hepatol. 2022;19(10):638–51.
7. Eslam M, Newsome PN, Sarin SK, Anstee QM, Targher G, Romero-Gomez M, et al. A new definition for metabolic dysfunction-associated fatty liver disease: an international expert consensus statement. J Hepatol. 2020;73(1):202–9.
8. Rinella ME, Lazarus JV, Ratziu V, Francque SM, Sanyal AJ, Kanwal F, et al. A multisociety Delphi consensus statement on new fatty liver disease nomenclature. J Hepatol. 2023;79(6):1542–56.
9. Kawaguchi T, Tsutsumi T, Nakano D, Torimura T. MAFLD: renovation of clinical practice and disease awareness of fatty liver. Hepatol Res. 2022;52(5):422–32.
10. Ayonrinde OT. Historical narrative from fatty liver in the nineteenth century to contemporary NAFLD - reconciling the present with the past. JHEP Rep. 2021;3(3):100261.
11. Gofton C, Upendran Y, Zheng MH, George J. MAFLD: how is it different from NAFLD? Clin Mol Hepatol. 2023;29(Suppl):S17–s31.
12. Connor CL. Fatty infiltration of the liver and the development of cirrhosis in diabetes and chronic alcoholism. Am J Pathol. 1938;14(3):347–64.
13. Leevy CM, Ryan CM, Fineberg JC. Diabetes mellitus and liver dysfunction; etiologic and therapeutic considerations. Am J Med. 1950;8(3):290–9.
14. Ludwig J, Viggiano TR, McGill DB, Oh BJ. Nonalcoholic steatohepatitis: Mayo Clinic experiences with a hitherto unnamed disease. Mayo Clin Proc. 1980;55(7):434–8.
15. Yilmaz Y. The heated debate over NAFLD renaming: an ongoing saga. Hepatol Forum. 2023;4(3):89–91.
16. Kaya E, Yilmaz Y. Metabolic-associated Fatty Liver Disease (MAFLD): a multi-systemic disease beyond the liver. J Clin Transl Hepatol. 2022;10(2):329–38.
17. Lin S, Huang J, Wang M, Kumar R, Liu Y, Liu S, et al. Comparison of MAFLD and NAFLD diagnostic criteria in real world. Liver Int. 2020;40(9):2082–9.
18. Pipitone RM, Ciccioli C, Infantino G, La Mantia C, Parisi S, Tulone A, et al. MAFLD: a multisystem disease. Ther Adv Endocrinol Metab. 2023;14:20420188221145549.
19. Pal SC, Méndez-Sánchez N. Insulin resistance and adipose tissue interactions as the cornerstone of metabolic (dysfunction)-associated fatty liver disease pathogenesis. World J Gastroenterol. 2023;29(25):3999–4008.
20. Zheng KI, Fan JG, Shi JP, Wong VW, Eslam M, George J, Zheng MH. From NAFLD to MAFLD: a "redefining" moment for fatty liver disease. Chin Med J. 2020;133(19):2271–3.
21. Nassir F, Rector RS, Hammoud GM, Ibdah JA. Pathogenesis and prevention of hepatic steatosis. Gastroenterol Hepatol (N Y). 2015;11(3):167–75.
22. Brunt EM, Wong VWS, Nobili V, Day CP, Sookoian S, Maher JJ, et al. Nonalcoholic fatty liver disease. Nat Rev Dis Primers. 2015;1(1):15080.
23. Ramírez-Mejía MM, Méndez-Sánchez N. What is in a name: from NAFLD to MAFLD and MASLD—unraveling the complexities and implications. Curr Hepatol Rep. 2023;22(4):221–7.
24. Buzzetti E, Pinzani M, Tsochatzis EA. The multiple-hit pathogenesis of non-alcoholic fatty liver disease (NAFLD). Metabolism. 2016;65(8):1038–48.
25. Loomba R, Friedman SL, Shulman GI. Mechanisms and disease consequences of nonalcoholic fatty liver disease. Cell. 2021;184(10):2537–64.
26. Ramírez-Mejía MM, Qi X, Abenavoli L, Romero-Gómez M, Eslam M, Méndez-Sánchez N. Metabolic dysfunction: the silenced connection with fatty liver disease. Ann Hepatol. 2023;28(6):101138.
27. Lim S, Kim JW, Targher G. Links between metabolic syndrome and metabolic dysfunction-associated fatty liver disease. Trends Endocrinol Metab. 2021;32(7):500–14.
28. Godoy-Matos AF, Silva Júnior WS, Valerio CM. NAFLD as a continuum: from obesity to metabolic syndrome and diabetes. Diabetol Metab Syndr. 2020;12:60.
29. Nguyen VH, Le MH, Cheung RC, Nguyen MH. Differential clinical characteristics and mortality outcomes in persons with NAFLD and/or MAFLD. Clin Gastroenterol Hepatol. 2021;19(10):2172–81.e6.
30. Chan WK, Chuah KH, Rajaram RB, Lim LL, Ratnasingam J, Vethakkan SR. Metabolic Dysfunction-Associated Steatotic Liver Disease (MASLD): a state-of-the-art review. J Obes Metab Syndr. 2023;32(3):197–213.
31. Guerra-Ruiz AR, Casals G, Iruzubieta P, Lalana M, Leis A, López RM, et al. Biochemical assessment

of metabolic associated fatty liver disease. Adv Lab Med. 2021;2(2):199–219.
32. Pal SC, Méndez-Sánchez N. Screening for MAFLD: who, when and how? Ther Adv Endocrinol Metab. 2023;14:20420188221145650.
33. Lekakis V, Papatheodoridis GV. Natural history of metabolic dysfunction-associated steatotic liver disease. Eur J Intern Med. 2023;122:3.
34. Ekstedt M, Nasr P, Kechagias S. Natural history of NAFLD/NASH. Curr Hepatol Rep. 2017;16(4):391–7.
35. Wree A, Broderick L, Canbay A, Hoffman HM, Feldstein AE. From NAFLD to NASH to cirrhosis-new insights into disease mechanisms. Nat Rev Gastroenterol Hepatol. 2013;10(11):627–36.
36. Bae SDW, George J, Qiao L. From MAFLD to hepatocellular carcinoma and everything in between. Chin Med J. 2022;135(5):547–56.
37. Shah PA, Patil R, Harrison SA. NAFLD-related hepatocellular carcinoma: the growing challenge. Hepatology. 2023;77(1):323–38.
38. Rinella ME, Neuschwander-Tetri BA, Siddiqui MS, Abdelmalek MF, Caldwell S, Barb D, et al. AASLD practice guidance on the clinical assessment and management of nonalcoholic fatty liver disease. Hepatology. 2023;77(5):1797–835.
39. Yamamura S, Eslam M, Kawaguchi T, Tsutsumi T, Nakano D, Yoshinaga S, et al. MAFLD identifies patients with significant hepatic fibrosis better than NAFLD. Liver Int. 2020;40(12):3018–30.
40. Ramírez-Mejía MM, Jiménez-Gutiérrez C, Eslam M, George J, Méndez-Sánchez N. Breaking new ground: MASLD vs. MAFLD-which holds the key for risk stratification? Hepatol Int. 2023;18:168.

# 2 Unveiling the MASLD Epidemic

Nahum Méndez-Sánchez, Mariana M. Ramírez-Mejía, and Xingshun Qi

## 2.1 Introduction

The epidemiology of metabolic dysfunction-associated steatotic liver disease (MASLD) varies across regions and populations and is influenced by a variety of genetic, environmental, and lifestyle factors [1]. Worldwide, the prevalence of the disease has increased dramatically, in parallel with rising rates of obesity, type 2 diabetes mellitus (T2DM), dyslipidemia, and metabolic syndrome [2]. Recent epidemiological data indicate that MASLD has become the most predominant cause of chronic liver disease (CLD) worldwide, affecting one third of the worldwide adult population [3].

N. Méndez-Sánchez (✉) · M. M. Ramírez-Mejía
Faculty of Medicine, National Autonomous University of Mexico, Mexico City, Mexico

Liver Research Unit, Medica Sur Clinic and Foundation, Mexico City, Mexico
e-mail: nmendez@medicasur.org.mx

X. Qi
Department of Gastroenterology, General Hospital of Northern Theater Command (formerly General Hospital of Shenyang Military Area), Shenyang, Liaoning Province, China

## 2.2 MASLD Epidemiology Over the Time

At the end of the twentieth century and the beginning of the twenty-first century it was difficult to determine the exact prevalence of MASLD due to the lack of diagnostic instruments with good sensitivity and specificity. Therefore the prevalence of MASLD varied according to the diagnostic method used (liver enzymes, imaging techniques or liver biopsy) [4]. At that time the prevalence of MASLD was divided according to the population studied, into unselected population and selected population, which referred to individuals with T2DM, metabolic syndrome, bariatric surgery, among others. The prevalence of MASLD in the unselected population ranged from 2.8% to 46%, while for the selected population it ranged from 33% to 99%, depending on the characteristics of the studies [5]. Over time, with the adoption of a sedentary lifestyle and the globalization of the Western diet, an increase in the prevalence of MASLD in developing countries began to be observed. The globalization of the Western diet, characterized by a high consumption of processed foods, saturated fats, and sugars, has played an important role in shaping the epidemiology of MASLD. These dietary habits, together with a sedentary lifestyle and reduced physical activity, contribute to weight gain, insulin resistance, and dyslipidemia, all of which are key



N. Méndez-Sánchez, X. Qi (eds.), *Metabolic Dysfunction-Associated Steatotic Liver Disease*,
https://doi.org/10.1007/978-981-97-9519-2_2

factors in the development and progression of the disease [6].

## 2.3 Global Burden of MASLD

### 2.3.1 Incidence and Prevalence

The incidence and prevalence of MASLD have risen substantially over the past few decades [7]. Recent research evidence indicates a dramatic 50.4% increase in the global prevalence of MASLD between 2006 and 2019. Prevalence rates reached 25.26% in 2006 and increased to 38% in 2019 [8]. This increase in prevalence highlights the growing burden of MASLD on public health systems worldwide. Nevertheless, the distribution of MASLD is heterogeneous and varies depending on the geographic region, ethnicity, genetic variants, and lifestyle factors (Fig. 2.1) [7]. Age and gender also play a key role in the epidemiology of MASLD. The disease predominantly affects adults, with a higher prevalence observed in middle-aged individuals [9]. Furthermore, although males have traditionally shown a slightly higher prevalence, rates among females tend to equalize after menopause, suggesting a potential protective effect of estrogen [10, 11]. Finally, ethnicity contribute to disparities in the prevalence of MASLD, with certain racial and ethnic groups, such as Hispanics, South Asians, and Pacific Islanders, showing increased susceptibility [12]. These variations may be attributed to genetic predispositions, cultural dietary patterns, and differences in lifestyle factors [13].

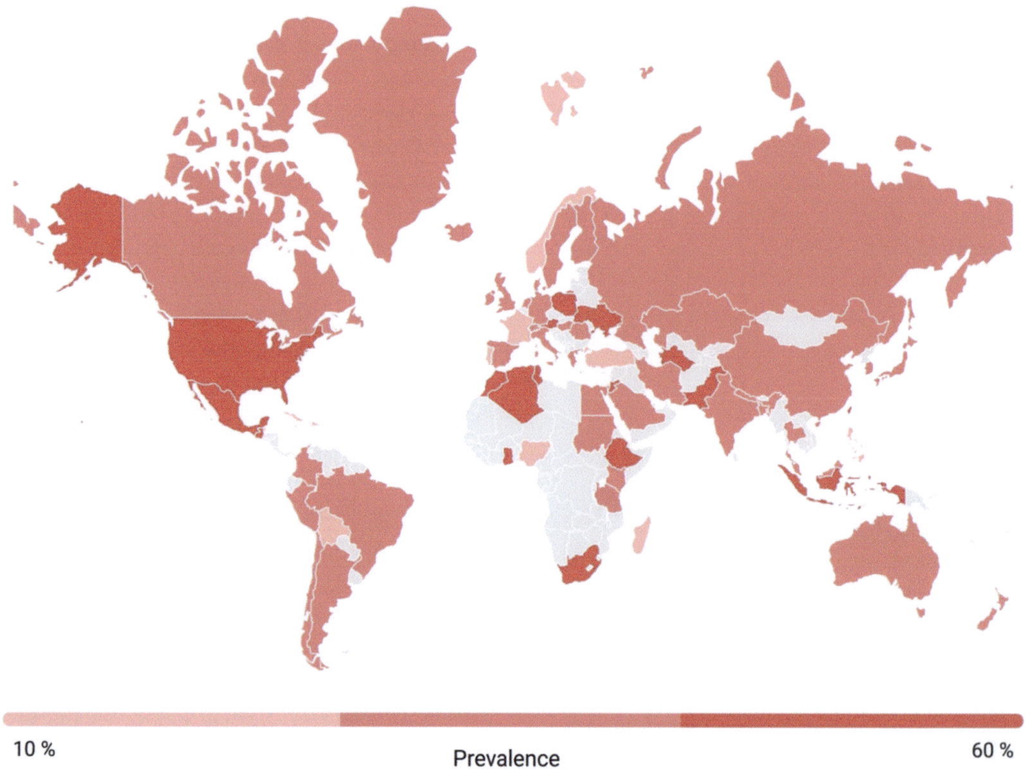


**Fig. 2.1** Prevalence of MASLD worldwide. This figure illustrates the worldwide distribution of the prevalence of metabolic dysfunction-associated steatotic liver disease (MASLD). Data from several epidemiological studies and meta-analyses are synthesized to describe the geographic variability and burden of MASLD in different regions of the world

### 2.3.2 Epidemiology of MASH and Liver Fibrosis

At least 20% of individuals with MASLD develop metabolic-associated steatohepatitis (MASH) a condition that significantly increases the risk of liver fibrosis, cirrhosis and associated complications such as hepatocellular carcinoma (HCC) [14]. The diagnosis of MASH is only made by liver biopsy, which makes it difficult to estimate its prevalence [15, 16]. Nevertheless, the global prevalence of MASH has been estimated to be 5.27%, based on the worldwide prevalence of MASLD [8]. Similar to MASLD, the prevalence of MASH varies according to geographic region, with the higher prevalence reported in Latin America (7.11%) and the lowest in Western Europe (4.02%) [8] (Fig. 2.2). As part of the natural history of MASLD, up to 25% of individuals will progress to liver fibrosis [17]. This progression is not uniform and depends on factors such as the severity of metabolic dysfunction, the presence of inflammation, and genetic predispositions [18]. Understanding the risk factors contributing to fibrosis development is crucial for identifying high-risk individuals and implementing targeted interventions [19].

### 2.3.3 Mortality

Mortality in MASLD represents a major concern, as the condition can progress to advanced stages of liver disease, including cirrhosis and HCC,

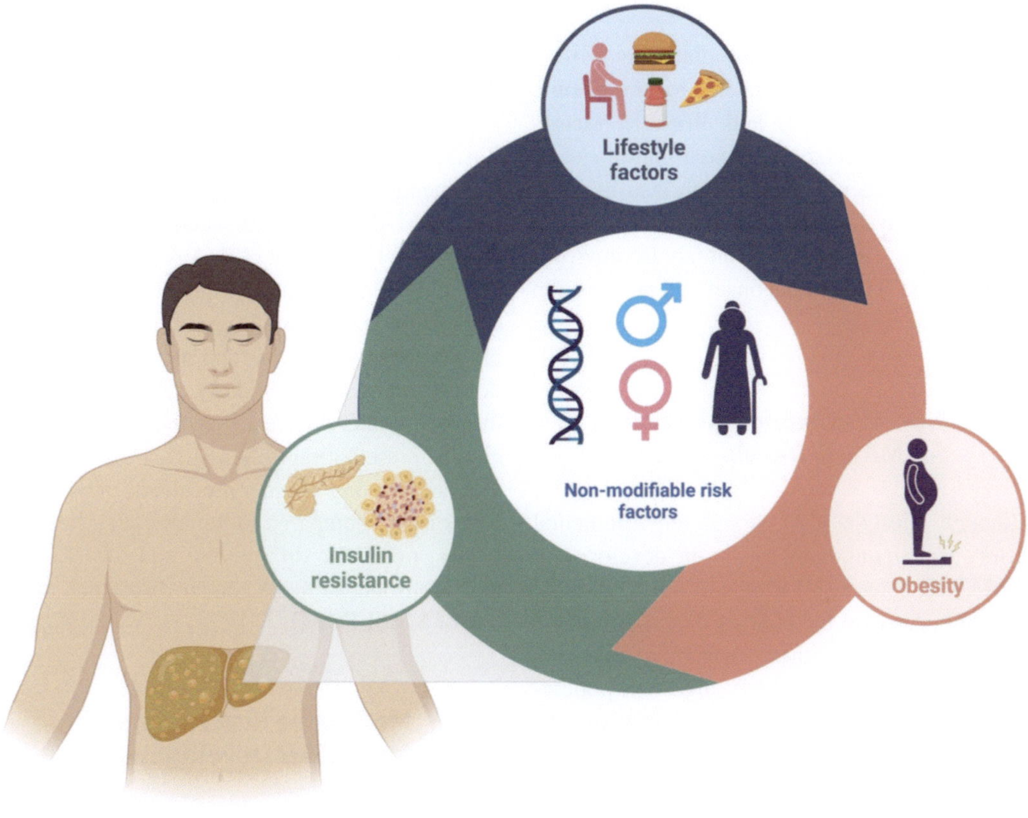


**Fig. 2.2** Risk factors associated with the development of MASLD. This figure describes the multifactorial nature of or metabolic dysfunction-associated steatotic liver disease (MASLD) illustrating the diversity of risk factors that contribute to its development. Key factors such as obesity, insulin resistance, dietary habits, sedentary lifestyle, and genetic predispositions are represented, highlighting the complex interplay of these elements in the pathogenesis of MASLD

leading to increased mortality rates [20]. Studies have demonstrated that people with MASLD have a higher mortality risk than the general population, specifically 1.7-fold higher risk of all-cause mortality [21, 22]. Moving toward cause-specific mortality it has been observed that individuals with MAFLD/MASLD have an increased risk for cardiovascular disease (CVD)-related mortality [21, 23]. Additionally, the association with liver fibrosis and cirrhosis in ELHGF/MASLD contributes significantly to the overall mortality burden. As the disease progresses, the risk of complications such as liver failure and portal hypertension increases, further elevating the risk of mortality [24, 25].

## 2.4 Risk Factors and Associated Comorbidities

MASLD is a multifactorial disorder, with a pathogenesis closely related to metabolic, genetic, environmental, and lifestyle factors (Fig. 2.2) [26]. Metabolic dysregulation lies at the heart of its development, with insulin resistance (IR), dyslipidemia, and obesity as the main drivers. This aberrant metabolic environment sets the stage for the onset and progression of MASLD [27].

### 2.4.1 Non-Modifiable Risk Factors for MASLD Development

Although lifestyle choices and environmental factors play an important role in the development of MASLD some risk factors are not modifiable and are intrinsic to the biology of the individual [28]. Understanding these non-modifiable risk factors is essential to identify high-risk populations and implement targeted preventive and screening measures [19].

#### 2.4.1.1 Genetic Predisposition and Ethnicity

Genetic factors contribute substantially to an individual's susceptibility to MASLD. Family studies and genome-wide association studies (GWAS) have identified numerous genetic variants associated with an increased risk of hepatic steatosis and its progression to more severe liver disease [29]. Polymorphisms in genes such as PNPLA3, TM6SF2, MBOAT7, and GCKR involved in lipid metabolism, insulin signaling, inflammation, and fibrogenesis have been implicated in the pathogenesis of MASLD [30]. These genetic predispositions may influence disease susceptibility, severity, and response to therapeutic interventions. Understanding an individual's genetic profile may help in designing personalized treatment strategies for MASLD [31]. Furthermore, the distribution of these genetic variants has been demonstrated to influence disparities in disease prevalence among different ethnic and racial groups [1]. Certain populations, such as those of Hispanic, South Asian, and Middle Eastern descent, have a higher prevalence of genetic variants associated with MASLD, contributing to disparities in disease burden [13].

#### 2.4.1.2 Age and Gender

Advancing age is associated with an increased risk of MASLD, and prevalence rates increase progressively with age [32]. Age-related changes in metabolic function, hormonal status, and body composition contribute to the increased susceptibility to hepatic steatosis and metabolic dysfunction observed in the elderly [33]. In addition, there are gender differences in the prevalence and clinical presentation of MASLD, with males traditionally having a higher prevalence of advanced liver disease compared to females [11]. Sex hormones, metabolic differences, and lifestyle factors contribute to these gender disparities in the risk of MASLD [34].

### 2.4.2 Modifiable Risk Factors for MASLD Development

#### 2.4.2.1 Obesity

Obesity is a multifaceted condition arising from a confluence of environmental, genetic, socioeconomic, and internal factors unique to each individual [35]. Prolonged imbalance between energy intake and expenditure precipitates metabolic disruptions, predominantly within adipose tissue. These metabolic dysregulations, compounded by nutrient overload and sedentary habits, are closely linked to the emergence of MASLD [36, 37].

#### 2.4.2.2 Insulin Resistance

IR, a key feature of the metabolic syndrome, plays a central role in the pathogenesis of MASLD. In normal physiological conditions, insulin plays a crucial role in the regulation of metabolic processes, including inhibition of lipolysis and gluconeogenesis in adipose tissue [38, 39]. As a consequence of the impairment of insulin action by IR, there is a dysregulation of lipid metabolism characterized by an increase in circulating free fatty acids (FFA). These elevated FFA levels, resulting from uncontrolled lipolysis in adipose tissue, contribute to the pathogenesis of MASLD [27].

#### 2.4.2.3 Lifestyle

Hypercaloric diets rich in sugars, refined carbohydrates, and saturated fats contribute to IR, dyslipidemia, and liver steatosis. Excessive consumption of processed foods, sugary drinks, and fried foods exacerbates metabolic dysfunction, predisposing individuals to MASLD [40]. Furthermore, physical inactivity is an important modifiable risk factor for MAFLD/MASLD. Sedentary lifestyles aggravate metabolic dysfunction, promote adiposity, and contribute to IR [41].

#### 2.4.2.4 Alcohol Consumption

Excessive alcohol consumption is a well-established risk factor for alcoholic fatty liver disease (ALD) [42]. Recent research highlights the importance of increased caloric intake from alcohol in the development of MASLD. Alcohol is inherently caloric, and its constant consumption can tip the energy balance into surplus, leading to weight gain and metabolic disturbances [43]. In addition, alcohol consumption can lead to IR by altering lipid metabolism, promoting increased lipid production and impairing the liver's ability to oxidize fatty acids [44].

### 2.4.3 MAFLD/MASLD Beyond the Liver

Beyond its primary liver effect, MASLD exert a significant impact on several extrahepatic organs and systems, contributing to a wide range of comorbidities. One of the most significant extrahepatic manifestations of MASLD is its association with cardiovascular disease (CVD). Epidemiological studies have consistently demonstrated an increased risk of atherosclerosis, coronary artery disease, myocardial infarction, and stroke in individuals with MASLD, implicating a higher rates of morbidity and mortality [45, 46]. Additionally, individuals with MASLD have a higher prevalence of chronic kidney disease (CKD) and an increased risk of developing progressive renal failure. Shared risk factors, such as IR, hypertension, and systemic inflammation, contribute to the pathogenesis of both MASLD and CKD [47, 48].

## 2.5 Epidemiology of MASLD by Regions

### 2.5.1 America

In North America, the disease has reached epidemic proportions, closely related to the increasing prevalence of obesity, T2DM and metabolic syndrome. In the United States, studies have reported a high prevalence of MASLD, with estimates ranging from 37.1% to 39.1% of the population. Hispanic and Latino populations in the Americas are particularly affected, with a higher prevalence compared to other ethnic groups [49]. Latin America is highly diverse, encompassing a wide range of ethnicities, cultures, and socioeconomic backgrounds. This diversity contributes to ethnic disparities in diet and lifestyle practices throughout the region. In addition, fragmented health systems and social inequalities further exacerbate these disparities. These factors influence the wide variability in the prevalence of MASLD in the region [50]. The current prevalence of MASLD in Latin America is 34.5% [51, 52]. In addition, the genetic composition in Latin

American is remarkably diverse, reflecting a heterogeneous ancestry influenced by admixture of Native American, European, and African populations. Finally, certain genetic variations, such as the I148M polymorphism of PNPLA3, are found at high frequencies in specific populations, Mexico exhibits a prevalence of 77%, Argentina follows closely with 63.7%, and Chile reports a prevalence of 59% [50]. These genetic variations contribute to the complex interplay of genetic and environmental factors underlying MASLD susceptibility and progression in Latin American populations.

### 2.5.2 Europe

Europe has also experienced a marked increase in the prevalence of MASLD, mirroring trends observed in North America [1]. Currently the prevalence of MASLD is 30.9%. Western European countries have reported significant rates of MASLD, especially in urban populations with high rates of obesity and metabolic dysfunction. Eastern European countries are also experiencing an increase in disease prevalence, although at a slightly lower rate [53]. Countries like Spain, Germany, Italy, and Turkey have reported significant rates of MASLD, 22.3%, 30%, 38.2%, and 48.4% respectively [3, 54, 55].

### 2.5.3 Asia

Asia represents a diverse landscape in terms of MASLD epidemiology, influenced by genetic, cultural, and socioeconomic factors. Rapid urbanization, industrialization, and dietary transitions have contributed to the increased prevalence of MASLD in many Asian countries [56]. Overall, the prevalence of MASLD in Asia is 30%, with Southeast Asia having the highest prevalence of 42%. Rapid urbanization, industrialization, and dietary transitions have contributed to the escalating prevalence of MASLD in many Asian countries, such as Iran, Taiwan, South Korea, and China [3].

### 2.5.4 Africa

The epidemiology of MASLD in Africa is less well studied than in other regions, but there is evidence to suggest an increasing prevalence, with a current prevalence of 13.5%. Studies in countries such as Ethiopia, South Africa, and Nigeria have revealed increasing rates of obesity and metabolic syndrome, which is likely contributing to the increasing burden of disease in these regions. However, more research is needed to better understand the epidemiology of the disease in the diverse populations of Africa [57, 58].

### 2.5.5 Pacific

The Pacific region, which includes countries such as Australia and New Zealand, faces a considerable burden of MASLD, consistent with trends observed in other developed nations. High rates of obesity, metabolic syndrome, and sedentary lifestyles contribute to the significant burden of disease in this region. In addition, indigenous Pacific Island populations may face unique challenges related to MASLD, influenced by socioeconomic disparities and cultural factors [50, 59].

## 2.6 Conclusions

In conclusion, the epidemiology of MASLD presents a complex interplay of genetic, environmental, and lifestyle factors, which has led to a dramatic increase in prevalence worldwide. MASLD has emerged as the most prevalent cause of chronic liver disease worldwide, affecting a substantial proportion of the adult population. The increasing prevalence of MASLD highlights the pressing need for robust public health strategies tailored to the complexities of the disease. These strategies should include preventive measures targeting modifiable risk factors such as obesity, IR, unhealthy eating habits, sedentary lifestyles, and excessive alcohol consumption. Educational campaigns promoting healthy lifestyles and early detection initiatives can play a key role in slowing the progression of the disease and mitigating its impact on individuals and healthcare systems.

## References


1. Younossi Z, Anstee QM, Marietti M, Hardy T, Henry L, Eslam M, et al. Global burden of NAFLD and NASH: trends, predictions, risk factors and prevention. Nat Rev Gastroenterol Hepatol. 2018;15(1):11–20.
2. Younossi Z, Tacke F, Arrese M, Chander Sharma B, Mostafa I, Bugianesi E, et al. Global perspectives on nonalcoholic fatty liver disease and nonalcoholic steatohepatitis. Hepatology. 2019;69(6):2672–82.
3. Teng ML, Ng CH, Huang DQ, Chan KE, Tan DJ, Lim WH, et al. Global incidence and prevalence of nonalcoholic fatty liver disease. Clin Mol Hepatol. 2023;29(Suppl):S32–s42.
4. Clark JM. The epidemiology of nonalcoholic fatty liver disease in adults. J Clin Gastroenterol. 2006;40(Suppl 1):S5–10.
5. Lazo M, Clark JM. The epidemiology of nonalcoholic fatty liver disease: a global perspective. Semin Liver Dis. 2008;28(4):339–50.
6. Loomba R, Sanyal AJ. The global NAFLD epidemic. Nat Rev Gastroenterol Hepatol. 2013;10(11):686–90.
7. Riazi K, Azhari H, Charette JH, Underwood FE, King JA, Afshar EE, et al. The prevalence and incidence of NAFLD worldwide: a systematic review and meta-analysis. Lancet Gastroenterol Hepatol. 2022;7(9):851–61.
8. Younossi ZM, Golabi P, Paik JM, Henry A, Van Dongen C, Henry L. The global epidemiology of nonalcoholic fatty liver disease (NAFLD) and nonalcoholic steatohepatitis (NASH): a systematic review. Hepatology. 2023;77(4):1335–47.
9. Henry L, Paik J, Younossi ZM. Review article: the epidemiologic burden of non-alcoholic fatty liver disease across the world. Aliment Pharmacol Ther. 2022;56(6):942–56.
10. Nagral A, Bangar M, Menezes S, Bhatia S, Butt N, Ghosh J, et al. Gender differences in nonalcoholic fatty liver disease. Euroasian J Hepatogastroenterol. 2022;12(Suppl 1):S19–s25.
11. Lonardo A, Nascimbeni F, Ballestri S, Fairweather D, Win S, Than TA, et al. Sex differences in nonalcoholic fatty liver disease: state of the art and identification of research gaps. Hepatology. 2019;70(4):1457–69.
12. Bonacini M, Kassamali F, Kari S, Lopez Barrera N, Kohla M. Racial differences in prevalence and severity of non-alcoholic fatty liver disease. World J Hepatol. 2021;13(7):763–73.
13. Riazi K, Swain MG, Congly SE, Kaplan GG, Shaheen AA. Race and ethnicity in Non-Alcoholic Fatty Liver Disease (NAFLD): a narrative review. Nutrients. 2022;14(21):4556.
14. Chan WK, Chuah KH, Rajaram RB, Lim LL, Ratnasingam J, Vethakkan SR. Metabolic dysfunction-associated Steatotic liver disease (MASLD): a state-of-the-art review. J Obes Metab Syndr. 2023;32(3):197–213.
15. Nalbantoglu IL, Brunt EM. Role of liver biopsy in nonalcoholic fatty liver disease. World J Gastroenterol. 2014;20(27):9026–37.
16. Sheka AC, Adeyi O, Thompson J, Hameed B, Crawford PA, Ikramuddin S. Nonalcoholic steatohepatitis: a review. JAMA. 2020;323(12):1175–83.
17. McCullough AJ. The clinical features, diagnosis and natural history of nonalcoholic fatty liver disease. Clin Liver Dis. 2004;8(3):521–33. viii
18. Singh S, Allen AM, Wang Z, Prokop LJ, Murad MH, Loomba R. Fibrosis progression in nonalcoholic fatty liver vs nonalcoholic steatohepatitis: a systematic review and meta-analysis of paired-biopsy studies. Clin Gastroenterol Hepatol. 2015;13(4):643–54.e9.
19. Huang TD, Behary J, Zekry A. Non-alcoholic fatty liver disease: a review of epidemiology, risk factors, diagnosis and management. Intern Med J. 2020;50(9):1038–47.
20. Bae SDW, George J, Qiao L. From MAFLD to hepatocellular carcinoma and everything in between. Chin Med J. 2022;135(5):547–56.
21. Nguyen VH, Le MH, Cheung RC, Nguyen MH. Differential clinical characteristics and mortality outcomes in persons with NAFLD and/or MAFLD. Clin Gastroenterol Hepatol. 2021;19(10):2172–81.e6.
22. Kim D, Konyn P, Sandhu KK, Dennis BB, Cheung AC, Ahmed A. Metabolic dysfunction-associated fatty liver disease is associated with increased all-cause mortality in the United States. J Hepatol. 2021;75(6):1284–91.
23. Zhao Q, Deng Y. Comparison of mortality outcomes in individuals with MASLD and/or MAFLD. J Hepatol. 2024;80(2):e62–e4.
24. Stepanova M, Rafiq N, Makhlouf H, Agrawal R, Kaur I, Younoszai Z, et al. Predictors of all-cause mortality and liver-related mortality in patients with non-alcoholic fatty liver disease (NAFLD). Dig Dis Sci. 2013;58(10):3017–23.
25. Ilyas F, Ali H, Patel P, Sarfraz S, Basuli D, Giammarino A, Satapathy SK. Increasing nonalcoholic fatty liver disease-related mortality rates in the United States from 1999 to 2022. Hepatol Commun. 2023;7(7):e00207.
26. Ramírez-Mejía MM, Méndez-Sánchez N. What is in a name: from NAFLD to MAFLD and MASLD—unraveling the complexities and implications. Curr Hepatol Rep. 2023;22(4):221–7.
27. Ramírez-Mejía MM, Qi X, Abenavoli L, Romero-Gómez M, Eslam M, Méndez-Sánchez N. Metabolic dysfunction: the silenced connection with fatty liver disease. Ann Hepatol. 2023;28(6):101138.
28. Juanola O, Martínez-López S, Francés R, Gómez-Hurtado I. Non-alcoholic fatty liver disease: metabolic, genetic, epigenetic and environmental risk factors. Int J Environ Res Public Health. 2021;18(10):5227.
29. Jonas W, Schürmann A. Genetic and epigenetic factors determining NAFLD risk. Mol Metab. 2021;50:101111.

30. Trépo E, Valenti L. Update on NAFLD genetics: from new variants to the clinic. J Hepatol. 2020;72(6):1196–209.
31. Eslam M, Valenti L, Romeo S. Genetics and epigenetics of NAFLD and NASH: clinical impact. J Hepatol. 2018;68(2):268–79.
32. Bertolotti M, Lonardo A, Mussi C, Baldelli E, Pellegrini E, Ballestri S, et al. Nonalcoholic fatty liver disease and aging: epidemiology to management. World J Gastroenterol. 2014;20(39):14185–204.
33. Guo J, Huang X, Dou L, Yan M, Shen T, Tang W, Li J. Aging and aging-related diseases: from molecular mechanisms to interventions and treatments. Signal Transduct Target Ther. 2022;7(1):391.
34. Eng PC, Forlano R, Tan T, Manousou P, Dhillo WS, Izzi-Engbeaya C. Non-alcoholic fatty liver disease in women—current knowledge and emerging concepts. JHEP Reports. 2023;5(10):100835.
35. Lin X, Li H. Obesity: epidemiology, pathophysiology, and therapeutics. Front Endocrinol (Lausanne). 2021;12:706978.
36. Jung UJ, Choi MS. Obesity and its metabolic complications: the role of adipokines and the relationship between obesity, inflammation, insulin resistance, dyslipidemia and nonalcoholic fatty liver disease. Int J Mol Sci. 2014;15(4):6184–223.
37. Vulchi J, Suryadevara V, Mohan P, Kamalanathan S, Sahoo J, Naik D, Selvarajan S. Obesity and metabolic dysfunction-associated fatty liver disease: understanding the intricate link. Journal of Translational Gastroenterology. 2023;1(2):74–86.
38. Pal SC, Méndez-Sánchez N. Insulin resistance and adipose tissue interactions as the cornerstone of metabolic (dysfunction)-associated fatty liver disease pathogenesis. World J Gastroenterol. 2023;29(25):3999–4008.
39. Pal SC, Eslam M, Mendez-Sanchez N. Detangling the interrelations between MAFLD, insulin resistance, and key hormones. Hormones (Athens). 2022;21(4):573–89.
40. Ristic-Medic D, Bajerska J, Vucic V. Crosstalk between dietary patterns, obesity and nonalcoholic fatty liver disease. World J Gastroenterol. 2022;28(27):3314–33.
41. Rector RS, Thyfault JP. Does physical inactivity cause nonalcoholic fatty liver disease? J Appl Physiol (1985). 2011;111(6):1828–35.
42. Seitz HK, Bataller R, Cortez-Pinto H, Gao B, Gual A, Lackner C, et al. Alcoholic liver disease. Nat Rev Dis Primers. 2018;4(1):16.
43. Sun FR, Wang BY. Alcohol and metabolic-associated fatty liver disease. J Clin Transl Hepatol. 2021;9(5):719–30.
44. Policarpo S, Carvalhana S, Craciun A, Crespo RR, Cortez-Pinto H. Do MAFLD patients with harmful alcohol consumption have a different dietary intake? Nutrients. 2022;14(7):1335.
45. Targher G, Byrne CD, Tilg H. NAFLD and increased risk of cardiovascular disease: clinical associations, pathophysiological mechanisms and pharmacological implications. Gut. 2020;69(9):1691–705.
46. Kasper P, Martin A, Lang S, Kütting F, Goeser T, Demir M, Steffen HM. NAFLD and cardiovascular diseases: a clinical review. Clin Res Cardiol. 2021;110(7):921–37.
47. Mantovani A, Lombardi R, Cattazzo F, Zusi C, Cappelli D, Dalbeni A. MAFLD and CKD: an updated narrative review. Int J Mol Sci. 2022;23(13):7007.
48. Wang TY, Wang RF, Bu ZY, Targher G, Byrne CD, Sun DQ, Zheng MH. Association of metabolic dysfunction-associated fatty liver disease with kidney disease. Nat Rev Nephrol. 2022;18(4):259–68.
49. Ciardullo S, Carbone M, Invernizzi P, Perseghin G. Exploring the landscape of steatotic liver disease in the general US population. Liver Int. 2023;43(11):2425–33.
50. Castellanos-Fernandez MI, Pal SC, Arrese M, Arab JP, George J, Méndez-Sánchez N. Nonalcoholic fatty liver disease in Latin America and Australia. Clin Liver Dis. 2023;27(2):301–15.
51. Arab JP, Díaz LA, Dirchwolf M, Mark HE, Lazarus JV, Vaughan E, et al. NAFLD: challenges and opportunities to address the public health problem in Latin America. Ann Hepatol. 2021;24:100359.
52. López-Velázquez JA, Silva-Vidal KV, Ponciano-Rodríguez G, Chávez-Tapia NC, Arrese M, Uribe M, Méndez-Sánchez N. The prevalence of nonalcoholic fatty liver disease in the Americas. Ann Hepatol. 2014;13(2):166–78.
53. Wong VW-S, Ekstedt M, Wong GL-H, Hagström H. Changing epidemiology, global trends and implications for outcomes of NAFLD. J Hepatol. 2023;79(3):842–52.
54. Cusacovich I, Sánchez-Lite I, Toribio B, González JM, Pérez-Rubio A, Andaluz-Ojeda D. Prevalence of nonalcoholic fatty liver disease in a Spanish town: a population-based study. Rev Clin Esp (Barc). 2023;223(7):396–404.
55. Canbay A, Kachru N, Haas JS, Meise D, Ozbay AB, Sowa JP. Healthcare resource utilization and costs among nonalcoholic fatty liver disease patients in Germany. Ann Transl Med. 2021;9(8):615.
56. Wong SW, Chan WK. Epidemiology of non-alcoholic fatty liver disease in Asia. Indian J Gastroenterol. 2020;39(1):1–8.
57. Paruk IM, Pirie FJ, Motala AA. Non-alcoholic fatty liver disease in Africa: a hidden danger. Glob Health Epidemiol Genom. 2019;4:e3.
58. Spearman CW, Afihene M, Betiku O, Bobat B, Cunha L, Kassianides C, et al. Epidemiology, risk factors, social determinants of health, and current management for non-alcoholic fatty liver disease in sub-Saharan Africa. Lancet Gastroenterol Hepatol. 2021;6(12):1036–46.
59. Wong MCS, Huang JLW, George J, Huang J, Leung C, Eslam M, et al. The changing epidemiology of liver diseases in the Asia-Pacific region. Nat Rev Gastroenterol Hepatol. 2019;16(1):57–73.

# 3 Decoding MASLD's Pathophysiology

Ludovico Abenavoli
and Giuseppe Guido Maria Scarlata

## Abbreviations

| | |
|---|---|
| FGF21 | Fibroblast growth factor 21 |
| FNDC5 | Fibronectin type III domain-containing protein 5 |
| GLUT | Glucose transporter |
| HCC | Hepatocellular carcinoma |
| HFHC | High fat/cholesterol |
| HFLC | High fat low carb |
| IFNL3/4 | Interferon lambda type 3 and 4 |
| IL | Interleukin |
| IRS1 | Insulin receptor substrate 1 |
| IRS2 | Insulin receptor substrate 2 |
| LPS | Lipopolysaccharide |
| MAFLD | Metabolic dysfunction-associated fatty liver disease |
| MASLD | Metabolic dysfunction-associated steatotic liver disease |
| MBOAT7 | Membrane domain-containing O-acyltransferase 7 |
| miRNA | Micro RNA |
| NAFLD | Nonalcoholic fatty liver disease |
| PNPLA3 | Patatin-like phospholipase domain-containing 3 |
| ROS | Reactive oxygen species |
| T2DM | Type 2 diabetes mellitus |
| TM6SF2 | Transmembrane 6 superfamily member 2 |
| TNF-α | Tumor necrosis factor-alfa |
| VLDL | Very low-density lipoproteins |

L. Abenavoli (✉) · G. G. M. Scarlata
Department of Health Sciences, Magna Graecia University of Catanzaro, Catanzaro, Italy
e-mail: l.abenavoli@unicz.it; giuseppeguidomaria.scarlata@unicz.it

## 3.1 Introduction

MASLD is a recent nomenclature that associates NAFLD with a condition of systemic metabolic dysfunction. It has been proposed in 2020 by an international expert group to better highlight the dysmetabolic comorbidities of NAFLD [13]. Diagnostic criteria include the detection of hepatic steatosis (with a diagnosis conducted by imaging, biomarkers, or histology) and at least one characteristic among overweight/obesity, type 2 diabetes mellitus (T2DM), and metabolic dysregulation. The last criterion requires the presence of at least two characteristics, including increased waist circumference, hypertension, hypertriglyceridemia, low levels of high-density lipoproteins, pre-diabetes, insulin resistance, and subclinical inflammation [8]. Several research teams evaluated this new scientific nomenclature through observational studies on large cohorts of patients. For example, MASLD patients showed higher levels of liver enzymes and more glucose and lipid-metabolism-related disorders. In this way, MASLD definition can specifically identify more patients at risk of developing cirrhosis and


N. Méndez-Sánchez, X. Qi (eds.), *Metabolic Dysfunction-Associated Steatotic Liver Disease*,
https://doi.org/10.1007/978-981-97-9519-2_3

liver cancer, as they are affected by metabolic syndrome [20]. Further investigations corroborated the important role of this new MASLD definition, as it identified patients with significant hepatic fibrosis or high liver stiffness better than the NAFLD criteria [39, 42]. Furthermore, MASLD and alcohol consumption were independently associated with the progression of atherosclerotic cardiovascular risk vs. the NAFLD group [38]. These evidences contribute to the MASLD definition acceptance in 2022 by the "Global multi-stakeholder consensus on the redefinition of fatty liver disease" [22]. At this point, several studies evaluated the prevalence in the general population (20–30%) and in patients with risk factors, such as inflammatory bowel diseases and overweight/obesity (40–50%) [3, 32]. In this regard, different diagnostic techniques are the main cause of this high epidemiological heterogeneity [1, 2]. The aim of this chapter is to explore the different pathogenetic ways that are involved in MAFLD development.

## 3.2 Exploring the Multifactorial Nature of MASLD Development

The pathogenesis of MASLD is influenced by several risk factors, such as T2DM, obesity, insulin resistance, a dysbiosis of the gut microbiota, and genetic and environmental factors. It is known as "multiple-hit" disease due to its multifactorial nature (Fig. 3.1). However, the key event in its development is the fat accumulation in >5% of hepatocytes, followed by the onset of several dysmetabolic comorbidities [30]. In physiological conditions the uptake of circulating lipids is regulated by the transporter fatty acid binding protein-1 in the hepatocyte plasma membrane through the transport of fatty acids into the cytoplasm. De novo lipogenesis converts acetyl-CoA to fatty acids and then esterifies and stores them as triglycerides. Peroxisome-activated receptor promoted fatty acid oxidation prevents hepatic fat accumulation via lipid metabolism processes. However, excess lipid intake or mitochondrial dysfunction promotes fatty acid oxidation in peroxisomes and cytochromes, producing reactive oxygen species (ROS). Hepatic transport of lipids occurs by storing them in the form of very low-density lipoproteins (VLDL) for storage in tissues. Pathogenetic events involving increased de novo hepatic lipogenesis or alterations in lipolysis processes underlie the accumulation of fat in the liver, responsible for the disease development [18]. Transcriptional factors regulate de novo lipogenesis, such as sterol regulatory element-binding transcription factor-1. Genes involved in this mechanism are upregulated during postprandial periods following a significant increase in glucose concentration and insulin secretion [46]. On the other hand, in insulin-resistant subjects, an increase in insulin due to increased lipolysis and fat intake promotes hepatic triglyceride synthesis [15]. In this way, the changes in gut microbiota composition are involved in MASLD pathogenesis. Gut microbiota is an ecosystem composed of over 35,000 bacterial species which performs several functions, such as nutrient and drug metabolism and antimicrobial protection, and it is involved in immunomodulation and the integrity of the gut barrier. A balance of the main Phyla, Bacteroidetes and Firmicutes, also known as eubiosis, grants the efficacy of these functions [31]. However, a gut microflora imbalance (or dysbiosis) has a substantial impact on the development of MASLD. Usually, there is a decrease in Bacteroidetes/Firmicutes ratio, with a reduction in abundance of *Clostridium*, *Rombutsia*, *Faecalibacterium* and *Blautia* genera, and an increase in abundance of *Actinobacteria*, *Proteobacteria*, *Prevotella*, *Fusobacterium*, *Escherichia*, *Lachnoclostridium* genera [1, 2]. The eubiosis of gut microbiota promotes the maintenance of tight junctions, consisting of several proteins, such as junctional adhesion molecules, occludin, claudin, tricellulin, and zonula occludens proteins [27]. However, a gut microbiota imbalance leads to increased intestinal permeability, better defined as leaky gut, causing the release of lipopolysaccharide (LPS) from Gram-negative bacteria outer membrane into the blood stream and passage to the liver through the portal vein [10]. LPS may act, bound

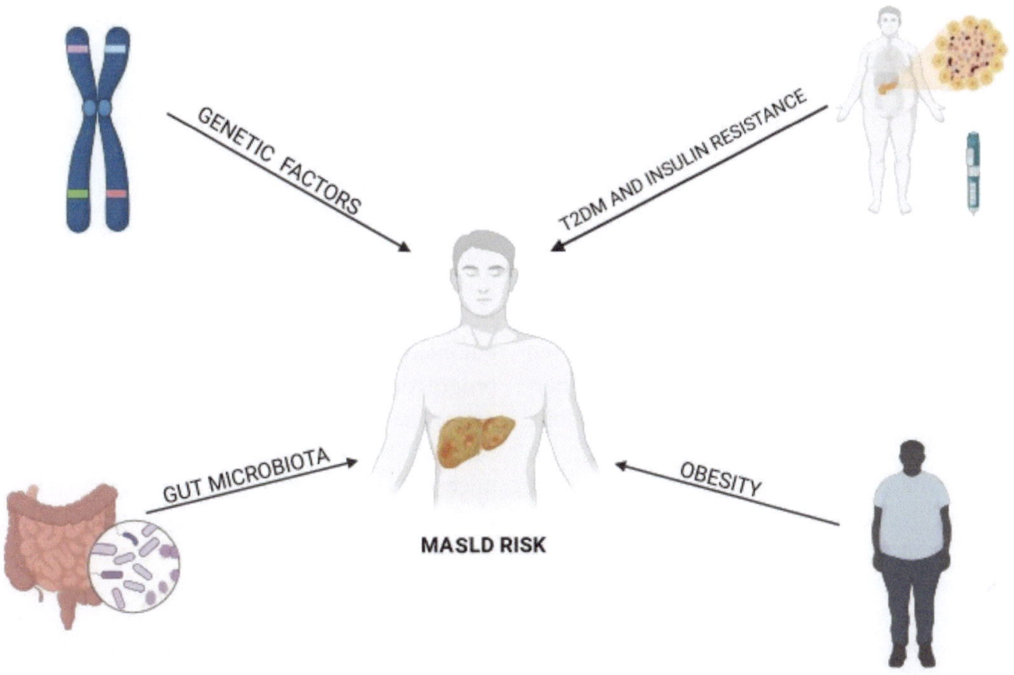


**Fig. 3.1** MASLD risk factors according to "multiple-hit" hypothesis

to the CD14 co-receptor, as a ligand for toll-like receptors resulting in the activation of the inflammatory cascade, including stress-activated protein phenoses, Jun amino N-terminal protein kinase, p38, interferon regulatory factor-3, and nuclear factor-jB, interleukin-6 (IL-6), and tumor necrosis factor-alfa (TNF-α), involved in insulin resistance, obesity and hepatic fat accumulation development [25]. This event can lead to the evolution of steatohepatitis into hepatocellular carcinoma (HCC). The gut microbiota is a main actor in the conversion of dietary choline into methylamines, a toxic compound. In case of increased intestinal permeability this compound can be absorbed in the liver, converted to trimethylamine-N-oxide resulting in inflammatory process and liver damage [9].

## 3.3 Impact of Diet

The term "diet" encompasses the collective food intake of individuals [47]. In this regard, the digestive system participates in the lysis of carbohydrates into short-chain fatty acids through fermentation, the lysis of proteins into amino acids, the synthesis of vitamins like vitamin K and the B vitamins, and the metabolism of polyphenols found in fruits and vegetables, such as flavonoids, stilbenes, lignans, and secoiridoids [34]. Diet plays a dual role in the development of MASLD: while a diet abundant in polyphenols, fiber, and omega-3 fatty acids offers protection, a diet high in saturated fat, red meat, and fried foods may predispose individuals to the disease [35]. Unhealthy foods, characterized by high calorie content and low nutritional value, are commonly referred to as "junk food". Excessive consumption of such foods, particularly prevalent among adolescents, can contribute to the onset of obesity and insulin resistance, significantly impacting quality of life [21]. For instance, mice fed a diet rich in trans-fat, fructose, and cholesterol developed fatty liver and subsequently HCC, particularly in the presence of obesity [17]. Conversely, the Mediterranean diet, conceived by Ancel Keys in the 1960s and predominantly practiced in Greece and Southern

Italy, emphasizes a low intake of saturated fat and a high consumption of vegetable oils. Its dietary pyramid recommends daily consumption of extra-virgin olive oil, fruits, vegetables, whole grains, bread, and legumes. Fish and shellfish are suggested several times a week, while eggs, poultry, and yogurt are recommended once a week. Meat and sweets are to be consumed sparingly. Additionally, this diet should be complemented by regular physical activity, adequate hydration, and moderate consumption of red wine [12]. The Mediterranean diet offers numerous health benefits by reducing metabolic comorbidities and consequently lowering the risk of stroke, heart failure, cardiovascular disease, and liver diseases [24]. These benefits are attributed to its composition, rich in polyphenols, particularly abundant in extra-virgin olive oil and wine, which possess antioxidant and anti-inflammatory properties, reducing levels of reactive oxygen species (ROS) and inhibiting proliferative pathways such as phosphatidylinositol 3-kinase, mitogen-activated protein kinases, and nuclear factor kappa B. Furthermore, vitamins C and E, along with flavonoids found in fruits and vegetables, help prevent DNA damage. Omega-3 fatty acids found in fish inhibit cell proliferation, inflammation, and tumor angiogenesis. Moreover, the diet's limited fat content restricts the development of hyperinsulinemia and obesity, thereby reducing hepatic fat accumulation [23]. In mice models fed high-fat diets, there was an increase in the abundance of the bacterial genera *Bacteroides* and *Clostridium* cluster XVIII, alongside a decrease in genera such as *Bifidobacterium, Prevotella, and Streptococcus*. This gut dysbiosis was associated with the production of secondary bile acids and an upregulation in the transcription of cytochrome P450 cholesterol 7 alpha-hydroxylase, which plays a role in bile acid synthesis in the liver. Elevated levels of total bile acids were observed in the plasma and feces of mice fed the STHD-01 diet, contributing to hepatic fat accumulation and the progression to HCC [41]. Similarly, increased dietary cholesterol could induce liver steatosis, steatohepatitis, fibrosis, and HCC in mice models fed a high-fat/high-cholesterol (HFHC) diet. The abundance of taxa such as Mucispirillum and Desulfovibrionaceae increased, while genera such as *Bacteroides* and *Bifidobacterium* decreased. Germ-free mice receiving fecal transplants from HFHC-fed mice exhibited lipid accumulation and liver inflammation. These findings suggest that a prolonged diet rich in cholesterol, combined with alterations in gut microbiota, may trigger the development and progression of MASLD-HCC. Authors investigating the metabolic phenotypes associated with MASLD-HCC analyzed serum metabolites of mice fed HFHC and high-fat low-carb (HFLC) diets. They found that bile acid metabolism was disrupted in mice fed the HFHC diet. Moreover, levels of LPS in the portal vein were higher in mice fed the HFHC diet compared to those fed the HFLC diet, indicating impaired intestinal barrier function. Additionally, mice fed a cholesterol-rich diet developed insulin resistance and oxidative stress, leading to activation of inflammatory mediators such as hepatic ROS, CD8+ T cells, natural killer T cells, and their associated cytokines [43]. Furthermore, excessive sugar consumption adversely affects gut microbiota composition, particularly fructose found in sweets and beverages. The predominance of acetate-producing gut bacteria, such as those of the *Bacteroides* genus, facilitates its conversion into Acetyl-CoA, contributing to hepatic lipogenesis and consequently, fatty liver formation [44]. High intake of saturated fats induces alterations in gut microbiota composition, reducing the abundance of genera such as *Bacteroides, Bifidobacterium*, and *Eubacterium*, thereby promoting insulin resistance commonly associated with MASLD. Conversely, omega-3 polyunsaturated fatty acids, present in some foods of the Mediterranean diet, mitigate hepatic triglyceride accumulation, insulin resistance, pro-inflammatory pathways, and promote gut microbiota balance [26]. A schematic representation of the impact of the diet in MASLD development is reported in Fig. 3.2.

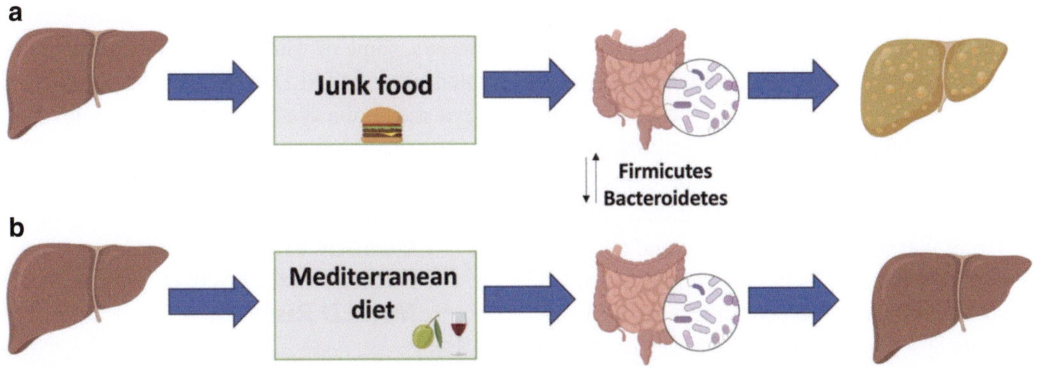


**Fig. 3.2** Impact of the junk food (**a**) and Mediterranean diet (**b**) in the MASLD development

## 3.4 Insulin Resistance and Metabolic Disturbances

Insulin is a helix-rich protein composed of 51 amino acids in two peptide chains (A and B) linked by two disulfide bonds. Its main function is to transport intracellular glucose to insulin-dependent cells and liver, muscle, and adipose tissues [16]. Moreover, it is involved in de novo lipogenesis. In brief, the binding of insulin to its own receptor triggers a phosphorylation process involving insulin receptor substrate 1/2 (Irs1/Irs2), activating the PI3K/Akt pathway. The ultimate goal of this process will be to activate the mTORC1/FoxO1/sterol regulatory element-binding protein 1c pathway. However, hyperinsulinemia downregulates hepatic Irs2 promoting insulin resistance. Glucose transporter (GLUT)-2 transports glucose into hepatocytes, but if glucose concentration increases, carbohydrate response element binding protein induces the expression of various lipogenic enzyme-related genes independently of insulin signaling. Elevated expression of hepatic Irs1 and downregulation of Irs2 lead to increased hyperinsulinemia resulting in increased de novo lipogenesis and development of steatosis [36]. Skeletal muscle contributes to blood glucose regulation through insulin-stimulated and GLUT4-mediated transport of glucose into skeletal muscle, promoting glycolysis and glycogen synthesis. In addition, skeletal muscle insulin resistance is widely found in T2DM. Indeed, excessive fatty acid intake promotes skeletal muscle insulin resistance along with increased intramyocellular lipids, leading to altered insulin signaling induced by lipid-derived metabolites [11]. Exercise significantly impacts insulin resistance, with a marked postprandial increase in muscle glycogenosynthesis and a reduction in hepatic triglycerides synthesis and de novo lipogenesis. Therefore, a proper lifestyle and constant physical activity are used for preventive and therapeutic purposes [29]. When T2DM develops in the context of insulin resistance, it may be an additional independent risk factor contributing to the progression of MASLD to liver cirrhosis [7]. T2DM is associated with an overproduction of pro-inflammatory cytokines, such as IL-1α, IL-6, IL-10, and IL-22. In this regard, a healthy microbiota counteracts this mechanism and the onset of T2DM and insulin resistance through the production of anti-inflammatory cytokines, such as IL-22 produced by *Roseburia intestinalis* and IL-10 produced by polysaccharide A of *Bacteroides fragilis*. Pre-clinical studies showed how the absence of the gene encoding IL-6 leads to a significant increase in the expression of defensins α3 and α4 in the intestine, creating an imbalance of the resident microflora and a pro-inflammatory environment [40]. Furthermore, the gut microbiota regulates insulin clearance, as observed from studies on germ-free mouse models subjected to an obesogenic diet rich in fat. These studies demonstrated an alteration in insulin clearance after 6 weeks of observation compared to mice treated with a control diet and with a healthy microbiota [14]. These evidences showed that insulin resistance and T2DM are linked to the increased intestinal permeability that characterizes patients with MASLD. T2DM accelerates disease progression, resulting in an increased risk of mortality from hepatic and extrahepatic complications, such as cardiovascular disease, nephropathy, and polyneuropathy [19]. Obesity is closely related to insulin resistance, as increased blood sugar leads to hyperglycemia and consequently to overweight. At the same time, obesity increases the pathogenesis of T2DM through stimulation of insulin resistance. Increased body mass index and decreased insulin receptor expression in visceral adipose tissue is inversely associated in obese individuals. The mechanism explaining this phenomenon is a downregulation of the visceral adipose tissue-specific insulin receptor, resulting in obesity-related dysfunction of adipose tissue cells. The reduction in insulin receptor stability is due to the activation of micro-RNA (miRNA)-128, which lowers insulin receptor expression in adipocytes [5]. In addition, obesity increases ROS formation in adipose tissue cells with related inflammatory process and increased insulin resistance [4]. However, 10–15% of the obese population has no cardiometabolic abnormalities. This finding has driven the notion of metabolically healthy obesity: a phenotype associated with normal levels of glucose, blood pressure, and lipid metabolism. Despite this, recent studies have shown obesity to be a driver of subclinical vascular inflammation, fatty liver, and fibrosis, independent of associated comorbidities [28]. Hypertension is generally associated with 40% of patients with MASLD. The occurrence of this comorbidity is attributable to several pathways: (i) increased sympathetic nervous system activation that stimulates hepatic VLDL-triglyceride production with deposition on the arterial wall, restricting blood flow and increasing blood pressure; (ii) rs5186 A1166C variant in the angiotensin type 1 receptor gene associated with hypertension in MASLD; (iii) systemic inflammation mediated by pro-inflammatory cytokines such as TNF-α and IL-6 resulting in increased blood pressure; (iv) hyperinsulinemia with increased blood pressure through a renin-angiotensin-aldosterone system-dependent mechanism in mice models [6]. These metabolic pathways, some of which have yet to be fully elucidated, allow MASLD to be defined as the expression of metabolic syndrome in patients with fatty liver.

## 3.5 Genetic and Epigenetic Factors Influencing MASLD Risk

Genetic and epigenetic factors are a risk factor for the development of MAFLD and for this reason are continually studied through different molecular biology approaches. Among these, the patatin-like phospholipase domain-containing 3 (PNPLA3) gene is one of the most studied genes worldwide, particularly its variant I148M (rs738409 C>G). This appears to predispose to the full spectrum of liver damage, ranging from simple steatosis to steatohepatitis and progressive fibrotic damage. The role of the PNPLA3 gene and the protein encoded by it remains unclear, and many studies attribute different functions to the I148M variant (rs738409 C>G); some attribute an acquired lipogenic function, others a loss of lipolytic function [37]. The transmembrane 6 superfamily member 2 (TM6SF2) is a membrane protein that is located in the cellular endoplasmic reticulum membrane and the endoplasmic reticulum-Golgi intermediate compartment. The TM6SF2 rs58542926 C>T variant was associated with liver steatosis and lower plasma cholesterol and triglycerides, especially in lean MASLD. Membrane domain-containing O-acyltransferase 7 (MBOAT7) is a protein located in the endoplasmic reticulum membrane with lysophospholipid acyltransferase activity. Recent studies have shown that carriers of the MBOAT7 variant (MBOAT7 rs641738 C>T) are associated with increased liver fat content, more severe liver damage, and an increased risk of liver fibrosis compared with genetically healthy subjects. Fibroblast growth factor 21 (FGF21) is a hepatokine that regulates metabolic homeostasis. The FGF21 rs838133 variant has been associated with an elevated serum FGF21 level and increased liver inflammation in individuals with MASLD. Interferon lambda type 3 and 4 (IFNL3/4) is a cytokine that is induced after viral infection by stimulating an immune and inflammatory pathway. Its variants rs12979860 and rs368234815 were associated with increased hepatic inflammation and severe fibrosis in patients with MASLD. Fibronectin type III domain-containing protein 5 (FNDC5) is a precursor of mycelin, which is cleaved to produce irisin from skeletal muscle. Its blood concentration is negatively associated with triglycerides content in obese subjects. A recent study showed that FNDC5 rs380 variant was associated with advanced steatosis but not inflammation or fibrosis in MASLD patients, as reported in Fig. 3.3. Although related to its pathogenesis, further studies could corroborate its role as a potential therapeutic target [45]. In recent years, several epigenetic studies have contributed to the elucidation of the pathophysiology of MASLD in different cohorts of patients. There is a strong association between DNA methylation and MASLD. Recent studies showed that a total of 66,247 CpG sites were differentially methylated in the advanced liver fibrosis group compared with that in the mild liver fibrosis group. There is also increased expression of hypomethylated genes compared with mild liver fibrosis patients. In addition, hypomethylation of cg08309687 was associated with MASLD and the development of T2DM. Histone methylation is also involved in the pathophysiology of MASLD. Histone demethylase, finger homeodomain plant 2 promotes increased de novo lipogenesis and hepatic fat content in mice with fatty liver and obesity. miRNAs are a class of non-coding RNAs that play important roles in regulating gene expression. In this way, 124 miRNA-103,125 miRNA-146b,126 miRNA-33, miRNA-130b-5p,122 miRNA-27a,123 miRNA-29c, 127 miRNA-7a,128 and miRNA-451,129 are strongly associated to MASLD development. For this reason, they are used as potentially diagnostic biomarkers. On the other hand, circular RNA may participate in the development and progression of liver steatosis by promoting hepatic fat accumulation. However, literature is lacking in regard to this topic [33].

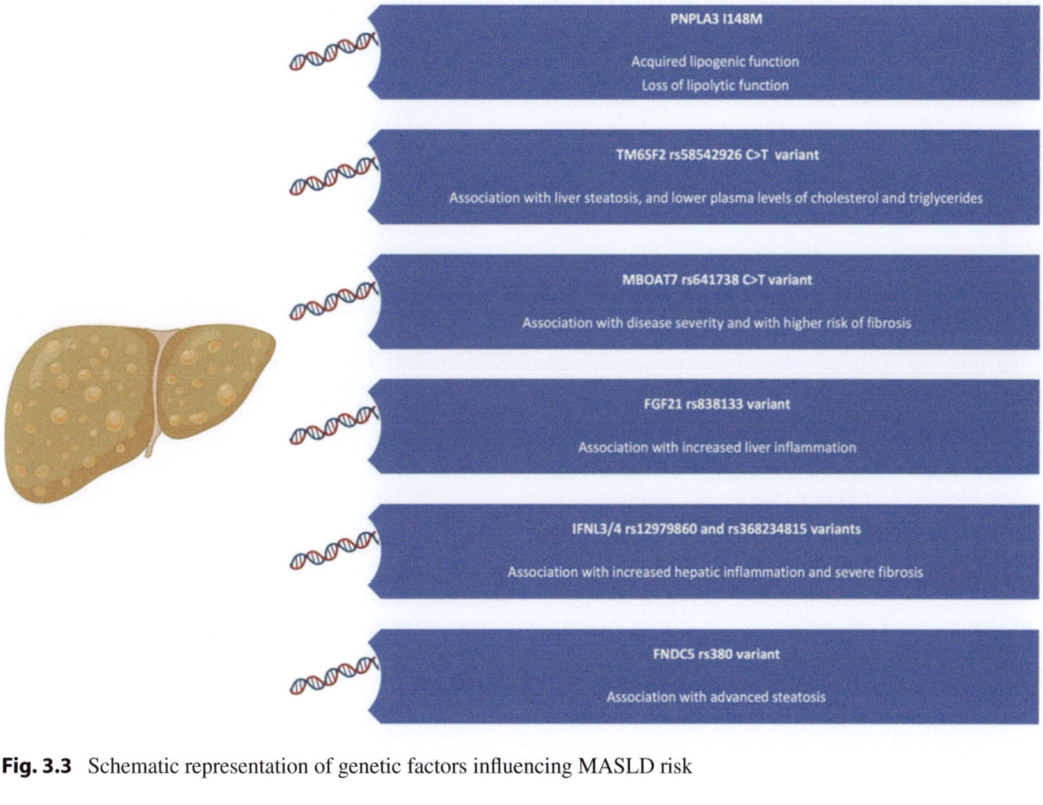


**Fig. 3.3** Schematic representation of genetic factors influencing MASLD risk

## 3.6 Conclusions

Totally decoding the pathogenesis of MASLD is still an open challenge for the scientific community because of the complex pathways involving several factors, including obesity, T2DM, insulin resistance, the gut microbiota composition, genetic and environmental factors, culminating in the "multiple-hit" hypothesis. On the other hand, this new nomenclature better defines the dysmetabolic comorbidities that afflict NAFLD patients and provides a correct diagnostic and therapeutic management. Diet plays a key role in the pathophysiology of fatty liver, modulating the composition of the gut microbiota and the occurrence of metabolic features. Among the many dietary regimens, the Mediterranean diet composed of foods with antioxidant and anti-inflammatory actions seems to be a real preventive and therapeutic measure. At the same time, continuous studies on genetic mutations and epigenetic DNA modifications involving MASLD could create robust diagnostic and therapeutic biomarkers in the near future. Overall, new efforts among clinicians and research are necessary to better define the complex interplay between fatty liver and metabolic dysregulation.

**Competing Interests** The authors have no conflicts of interest to declare that are relevant to the content of this chapter.

## References

1. Abenavoli L, Scarlata GGM, Scarpellini E, Boccuto L, Spagnuolo R, Tilocca B, et al. Metabolic-dysfunction-associated fatty liver disease and gut microbiota: from fatty liver to dysmetabolic syndrome. Medicina. 2023a;59(3):594. https://doi.org/10.3390/medicina59030594.
2. Abenavoli L, Spagnuolo R, Scarlata GGM, Scarpellini E, Boccuto L, Luzza F. Ultrasound prevalence and clinical features of nonalcoholic fatty liver disease in patients with inflammatory bowel diseases: a real-life cross-sectional study. Medicina. 2023b;59(11):1935. https://doi.org/10.3390/medicina59111935.
3. Abenavoli L, Scarlata GG, Spagnuolo R, Luzza F. Can dysmetabolic comorbidities carry hepatic fat accumulation in patients with inflammatory bowel diseases? Minerva Gastroenterol (Torino). 2024; https://doi.org/10.23736/S2724-5985.23.03617-3.
4. Ahima RS. Connecting obesity, aging and diabetes. Nat Med. 2009;15(9):996–7. https://doi.org/10.1038/nm0909-996.
5. Arcidiacono B, Chiefari E, Foryst-Ludwig A, Currò G, Navarra G, Brunetti FS, et al. Obesity-related hypoxia via mir-128 decreases insulin-receptor expression in human and mouse adipose tissue promoting systemic insulin resistance. EBioMedicine. 2020;59:102912. https://doi.org/10.1016/j.ebiom.2020.102912.
6. Badmus OO, Hinds TD, Stec DE. Mechanisms linking metabolic-associated fatty liver disease (MAFLD) to cardiovascular disease. Curr Hypertens Rep. 2023;25(8):151–62. https://doi.org/10.1007/s11906-023-01242-8.
7. Bhatt HB, Smith RJ. Fatty liver disease in diabetes mellitus. Hepatobiliary Surg Nutr. 2015;4(2):101–8. https://doi.org/10.3978/j.issn.2304-3881.2015.01.03.
8. Bianco C, Romeo S, Petta S, Long MT, Valenti L. Mafld vs NAFLD: let the contest begin! Liver Int. 2020;40(9):2079–81. https://doi.org/10.1111/liv.14620.
9. Buzzetti E, Pinzani M, Tsochatzis EA. The multiple-hit pathogenesis of non-alcoholic fatty liver disease (NAFLD). Metabolism. 2016;65(8):1038–48. https://doi.org/10.1016/j.metabol.2015.12.012.
10. Camilleri M. Leaky gut: mechanisms, measurement and clinical implications in humans. Gut. 2019;68(8):1516–26. https://doi.org/10.1136/gutjnl-2019-318427.
11. Cusi K. Role of obesity and lipotoxicity in the development of nonalcoholic steatohepatitis: pathophysiology and clinical implications. Gastroenterology. 2012;142(4):711. https://doi.org/10.1053/j.gastro.2012.02.003.
12. Davis C, Bryan J, Hodgson J, Murphy K. Definition of the Mediterranean diet; a literature review. Nutrients. 2015;7(11):9139–53. https://doi.org/10.3390/nu7115459.
13. Eslam M, Newsome PN, Sarin SK, Anstee QM, Targher G, Romero-Gomez M, et al. A new definition for metabolic dysfunction-associated fatty liver disease: an international expert consensus statement. J Hepatol. 2020;73(1):202–9. https://doi.org/10.1016/j.jhep.2020.03.039.
14. Foley KP, Zlitni S, Duggan BM, Barra NG, Anhê FF, Cavallari JF, et al. Gut microbiota impairs insulin clearance in obese mice. Mol Metab. 2020;42:101067. https://doi.org/10.1016/j.molmet.2020.101067.
15. Gaggini M, Morelli M, Buzzigoli E, DeFronzo R, Bugianesi E, Gastaldelli A. Non-alcoholic fatty liver disease (NAFLD) and its connection with insulin resistance, dyslipidemia, atherosclerosis and coronary heart disease. Nutrients. 2013;5(5):1544–60. https://doi.org/10.3390/nu5051544.
16. Hua Q. Insulin: a small protein with a long journey. Protein Cell. 2010;1(6):537–51. https://doi.org/10.1007/s13238-010-0069-z.
17. Hymel E, Vlock E, Fisher KW, Farazi PA. Differential progression of unhealthy diet-induced hepatocellular carcinoma in obese and non-obese mice. PLoS One.

2022;17(8):e0272623. https://doi.org/10.1371/journal.pone.0272623.
18. Ipsen DH, Lykkesfeldt J, Tveden-Nyborg P. Molecular mechanisms of hepatic lipid accumulation in non-alcoholic fatty liver disease. Cell Mol Life Sci. 2018;75(18):3313–27. https://doi.org/10.1007/s00018-018-2860-6.
19. Kaya E, Yilmaz Y. Metabolic-associated fatty liver disease (MAFLD): a multi-systemic disease beyond the liver. J Clin Transl Hepatol. 2021;10(2):329–38. https://doi.org/10.14218/jcth.2021.00178.
20. Lin S, Huang J, Wang M, Kumar R, Liu Y, Liu S, et al. Comparison of MAFLD and NAFLD diagnostic criteria in Real World. Liver Int. 2020;40(9):2082–9. https://doi.org/10.1111/liv.14548.
21. Malmir H, Mahdavi FS, Ejtahed HS, Kazemian E, Chaharrahi A, Mohammadian Khonsari N, et al. Junk food consumption and psychological distress in children and adolescents: a systematic review and meta-analysis. Nutr Neurosci. 2022;26(9):807–27. https://doi.org/10.1080/1028415x.2022.2094856.
22. Méndez-Sánchez N, Bugianesi E, Gish RG, Lammert F, Tilg H, Nguyen MH, et al. Global multi-stakeholder endorsement of the MAFLD definition. Lancet Gastroenterol Hepatol. 2022;7(5):388–90. https://doi.org/10.1016/s2468-1253(22)00062-0.
23. Mentella MC, Scaldaferri F, Ricci C, Gasbarrini A, Miggiano GAD. Cancer and mediterranean diet: a review. Nutrients. 2019;11(9):2059. https://doi.org/10.3390/nu11092059.
24. Merra G, Noce A, Marrone G, Cintoni M, Tarsitano MG, Capacci A, et al. Influence of mediterranean diet on human gut microbiota. Nutrients. 2020;13(1):7. https://doi.org/10.3390/nu13010007.
25. Miele L, Valenza V, La Torre G, Montalto M, Cammarota G, Ricci R, et al. Increased intestinal permeability and tight junction alterations in nonalcoholic fatty liver disease. Hepatology. 2009;49(6):1877–87. https://doi.org/10.1002/hep.22848.
26. Moussa I, Day RS, Li R, Kaseb A, Jalal PK, Daniel-MacDougall C, et al. Association of dietary fat intake and hepatocellular carcinoma among us adults. Cancer Med. 2021;10(20):7308–19. https://doi.org/10.1002/cam4.4256.
27. Odenwald MA, Choi W, Kuo W-T, Singh G, Sailer A, Wang Y, et al. The scaffolding protein ZO-1 coordinates actomyosin and epithelial apical specializations in vitro and in vivo. J Biol Chem. 2018;293(45):17317–35. https://doi.org/10.1074/jbc.ra118.003908.
28. Pan Z, Eslam M. Metabolically healthy obese and MAFLD: does weight status alone matter? Hepatol Int. 2022;16(6):1253–5. https://doi.org/10.1007/s12072-022-10433-5.
29. Rabøl R, Petersen KF, Dufour S, Flannery C, Shulman GI. Reversal of muscle insulin resistance with exercise reduces postprandial hepatic de novo lipogenesis in insulin resistant individuals. Proc Natl Acad Sci. 2011;108(33):13705–9. https://doi.org/10.1073/pnas.1110105108.
30. Ramírez-Mejía MM, Qi X, Abenavoli L, Romero-Gómez M, Eslam M, Méndez-Sánchez N. Metabolic dysfunction: the silenced connection with fatty liver disease. Ann Hepatol. 2023;28(6):101138. https://doi.org/10.1016/j.aohep.2023.101138.
31. Rinninella E, Raoul P, Cintoni M, Franceschi F, Miggiano G, Gasbarrini A, et al. What is the healthy gut microbiota composition? A changing ecosystem across age, environment, diet, and diseases. Microorganisms. 2019;7(1):14. https://doi.org/10.3390/microorganisms7010014.
32. Rodriguez-Duque JC, Calleja JL, Iruzubieta P, Hernández-Conde M, Rivas-Rivas C, Vera MI, et al. Increased risk of MAFLD and liver fibrosis in inflammatory bowel disease independent of classic metabolic risk factors. Clin Gastroenterol Hepatol. 2023;21(2):406. https://doi.org/10.1016/j.cgh.2022.01.039.
33. Rodríguez-Sanabria JS, Escutia-Gutiérrez R, Rosas-Campos R, Armendáriz-Borunda JS, Sandoval-Rodríguez A. An update in epigenetics in metabolic-associated fatty liver disease. Front Med. 2022;8:8. https://doi.org/10.3389/fmed.2021.770504.
34. Rowland I, Gibson G, Heinken A, Scott K, Swann J, Thiele I, et al. Gut microbiota functions: metabolism of nutrients and other food components. Eur J Nutr. 2017;57(1):1–24. https://doi.org/10.1007/s00394-017-1445-8.
35. Ruiz-Margáin A, Román-Calleja BM, Moreno-Guillén P, González-Regueiro JA, Kúsulas-Delint D, Campos-Murguía A, et al. Nutritional therapy for hepatocellular carcinoma. World J Gastrointest Oncol. 2021;13(10):1440–52. https://doi.org/10.4251/wjgo.v13.i10.1440.
36. Sakurai Y, Kubota N, Yamauchi T, Kadowaki T. Role of insulin resistance in MAFLD. Int J Mol Sci. 2021;22(8):4156. https://doi.org/10.3390/ijms22084156.
37. Spagnuolo R, Abenavoli L, Corea A, Larussa T, Mancina RM, Cosco C, et al. Multifaceted pathogenesis of liver steatosis in inflammatory bowel disease: a systematic review. Eur Rev Med Pharmacol Sci. 2021;25(18):5818–25. https://doi.org/10.26355/eurrev_202109_26800.
38. Tsutsumi T, Eslam M, Kawaguchi T, Yamamura S, Kawaguchi A, Nakano D, et al. MAFLD better predicts the progression of atherosclerotic cardiovascular risk than NAFLD: generalized estimating equation approach. Hepatol Res. 2021;51(11):1115–28. https://doi.org/10.1111/hepr.13685.
39. van Kleef LA, Ayada I, Alferink LJM, Pan Q, de Knegt RJ. Metabolic dysfunction–associated fatty liver disease improves detection of high liver stiffness: the Rotterdam study. Hepatology. 2021;75(2):419–29. https://doi.org/10.1002/hep.32131.
40. Wu S, Zhang Y, Ma J, Liu Y, Li W, Wang T, et al. Interleukin-6 absence triggers intestinal microbiota dysbiosis and mucosal immunity in mice. Cytokine. 2022;153:155841. https://doi.org/10.1016/j.cyto.2022.155841.

41. Yamada S, Takashina Y, Watanabe M, Nagamine R, Saito Y, Kamada N, et al. Bile acid metabolism regulated by the gut microbiota promotes non-alcoholic steatohepatitis-associated hepatocellular carcinoma in mice. Oncotarget. 2018;9(11):9925–39. https://doi.org/10.18632/oncotarget.24066.
42. Yamamura S, Eslam M, Kawaguchi T, Tsutsumi T, Nakano D, Yoshinaga S, et al. MAFLD identifies patients with significant hepatic fibrosis better than NAFLD. Liver Int. 2020;40(12):3018–30. https://doi.org/10.1111/liv.14675.
43. Zhang X, Coker OO, Chu ES, Fu K, Lau HC, Wang Y-X, et al. Dietary cholesterol drives fatty liver-associated liver cancer by modulating gut microbiota and metabolites. Gut. 2020;70(4):761–74. https://doi.org/10.1136/gutjnl-2019-319664.
44. Zhao S, Jang C, Liu J, Uehara K, Gilbert M, Izzo L, et al. Dietary fructose feeds hepatic lipogenesis via microbiota-derived acetate. Nature. 2020;579(7800):586–91. https://doi.org/10.1038/s41586-020-2101-7.
45. Zhu X, Xia M, Gao X. Update on genetics and epigenetics in metabolic associated fatty liver disease. Ther Adv Endocrinol Metab. 2022;13:204201882211321. https://doi.org/10.1177/20420188221132138.
46. Zhu Z, Zhang X, Pan Q, Zhang L, Chai J. In-depth analysis of de novo lipogenesis in non-alcoholic fatty liver disease: mechanism and pharmacological interventions. Liver Res. 2023;7(4):285–95. https://doi.org/10.1016/j.livres.2023.11.003.
47. Zohoori FV. Chapter 1: Nutrition and diet. Monogr Oral Sci. 2019;28:1–13. https://doi.org/10.1159/000455365.

# 4 Liver Steatosis: From Lipotoxicity to Cellular Damage

Tobias Puengel and Frank Tacke

Metabolic dysfunction-associated steatotic liver disease (MASLD) represents the most common cause of chronic liver disease [1]. MASLD is defined by hepatic steatosis in the presence of cardiometabolic risk factors (i.e., obesity, type 2 diabetes/glucose intolerance, hypertension, dyslipidemia), and its prevalence is expected to rise further in the near future, therefore representing a major global health burden [2, 3]. Of note, MASLD—formerly termed "Nonalcoholic fatty liver disease (NAFLD)"—allows the consumption of alcohol amounts up to 140 g/wk. for female and 210 g/wk. for male individuals [4]. Chronic, low-grade, sterile inflammation, which is orchestrated by parenchymal (mainly hepatocytes) and non-parenchymal resident or freshly infiltrated immune cells (e.g., macrophages, neutrophils, hepatic stellate cells [HSCs]), is the key driver of progression to metabolic dysfunction-associated steatohepatitis (MASH; formerly referred to as nonalcoholic steatohepatitis [NASH]) and liver fibrosis [5, 6]. Meta-analyses reveal that progression of fibrosis is influenced by extrinsic (e.g., genetics, sex, age) and intrinsic (e.g., lifestyle factors, dietary habits, gut microbiota) risk factors [7], while fibrosis stage correlates with disease-related morbidity and mortality among MASH patients and is associated with liver cirrhosis or hepatocellular carcinoma (HCC) [8, 9]. Given that heterogeneity of MASLD in respect of modifiable and non-modifiable factors or extrahepatic disease drivers contributing to conditions like MASLD such as in the gastrointestinal tract, adipose tissue, or the endocrine system, there is ongoing exploration into targeting these mediators for the treatment of MASH. Although extensive pathomechanistic insights over the last decades led to the successful identification of pharmacologic targets impeding the development of promising drug candidates, most advanced approaches particularly focus on metabolic pathways to mitigate the detrimental effects on hepatocytes, thereby dampening subsequent inflammatory and fibrogenic signals indirectly [10]. This had led to the approval of the first MASH-targeting therapy, resmetirom, as discussed below. The in-depth understanding of metabolic, inflammatory and fibrogenic pathways in MASLD/MASH is expected to fuel the development of further, even more effective therapeutics.

T. Puengel
Department of Hepatology & Gastroenterology, Charité - Universitätsmedizin Berlin, Campus Virchow-Klinikum and Campus Charité Mitte, Berlin, Germany

Berlin Institute of Health, Berlin, Germany
e-mail: tobias.puengel@charite.de

F. Tacke (✉)
Department of Hepatology & Gastroenterology, Charité - Universitätsmedizin Berlin, Campus Virchow-Klinikum and Campus Charité Mitte, Berlin, Germany
e-mail: frank.tacke@charite.de



N. Méndez-Sánchez, X. Qi (eds.), *Metabolic Dysfunction-Associated Steatotic Liver Disease*,
https://doi.org/10.1007/978-981-97-9519-2_4

## 4.1 Dysregulated Lipid and Carbohydrate Metabolism Promotes Hepatic Steatosis

In homeostasis, the liver crucially balances the uptake, synthesis and systemic distribution of lipids as a source of energy supply for metabolically active tissues such as the skeletal or cardiac muscle [11]. Under physiologic conditions the hepatic triglyceride (TG) content averages approximately less than 5% of the total liver volume, although the liver regularly processes a large amount of fatty acids derived from our diet or other nutrient storage organs like adipose tissue [12, 13]. While insulin actions suppress lipolysis in the fed state, during fasting lipolysis generates endogenous fatty acids, which are released from the adipose tissue into the systemic circulation. Especially during disease states the relatively small proportion of dietary fatty acids generated from lipolysis of TG-rich lipoproteins such as apolipoprotein B-containing lipoproteins, chylomicrons or very low-density lipoprotein (VLDL) particles is increased [11, 13]. Hepatic steatosis as a result of excessive lipid accumulation is a hallmark during development of MASLD and its progression to MASH. In consequence, MASLD evolved as the major driver of liver-related morbidity and mortality, representing one of the leading causes for liver transplantation [14, 15]. Excessive energy substrates such as carbohydrates or dietary fats lead to increased hepatic de novo lipogenesis (DNL), while free fatty acids are released from inflamed and metabolically dysfunctional adipose tissue, which additionally accumulate in the liver. TGs are insoluble molecules comprising free fatty acids—therefore, enabling effective intracellular storage as lipid droplets or transport via lipoproteins throughout the body [12]. In the course of MASLD, once the hepatic lipid storage capacity is overwrought due to disproportionate fatty acid oxidation and insufficient secretion of VLDL molecules, metabolic injury exceeds (Fig. 4.1).

Evidence indicates that hepatic DNL plays a pivotal role in the course and progression of MASLD. Thus, well-characterized enzymes catalyzing the different steps of TG formation represent promising targets for compounds aiming at correcting malfunctioning metabolic pathways to ameliorate metabolic disturbances and cellular stress signals [16, 17]. Lead compounds demonstrating liver fat lowering efficacy in phase II clinical studies directly modulating lipogenesis target a variety of essential enzymes involved in DNL such as (i) stearoyl-coenzyme A desaturase 1 (SCD1), (ii) acetyl-CoA carboxylase (ACC), (iii) fatty acid synthase (FAS) or (iv) diacylglycerol O-acyltransferase 2 (DGAT2). (i) SCD1 acts

**Fig. 4.1** From metabolic injury to cellular damage, inflammation and liver fibrosis. In MASLD and MASH, metabolic dysregulation occurs due to a complex interplay of non-modifiable and modifiable, intra- and extrahepatic mediators stimulating a series of harmful processes within hepatocytes including ER stress, oxidative stress and mitochondrial dysfunction. Excessive accumulation of fatty acids and increased de novo lipogenesis (DNL) results in lipotoxicity, prompting the release of stress signals and initiation of cell death pathways in metabolically strained hepatocytes, which in turn trigger immune responses, sparking inflammation and fibrogenesis. Profibrogenic factors and cellular crosstalk prompt activation and transdifferentiation of quiescent HSCs to scar tissue producing myofibroblasts. Once metabolic injury subsides pro-resolving factors stimulate reversion of myofibroblasts to a "quiescent"-like HSC phenotype and elimination of activated HSCs resulting in tissue repair. Abbreviations: ATP, adenosine triphosphate; CCL, chemokine (C–C motif) ligand; IL, interleukin; DAMPs, damage-associated molecular patterns; ER, endoplasmic reticulum; EVs, extracellular vesicles; FFA, free fatty acids; FGF, fibroblast growth factor; FXR, farnesoid X receptor; GIP, glucose-dependent insulinotropic polypeptide; GLP-1, glucagon-like peptide 1; HSC, hepatic stellate cell; LPS, lipopolysaccharide; LXR, liver X receptors; MASH, metabolic dysfunction-associated steatohepatitis; MASLD, metabolic dysfunction-associated steatotic liver disease; MMP, matrix metalloproteinases; PAMPs, pathogen-associated molecular patterns; PPAR, peroxisome proliferator-activated receptor; ROS, reactive oxygen species; TIMP, tissue inhibitor of matrix metalloproteinases; TNF, tumor necrosis factor; THR, thyroid hormone receptor. The figure was created with BioRender.com

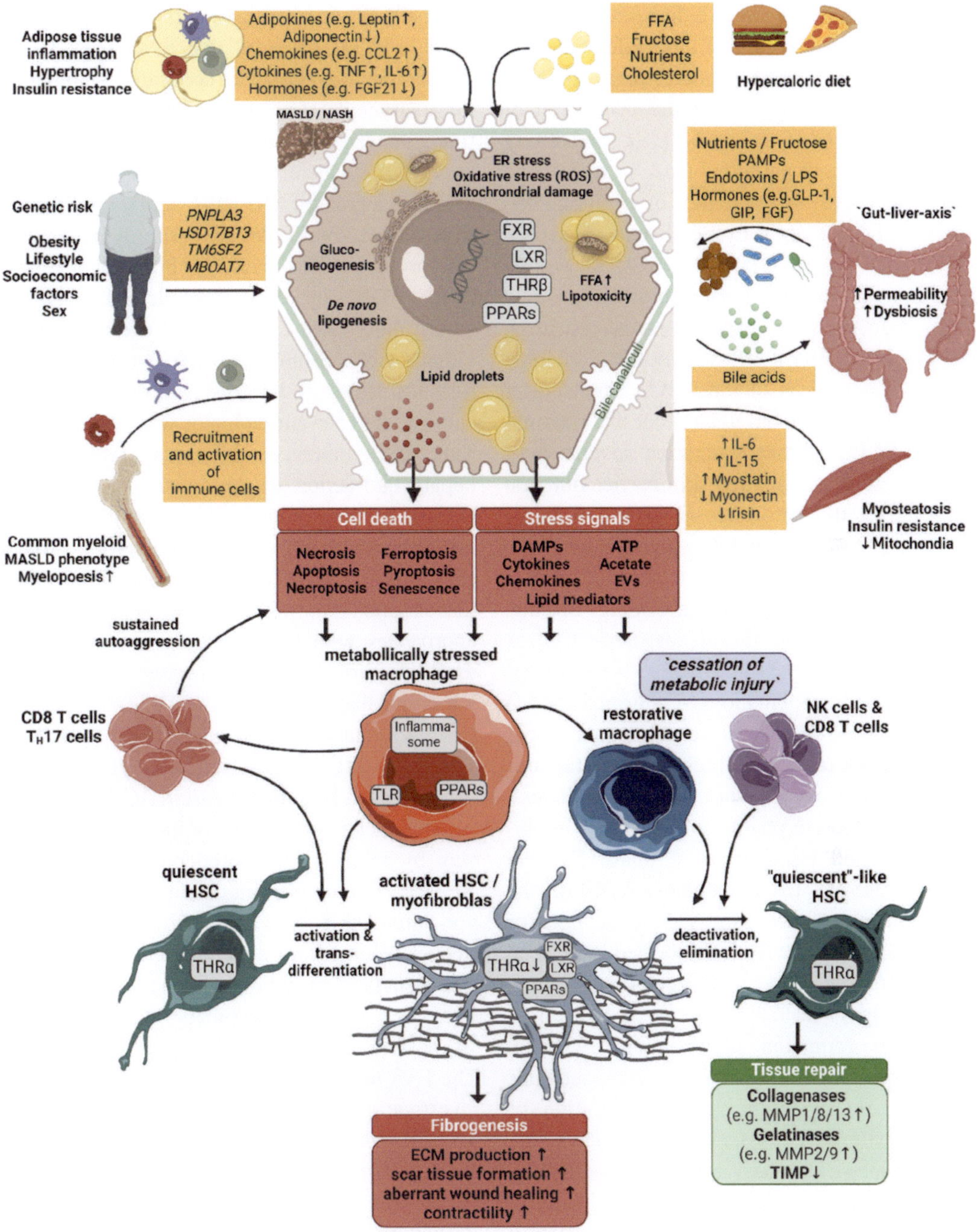
Adipose tissue inflammation
Hypertrophy
Insulin resistance
Adipokines (e.g. Leptin↑, Adiponectin↓)
Chemokines (e.g. CCL2↑)
Cytokines (e.g. TNF↑, IL-6↑)
Hormones (e.g. FGF21↓)
FFA
Fructose
Nutrients
Cholesterol
Hypercaloric diet
MASLD / NASH
ER stress
Oxidative stress (ROS)
Mitochrondrial damage
Genetic risk
Obesity
Lifestyle
Socioeconomic factors
Sex
PNPLA3
HSD17B13
TM6SF2
MBOAT7
Gluco-neogenesis
De novo lipogenesis
FXR
LXR
THRβ
PPARs
FFA↑
Lipotoxicity
Lipid droplets
Bile canaliculi
Nutrients / Fructose
PAMPs
Endotoxins / LPS
Hormones (e.g.GLP-1, GIP, FGF)
`Gut-liver-axis`
↑Permeability
↑Dysbiosis
Bile acids
Recruitment and activation of immune cells
Common myeloid
MASLD phenotype
Myelopoesis↑
↑IL-6
↑IL-15
↑Myostatin
↓Myonectin
↓Irisin
Myosteatosis
Insulin resistance
↓Mitochondia
Cell death
Necrosis
Apoptosis
Necroptosis
Ferroptosis
Pyroptosis
Senescence
Stress signals
DAMPs
Cytokines
Chemokines
ATP
Acetate
EVs
Lipid mediators
sustained autoaggression
metabollically stressed macrophage
`cessation of metabolic injury`
CD8 T cells
$T_H$17 cells
Inflamma-some
TLR
PPARs
restorative macrophage
NK cells & CD8 T cells
quiescent HSC
activated HSC / myofibroblas
"quiescent"-like HSC
activation & trans-differentiation
THRα
THRα↓
FXR
LXR
PPARs
deactivation, elimination
THRα
Tissue repair
Collagenases
(e.g. MMP1/8/13↑)
Gelatinases
(e.g. MMP2/9↑)
TIMP↓
Fibrogenesis
ECM production ↑
scar tissue formation ↑
aberrant wound healing ↑
contractility ↑

as key metabolic regulator either directing fatty acids towards β oxidation or intracellular storage by formation of TGs [18]. Interestingly, SCD1 is the rate limiting enzyme of the generation of monounsaturated fatty acids [18], converting stearoyl-CoA and palmitoyl-CoA to oleate and palmitoleate [19]. In the context of metabolic diseases, SCD1 activity is dysregulated—thus, contributing to progression of MASLD to MASH [20]. In addition, preclinical studies demonstrate that a reduced SCD1 expression resulted in an increased cholesterol efflux from the liver most likely via activation of the ABCA1 transporter [21]. Moreover, one has to consider that pharmacologic SCD1 inhibitors reported adverse drug reactions such as impaired skin barrier function or accelerated atherosclerosis in experimental MASLD [22, 23]. Aramchol, which is a synthetic fatty acid–bile acid conjugate (FABAC), inhibits SCD1 activity potentially amending obesity, hepatic steatosis, and insulin resistance [22]. A phase IIb clinical trial (NCT02279524) evaluated efficacy of aramchol in biopsy-confirmed MASH patients with F2–F3 fibrosis revealing modest but nonsignificant reduction in relative liver fat content as well as fibrosis stage [24]. Nonetheless, beneficial effects of pharmacologic SDC1 inhibition suggested initiation of a phase III trial (NCT04104321). (ii) In humans, ACC1 is the predominant isoform expressed in the liver or adipose tissue, while ACC2 is located in skeletal and heart muscle tissue. ACC regulates the transition from lipogenic to oxidative metabolism catalyzing the formation of malonyl-CoA from acetyl-CoA, which acts as an important activator of fatty acid oxidation through inhibition of carnitine palmitoyl transferase 1 (CPT1) as CPT1 allocates long-chain fatty acids to mitochondria for β oxidation. Therefore, pharmacologic inhibition of ACC suppresses DNL and stimulates β oxidation of fatty acids potentially reducing hepatic lipid accumulation and subsequent lipotoxicity [11]. Interestingly, experimental rodent models of MASLD and MASH suggest targeting both ACC isoforms is favorable to effectively ameliorate steatosis and insulin sensitivity and improve hepatic lipid handling [25, 26]. To date, four ACC inhibitors have been evaluated in clinical trials. While investigation of two compounds have been discontinued due to unwanted side effects (decline in platelet count due to impaired megakaryocyte demarcation membrane formation upon DNL inhibition [27] and significant hypertriglyceridemia most likely as a result of adaptive increased SREBP-1 activity [28]), two liver-directed molecules are currently under clinical investigation (phase II). Firsocostat nearly blocked DNL in a dose-dependent manner and significantly lowered hepatic fat content in individuals with presumed MASH (NCT02876796) [29, 30]. However, improvement of liver fibrosis as a patient relevant endpoint was not achieved. The ACC inhibitor clesacostat reduced the hepatic fat fraction in a dose- and time-dependent manner but also culminated in hypertriglyceridemia (NCT03248882) [31, 32]. Therefore, clinical evaluation of clesacostat as monotherapy was discontinued proposing combinational approaches with lipid-lowering agents such as diacylglycerol O-acyltransferase 2 (DGAT2) inhibitors like ervogastat (NCT04321031) [33]. (iii) FAS catalyzes the formation of palmitate, a saturated fatty acid, from acetyl-CoA and malonyl-CoA [34]. In contrast to ACC inhibitors, which target an earlier step of the lipogenic pathway by inhibiting the production of malonyl-CoA, FAS inhibition modulates DNL but does not stimulate β oxidation of fatty acids [35]. Recent results from experimental MASH indicate beneficial metabolic potency ameliorating steatosis as well as inflammation and liver fibrosis, postulating multimodal efficacy in vivo [36]. The FAS inhibitor TVB-2640 is currently under investigation in MASH patients with F2–F3 fibrosis—results on histologic endpoints after 1 year of treatment are anticipated to be published soon (phase IIb study NCT04906421). Earlier studies observed that already a relatively modest DNL inhibition upon administration moderately reduced liver fat content and improved liver injury markers suggesting a greater dose-dependent efficacy potential as well as a sufficient safety window. (iv) Esterification of diacylglycerol with a fatty acid-CoA is the final step of TG synthesis catalyzed by DGAT. While DGAT1 is predominantly expressed in the intestine and involved in absorption of dietary fats [37], DGAT2 is expressed in metabolically active tissues such as the liver or adipose tissue [38]. Mechanistically, DGAT2 fosters lipid storage in hepatocytes through incorporation of fatty acids from DNL into TGs [39]. Therefore, pharmacologic antagonism is supposed to reduce the hepatocyte lipid burden. Preclinical studies revealed that targeting the final step of TG formation by inhibition of DGAT2 did not result in accumulation of preceding substrates most likely through counteracting reduced expression of molecules such as SREBP involved in lipogenesis and oxidative signaling [40, 41]. Moreover, pharmacologic modulation of DGAT2 in experimental MASLD and MASH ameliorated hepatic steatosis and fibrosis as well as—in contrast to ACC inhibitors [28]—decreased circulating TGs [31, 42]. A small molecule (ervogastat; PF-06865571) effectively inhibiting DGAT2 is currently under investigation in a phase 2b clinical trial (NCT04839393) for treatment of MASLD and has already demonstrated a significant reduction of liver fat [43–45]. More recently, another phase 2b clinical study (NCT03334214) reported beneficial fat reducing effects in patients with type 2 diabetes and MASLD by administration of a gene silencing approach (IONIS-DGAT2rx, once weekly via subcutaneous injection) [46]. Nonetheless, while those pharmacologic approaches report promising reduction in liver fat, clinical trials are still in a preliminary stage for example lacking liver biopsy endpoints (NCT04321031; NCT04932512). In summary, lead compounds directly modulating lipidomic pathways indicate sufficient efficacy in lowering liver fat content in clinical trials, reporting a close association between the degree of DNL inhibition and improvement of hepatic fat content. Interestingly, an ongoing clinical trial (NCT04321031) is currently testing a combinational approach modulating different steps of the DNL, testing ervogastat (DGAT2 inhibition) in coadministration with clesacostat (ACC inhibition) to overcome negative side effects of ACC inhibitor monotherapy elevating circulating TGs. However, as MASLD is a multidimensional disease beneficial metabolic effects might be insufficient especially for the treatment of advanced disease stages and progressed fibrosis. Therefore, DNL inhibitors are anticipated to be interesting agents for combination with other therapeutic agents that modulate different disease drivers.

Evidence is available indicating that excessive fructose consumption, which is commonly incorporated in beverages and highly processed foods, can be considered as an important contributor to lipogenesis as well as obesity, steatosis and insulin resistance [47, 48]. Excessive dietary fructose may already affect the gut microbiota causing dysbiosis, gut barrier dysfunction and increasing nutrient absorption [49, 50]. Interestingly, the consumption of sugar-sweetened beverages is associated with an increased rate of liver-related mortality and liver cancer [51]. The liver is the primary organ confronted with an overload of fructose and gut-derived fructose metabolites. Based on the unique aspects of fructose metabolism, fructose can drive hepatic DNL and modulate the activation status of hepatocytes as well as immune cells in the liver [48, 52]. The close association between excessive fructose consumption and MASLD progression triggered the development of compounds modulating fructose absorption and metabolism. Fructokinase, or ketohexokinase (KHK) catalyzes the conversion of fructose to fructose-1-phosphate—therefore, representing a potential target for the treatment of MASLD and MASH. While preclinical studies evaluating the potential of KHK inhibitors such as PF-06835919 encouraged the progression to clinical assessment [53], all clinical trials testing those compounds in individuals with type 2 diabetes or MASLD have been discontinued because of relatively modest effects on hepatic fat content and glycemic control (NCT03256526, NCT03969719) [54, 55]. Moreover, genome-wide association studies conducted in large cohorts have identified susceptibility genes such as PNPLA3, MBOAT7, and TM6SF2, that significantly influence key metabolic pathways within hepatocytes (e.g., processing of excessive lipids and carbohydrates) and thus, contributing to MASLD and MASH [56, 57]. Therefore, gene modifying strategies including RNA-based techniques, small molecules or aiming at downstream targets qualify as promising anti-MASH approaches, which are currently under clinical investigation [58, 59].

## 4.2 Lipotoxicity and Nuclear Receptors Impact Liver Health

Lipotoxicity is key feature during progression of MASLD from steatosis to MASH and liver fibrosis, which can be determined by overload of fatty acids and triglycerides in hepatocytes triggering the generation of injurious lipid metabolites [60]. In turn, hepatocellular metabolic dysfunction leads to onset of mitochondrial dysfunction, endoplasmic reticulum (ER) stress and increased lipid oxidation as well as subsequent production of oxidative stress signals (e.g., reactive oxygen species [ROS]) (Fig. 4.1) [61]. Fatty acids are processed into fatty acyl-CoAs in the cytoplasm, transported to the mitochondria, where they are further degraded to acetyl-CoA through fatty acid oxidation [62]. Overactivation of fatty acid oxidation and subsequent tricarboxylic acid cycle generate an electron overflow through the electron transport chain triggering activation of molecular oxygen to form superoxide and hydrogen peroxide initiating lipid peroxidation. Of note, saturated fatty acids remain a more hepatotoxic potential than unsaturated species most likely due to certain metabolic aspects as unsaturated fatty acids are esterified more efficiently through peroxisomal β oxidation into TGs [63]. Moreover, unsaturated fatty acids, specifically long-chain omega-3 fatty acids, hold the potential to beneficially regulate driving pathways of MASLD progression or directly counteract fatty acid induced hepatotoxicity [10]. However, therapeutic efficacy is limited by susceptibility to peroxidation and degradation—consequently leading to the development of structurally engineered fatty acids such as icosabutate [64]. Those modified polyunsaturated fatty acids resist hepatocyte uptake and peroxidative processes, thereby maintaining the beneficial metabolic effects of long-chain omega-3 fatty acids [64]. Hepatoprotective effects in patients with elevated circulating lipids suggest the concept of structurally engineered fatty acids as a novel approach for the treatment of MASLD [10].

Metabolic liver injury can be influenced by a variety of intrahepatic but also extrahepatic stimuli highlighting the concept of a multidimensional disease. For instance, oxidative stress in other metabolic tissues such as adipose or muscle tissue as a consequence of hyperglycemia and insulin resistance known in diabetic individuals may contribute to hepatic lipotoxicity [65]. Moreover, abovementioned ACC inhibition subsequently results in reduced lipotoxicity by suppressing DNL and stimulating fatty acid oxidation [11]. In this context, fatty acid oxidation can further be modulated by nuclear receptor signaling such as thyroid hormone receptor beta (THRβ), farnesoid X receptors (FXRs) or peroxisome proliferator-activated receptors (PPARs) or liver X receptors (LXRs). Nuclear receptors are triggered by different ligands including lipids, bile acids or hormones initiating expression of transcription factors that are involved in metabolic relevant processes such as lipid or glucose handling [66, 67]. Thyroid hormones are essentially involved in systemic and local energy metabolism influencing lipid (e.g., uptake of fatty acids, DNL, lipolysis or fatty acid oxidation) and glucose (e.g., glycolysis, gluconeogenesis, glycogen synthesis, and glycogenolysis) metabolism in the liver and thereby, represent important modifiers of metabolic disease drivers [68].

Thyroid hormone actions are mediated via THRα and β, which display a distinct tissue and cell-type specific distribution. Thyroid hormone signaling is either directed via gene transcription as nuclear transcription factors (type 1 signaling) or via activation of intracellular signaling cascades (type 3 signaling), which is the predominant mode of action influencing hepatic lipid or glucose handling [69]. Robust evidence is available demonstrating that clinical hypothyroidism is associated with dysregulated lipid profiles (increase of total cholesterol, LDL-cholesterol and plasma triglycerides) [68, 70]. In turn, thyroid hormone replacement therapy by levothyroxine in overt hypothyroid patients can alleviate dyslipidemia. However, simple pharmacologic substitution of thyroid hormones potentially induces adverse effects similar to hyperthyroid states (e.g., cardiac arrhythmia, bone demineralization, sleep disorders or hair loss). Nonetheless, as unwanted side effects can predominantly be attributed to THRα-mediated signaling, THRβ-selective compounds such as the THRβ mimetic resmetirom may provide thyroid hormone-related benefits for MASLD patients [10]. Resmetirom (MGL-3196, Rezdiffra) has been evaluated for the treatment of MASH and liver fibrosis in the phase 3 MAESTRO-NASH trial (NCT03900429). Latest results from a preplanned interim analysis have recently been published demonstrating MASH resolution and at least one stage improvement of liver fibrosis [71], corroborating the concept of targeting THRs to modulate TH activities. Encouraging results from the phase III MAESTRO trials evaluating the THRβ-selective thyromimetic resmetirom now led to approval by the U.S. Food and Drug Administration (FDA) as the first and so far only medication for the indication of non-cirrhotic MASH with moderate to advanced liver fibrosis [71, 72]. Of note, within the US label, performing a liver biopsy is not mandatory for the diagnosis of MASH and subsequent prescription of resmetirom. The recommended dosage is 80 mg or 100 mg orally once daily depending on the patient's weight (</> 100 kg). The European Medicines Agency (EMA) recently announced that marketing authorization application for resmetirom has been validated, so that final approval for the treatment of MASH and liver fibrosis by the EMA can be expected at the beginning of 2025 [73]. Yet, future studies need to elucidate the exact mode of action of THRβ agonism. In this context, more insights regarding systemic versus local as well as cell type-specific thyroid hormone actions are of utmost interest to develop and test novel thyroid hormone-based therapeutic approaches. Strategies modulating the thyroid hormone availability in the liver beyond directly targeting THRs are currently under investigation including targets such as thyroid hormone metabolizing enzymes (e.g., deionidase 1/3) or thyroid hormone transporters (e.g., monocarboxylate transporter 8 [MCT8] or sodium/bile acid cotransporter [NTCP]) [68, 74, 75].

FXR is expressed in many tissues, including kidney, stomach, intestine, gall bladder, liver, and adipose tissue representing the most important nuclear receptor for the maintenance of bile acids, which can subsequently modulate metabolic pathways locally or on long distance and is involved in lipid and glucose metabolism (e.g., hepatic glycogenolysis, gluconeogenesis, DNL, fatty acid oxidation) as well as immune responses [76, 77]. Bile acids display soluble mediators, which are metabolized by the gut microbiota, potentially acting as metabolically relevant hormones via enterohepatic circulation and exerting immunologic functions. Evidence supports the concept that disruption of FXR signaling can be linked with several entities of metabolic and liver diseases including MASLD. Thus, FXR is considered a promising target for the treatment of metabolic disease. However, available data regarding FXR signaling in MASH are inconsistent. FXR deletion was associated with insulin resistance, elevated plasma triglycerides, cholesterol levels and hepatic steatosis. On the contrary, intestinal microbiota composition significantly contributed in an FXR-dependent fashion to development of obesity in a dietary mouse model. Positive effects of pharmacologic FXR agonism dampening obesity, hepatic steatosis, and fibrosis support the concept of therapeutic FXR modification and initiation of clinical trials [67, 78]. In MASH patients, FXR signaling leads to increasing bile acid levels, changes in the bile acid composition as a consequence of insulin resistance, intestinal dysbiosis and impaired hepatocyte excretion potentially explaining bile acid-associated hepatotoxicity. In turn, one could speculate that beneficial effects of FXR agonism might display a consequence of restored bile acid balance. A recent phase 2 clinical trial reported that the small molecule FXR agonist cilofexor resulted in reduction of steatosis and fibrosis in MASH patients. Obeticholic acid (OCA) is an FXR agonist that has been extensively investigated in MASLD demonstrating multiple beneficial metabolic effects. Administration of OCA for 72 weeks in adult MASH patients in the phase 2 FLINT trial (NCT01265498) effectively improved histological disease features [79]. Post-hoc analyses demonstrated additional effects of OCA reducing obesity and serum aminotransferase levels. However, the authors observed increasing levels of plasma lipids such as low-density lipoprotein-C (LDL-C) and hemoglobin A1c levels (HbA1c) compared to placebo groups, which could be reversed by additional treatment with atorvastatin (NCT02633956) [80, 81]. A phase 3 clinical trial (REGENERATE, NCT02548351) with OCA in adult MASH patients has recently been terminated. The interim analysis showed improvement of fibrosis while the primary outcome of MASH resolution was not met [82]. This was confirmed in an independent, more stringent pathological analysis requested by regulatory agencies, which confirmed a significant improvement of hepatic fibrosis [83]. Nonetheless, these data did not lead to provisional approval of OCA in this indication.

PPARs can act as lipid sensors responsive to fatty acids and derivates. Activated PPARs modulate tissue-specific transcriptomic profiles enabling complex adaptation to dietary changes or metabolic injury—thus, regulating several key pathways involved in MASH progression [84]. The PPAR family comprises three isotypes, PPARα, β/δ, and γ, that display distinct cell-type-specific expression profiles potentially resulting in complementary actions in the pathogenesis of MASLD [67]. PPARα represents the predominant isoform in the liver, particularly in mice, which is involved in fatty acid oxidation, lipid transport, gluconeo- or ketogenesis and correlates with the presence of MASH [85]. PPARγ actions are mainly exerted in adipose tissue regulating adipocyte differentiation, lipid and glucose metabolism, thereby promoting oxidation of fatty acids and storage as triglycerides. The functions of PPARβ/δ in metabolic disease are less clear, whereas promotion of hepatic fatty acid oxidation is reported. Preclinical studies modulating PPAR activities revealed beneficial metabolic potential corroborating evaluation of different PPAR-targeted interventions for the treatment of MASH. Available PPAR agonists are chemically distinct and hence exhibit various pharmacokinetic and pharmacodynamic properties leading to compound-specific responses, suggesting necessity of individual efficacy and safety assessments [84]. While multiple single and dual (e.g., elafibranor [α/δ] or saroglitazar [α/γ]) PPAR agonists have demonstrated robust anti-MASH activity in several preclinical models, clinical efficacy assessed on histological endpoints have been reported to be rather modest [85–87]. Whereas, simultaneous activation of several PPAR isotypes or pan-PPAR agonists (e.g., lanifibranor) result in pleiotropic actions across different organs and cell types enhancing therapeutic synergies of PPAR modulation in the course of MASLD and progression to MASH and fibrosis [84, 85]. The phase 2b NATIVE trial (NCT03459079) evaluated effectiveness of lanifibranor in MASH patients reporting dose-dependent successful achievement on histological (MASH resolution and regression of fibrosis stage) and composite endpoints [88]. Moreover, lanifibranor improved glucose control and lipid handling as indicated by decreased triglycerides and increased HDL-cholesterol. Those positive results corroborate the concept of pan-PPAR agonism for the treatment of MASLD and supported the initiation of a phase 3 clinical study (NCT04849728) that is currently ongoing. Of note, as cardiovascular events represent a leading cause of morbidity and mortality in MASLD patients, preclinical as well as clinical trials reported PPAR-directed amelioration of intra- and extrahepatic vascular dysfunction in MASH [84]. However, even the large clinical trials are not usually neither designed nor powered enough to measure cardiovascular benefits, encouraging the implementation of cardiovascular disease-related endpoints in future MASH trials [89].

LXR comprises two isoforms, namely LXRα and LXRβ, governing hepatic triglyceride and cholesterol metabolism [67]. Within hepatic processes, LXR plays a dual role: it governs fatty acid metabolism by stimulating the expressions of SREBP1c, SCD1, and fatty acid synthase, with particular emphasis on SREBP-1c, often hailed as a primary controller of lipid synthesis. LXR signaling orchestrates alterations in energy storage by activating triglyceride and fatty acid synthesis. Concurrently, LXR fosters cholesterol efflux while diminishing cholesterol synthesis and uptake. In the context of MASLD, LXR is believed to harbor contradictory functions. Although its expression reportedly escalates with the severity of MASH and fibrosis [90], potentially exacerbating obesity and steatosis, it also demonstrates anti-inflammatory properties and aids in mitigating hypercholesterolemia. Consequently, the precise role of LXR in MASH remains ambiguous. Despite the development of numerous selective LXR agonists, further data are requisite before contemplating their therapeutic application in MASLD [10, 67].

## 4.3 Gut-Liver Axis: Role of the Microbiome and Incretins

The gastrointestinal tract stands as the most expansive mucosal surface within the human body and subject to constant exposure to dietary antigens and microbes [76]. Nutrients from our diet play a pivotal role in influencing both the composition and functionality of the gut microbiome. The gastrointestinal barrier is fortified by a complex orchestration of epithelial and endothelial cells, along with elements of innate and adaptive immunity and their respective mediators. Together, these components orchestrate the body's intricate defense mechanisms against the challenges posed by this dynamic environment. MASLD is a multidimensional disease fuelled by complex interorgan crosstalk. Multiple signals (e.g., lipids, hormones, cytokines, chemokines) derived from metabolically active tissues such as adipose tissue, skeletal muscle or the intestine influence dysregulated metabolic pathways in the liver [76, 91–94]. In this context, gut and the liver assemble as an important anatomically and functionally linked entity, which can be referred to as "gut-liver axis", connecting an altered intestinal state (e.g., dysbiosis, gut-barrier permeability) to metabolic injury in the pathogenesis of MASLD as well as other liver disease entities (Fig. 4.1) [76]. Gut-associated signals include nutritional factors, gut-derived hormones, bile acids as well as bacterial metabolites (e.g., trimethylamine, ethanol) and antigens (e.g., lipopolysaccharide) regulating metabolism and various immune responses [10, 76]. Most importantly, deeper insights into the bidirectional interplay between the gut and liver under healthy as well as diseased conditions offer opportunities for novel therapeutic approaches targeting the gut-liver axis and beyond [10, 76]. Ample preclinical evidence supports microbiota interventions to reduce metabolic injury. Conceptually, reversing gut dysbiosis modulating the composition of the microbiome in MASLD using antibiotics, probiotics or fecal microbiota transplantation to reduce inflammatory signals and reverse perturbations in gut barrier function subsequently ameliorating metabolic injury [10]. However, clinical evidence for long-term anti-inflammatory or antifibrotic effects as clinically relevant endpoints is lacking [95]. Nonetheless, precision microbiome-centered therapies, including engineered bacteria, postbiotics and phages, may provide a promising avenue for more individualized treatments in MASLD [96].

Several pharmacologic compounds targeting or directly mimicking beneficial effects of gut-derived, endogenous, metabolically relevant hormones are currently under evaluation in advanced clinical trials or already in clinical use for metabolic diseases [10, 97]. Combinations of incretins offer the potential for greater weight loss, as well as acting via synergistic mechanisms to enhance beneficial effects on liver injury. As GLP-1 receptor agonists have been licensed for the treatment of diabetes and obesity, they were one of the first drug types to be evaluated in patients with MASH, and successful phase IIa and IIb studies have resulted in progression to phase III clinical trials [98]. Alongside GLP-1 receptor agonists, newer combinations with glucagon agonists and/or glucose-dependent insulinotropic peptide (GIP) agonists have been explored in related patient groups with evidence of improvements in weight, insulin resistance and noninvasive liver parameters [98]:

- GLP-1 receptor agonists (e.g., semaglutide or liraglutide).
- GLP-1/glucagon dual agonists (e.g., cotadutide, survodutide or efinopegdutide).
- GLP-1/GIP (glucose-dependent insulinotropic polypeptide) dual agonists (e.g., tirzepatide).
- GLP-1/GIP/glucagon triple agonists (e.g., retatrutide).

There is also uncertainty regarding the optimal ratio of glucagon and GIP agonism to GLP-1 agonism in combination agents, and as to whether GIP agonism or antagonism is the optimal approach. Finally, there are also multiple hypothetical permutations combining gut hormone agonists with other emerging assets in the field. Modulation of gut-derived hormones can beneficially influence energy availability predominantly via improving hepatocyte metabolism [10]. Since the launch of the first GLP-1 agonists, namely exenatide in 2005, interest in GLP-1 agonists has soared beyond managing glucose sensitivity in type 2 diabetes including associated conditions like obesity, cardiovascular disease, diabetic kidney disease, and more recently, MASH [6, 98]. Initially, research focused on how GLP-1-induced weight loss impacts hepatic steatosis and inflammation in MASH. With the arrival of dual and triple agonists additionally targeting glucagon and GIP receptors, attention has shifted to potential synergistic effects on different disease drivers. GLP-1, synthesized predominantly in intestinal endocrine cells located in the distal ileum and colon but also distributed in the jejunum and duodenum, exerts its influence across several organs. Within the pancreas, it triggers beta cells to release insulin in a glucose-dependent manner while simultaneously suppressing glucagon secretion from alpha cells. These effects, observed with GLP-1 agonist therapy, are linked to improved glucose regulation and a decrease in liver fat content in individuals with MASH. Human studies indicate that GLP-1 enhances brain glucose clearance and reduces the anticipation of food reward, potentially leading to a decrease in overall food intake [99, 100].

Consequently, it can be surmised that the impact of GLP-1 on MASH is likely indirect, possibly stemming from a reduction in calorie intake, body weight and insulin resistance, all contributing to the attenuation of liver lipid accumulation and subsequent hepatic inflammation. The LEAD studies investigated liraglutide's efficacy in treating both type 2 diabetes and obesity. Subanalyses of these studies demonstrated its positive impact on metabolic liver injury [101]. Further clinical evaluation in individuals with biopsy-proven MASH revealed that liraglutide achieved histological MASH resolution without worsening of fibrosis [102] and ameliorated metabolic dysfunction, insulin resistance and lipotoxicity (LEAN; NCT01237119) [103]. The LEAN study led to initiation of the phase IIb SEMA-NASH study evaluating semaglutide for the treatment of MASLD and MASH (NCT02970942) [104]. The study met its primary endpoint of MASH resolution without worsening of liver fibrosis, while the secondary endpoint of histologic fibrosis improvement was not met. Nonetheless, therapeutic application of semaglutide led to a dose-dependent, slower progression of liver fibrosis than placebo suggesting that weight loss is the predominant driver of efficacy of GLP-1 receptor agonists in patients with MASH. Nonetheless, insufficient antifibrotic efficacy reflects the duration of treatment needed and the lack of statistical power for fibrosis in the phase IIb study corroborating further evaluation of semaglutide in a larger phase 3 clinical trial (ESSENCE; NCT04822181). First interim results regarding histological end-points can be expected in early 2024. A future milestone might be the evolution from subcutaneous to oral application that is supposed to be more cost effective and acceptable to patients [105]. Moreover, semaglutide has been safe and well tolerated in compensated MASH cirrhosis, while primary endpoints were not met (NCT03987451) [106].

Glucagon, primarily synthesized in pancreatic alpha cells, with a lesser amount potentially produced in the small intestine, plays a pivotal role in metabolic regulation [98]. Elevated levels of glucagon stimulate gluconeogenesis and glycogenolysis, while simultaneously curbing hepatic lipid formation. Although glucagon stimulates insulin secretion from beta cells, its potency pales in comparison to GLP-1 possibly due to its weak GLP-1 receptor binding. Concerning liver function, glucagon serves various purposes, including promoting mitochondrial turnover/function as well as mitigating oxidative stress, hepatic lipogenesis, and steatosis. It also significantly reduces hepatic glycogen reserves while triggering gluconeogenesis. Experimental evidence in humans suggests a modest immediate impact on energy expenditure, whereas prolonged GLP-1/glucagon dual agonism affects energy intake, possibly mediated through central nervous system GLP-1 receptors [98, 107]. However, acute hyperglycemia associated with glucagon agonism, especially considering higher prevalence of type 2 diabetes in MASH patients, raises concerns about its safety and efficacy as a monotherapy with this indication. Moreover, prolonged glucagon treatment may enhance hepatic insulin sensitivity by augmenting insulin activity over time [108]. Nonetheless, combination with GLP-1-targeted strategies appears to alleviate glucagon-induced hyperglycemia without compromising the other beneficial glucagon-dependent effects. Cotadutide, a balanced GLP-1/glucagon dual agonist, is currently under investigation in a phase 2b/3 clinical trial in non-cirrhotic MASH patients (NCT05364931). Previous investigations in patients with type 2 diabetes and chronic kidney disease demonstrated that cotadutide significantly affected hepatic glycogen synthesis and resulted in reduced hepatic fat fraction and noninvasive fibrosis assessment (NCT03550378; NCT03235050) [109, 110]. Due to study reports reduction of liver fat has been confirmed in a dose finding study of cotadutide in obese subjects with MASLD and MASH (NCT04019561) [98] corroborating recent initiation of a consecutive phase 2b/3 clinical study (NCT05364931). Survodutide (BI456906) is another promising GLP-1/glucagon dual agonist, that has shown weight reduction and improved glycemic control in patients with type 2 diabetes and obesity, which is currently also under investigation in MASH patients (NCT04771273; phase 2) [98, 111]. In a phase 2a study, the GLP-1/glucagon agonist efinopegdutide was more efficacious in reducing liver fat compared to semaglutide [112].

K cells found in the intestinal epithelium, mainly in the proximal duodenum, secrete GIP in response to dietary fat stimulation. GIP primarily impacts adipokine secretion and enhances the storage capacity of adipose tissue. Truncated GIP has been identified in pancreatic tissue, potentially influencing alpha/beta cell communication. Notably, GIP can prompt glucagon secretion even in hyperglycemic patients [113]. The presence of GIP receptors in the central nervous system suggests their involvement in regulating body weight and food intake, sparking debates on whether GIP antagonism or agonism is preferable for targeting these receptors [98, 114]. Preclinical studies indicate that GIP promotes lipid accumulation in the liver, while genetically modified mice ($GIP^{-/-}$) exhibit reduced liver fat [115]. The GLP-1/GIP dual agonist tirzepatide is currently tested in a phase 2 clinical trial evaluating effectiveness in MASH patients (SYNERGY-NASH; NCT04166773). Available clinical data from the SURMOUNT-1 trial evaluating tirzepatide in obese individuals reported significant weight loss [116] and analysis of a subpopulation of the SURPASS-3 trial additionally demonstrated that tirzepatide reduced liver fat and alleviated liver injury [117]. Determining the ideal ratio of triagonist molecules remains a subject of ongoing investigation. Based on promising preclinical data, the initial molecule in this class, retatrutide, has recently commenced clinical development [118–120].

Fibrobast growth factors (FGFs) are a family of 23 molecules, which are involved in various systemic signaling cascades comprising cell differentiation, angiogenesis as well as wound healing processes and energy homeostasis, gaining organ specificity through FGF receptor tissue distribution. The FGF-15/−19 axis is upregulated via FXR signaling in enterocytes. FGF19 is an enterokine that reaches the liver via portal circulation and binds to the FGF receptor 4/β-klotho, which thereby represses bile acid synthesis and gluconeogenesis in the liver. Preclinical studies corroborate FXR-FGF-15/−19 regulation favoring liver regeneration. In detail, induction of FGF15/19 was shown to dampen steatosis, inflammation, and fibrosis in experimental MASH [121, 122]. The humanized FGF19 analogue aldafermin significantly ameliorated histological features, imaging scores and serum markers in a phase 2b clinical trial in biopsy-proven MASH patients (NCT02443116) [123]. However, aldafermin did not improve fibrosis stage in a biopsy-controlled phase 2b clinical trial (ALPINE 2/3) in non-cirrhotic

MASH patients, despite positive effects on a number of secondary endpoints, leading to the discontinuation of drug development with this indication (NCT03912532) [124, 125]. More recently, it was reported that treatment with aldafermin in patients with compensated MASH cirrhosis achieved significant reduction in the "enhanced liver fibrosis" (ELF) score as a potential surrogate for clinical benefit (ALPINE 4; NCT04210245) [126].

FGF21 is one more representative of the FGF family, which is a systemically circulating endocrine hormone expressed in various tissues such as the liver and crucially involved in energy metabolism of predominantly hepatic and adipose tissue. Available data indicate that hepatic FGF21 expression is stimulated as a response to metabolic disturbance (e.g., lipolysis, ketogenesis). FGF21 is attributed with beneficial activities such as increasing energy expenditure, alleviating glycemic control, improving lipid handling and reducing hepatic stress signals. In detail, FGF21 stimulates glucose uptake in adipocytes thereby beneficially influencing insulin sensitivity and reducing hepatic fat content [67]. However, the precise role of FGF21 during the pathogenesis of MASLD and progression to MASH/fibrosis remains ambiguous. Interestingly, the majority of studies report that elevated serum levels are associated with MASLD and other metabolic diseases such as type 2 diabetes correlating with MASH severity [10, 127]. On the contrary, endogenous relative FGF21 deficiency was found to predispose particularly pediatric patients to obesity, insulin resistance and MASLD, possibly indicating variations of FGF21 activity depending on age or sex-hormone levels [128]. Beneficial potency led to the development and subsequent improvement of multiple engineered FGF21 agonistic molecules such as efruxifermin, pegozafermin or pegbelfermin, which have been investigated intensively in preclinical and clinical studies [129, 130]. FGF21 agonism has been linked to beneficial metabolic effects amending obesity, reducing liver fat and improving insulin resistance. The FALCON program (NCT03486899; NCT03486912) evaluated efficacy of the pegylated FGF21 analogue pegbelfermin in patients with MASH-fibrosis and -cirrhosis ameliorating hepatic steatosis and surrogate markers of liver fibrosis. However, despite liver biopsy revealed improvement of advanced liver fibrosis (stage F3), primary endpoints were not met for either study leading to early discontinuation of the clinical development of the FGF21 agonist pegbelfermin for the treatment of MASH [131–134]. One hypothesis for the disappointing study results might be explained by the limited activity of pegbelfermin against adipose tissue FGF receptors, as evidenced by only slight increases of the downstream molecule adiponectin compared to findings with other FGF21 analogues such as efruxifermin. Recent findings give evidence that the FGF21 analogue efruxifermin in particular improved glycemic control, resolved MASH and expands antifibrotic efficacy—thus, representing a promising option for the treatment of MASH and liver fibrosis or cirrhosis (HARMONY; NCT04767529) [129, 135, 136]. In line, other adapted compounds such as pegozafermin, which is a long-acting glycopegylated molecule with improved half-life, entered clinical stage and demonstrated antifibrotic potency, suggesting further evaluation in a phase 3 clinical trial for the indication of MASH (ENLIVEN; NCT04929483) [137, 138]. Despite the clear efficacy signals observed in the efruxifermin and pegoazefermin trials, long-term safety (e.g., relevance of anti-drug antibodies, bone density) has currently not been demonstrated for these compounds.

As many new potential drug targets emerge, combinatorial treatment strategies might reveal additive beneficial effects in contrast to single drug treatments, helping to overcome limitations of monotherapies and sustain therapeutic benefits. When evaluating combination therapy, it is essential to weigh its effectiveness against the heightened potential for side effects, interactions between drugs, and associated expenses. The efficacy of the FXR agonist cilofexor and the ACC inhibitor firsocostat were evaluated as monotherapies and coadministration in advanced MASH in the phase 2b ATLAS trial (NCT03449446). While no treatment arm in the trial achieved statistical significance against the primary endpoint (at least one stage improvement in fibrosis or MASH resolution), a numerically higher percentage of patients in the combination group achieved fibrosis reduction. Moreover, a fixed combination of firsocostat and cilofexor coadministered with the GLP-1 receptor agonist semaglutide is currently being evaluated in compensated MASH cirrhosis (WAYFIND; NCT04971785). Coadministration of the ACC inhibitor firsocostat and the GLP-1 receptor agonist semaglutide was evaluated in an open label phase II trial (NCT03987074) resulting in a significantly greater relative reduction in liver fat content and improving markers of liver injury and noninvasive liver stiffness compared to monotherapy [139]. Considering that incretin agonists primarily act via weight loss, the initial combinations could prioritize agents known for direct impact on fibrosis, such as FGF21 and pan-PPAR agonists [10]. Additional therapy with efruxifermin in patients with MASH and type 2 diabetes that already receive a GLP-1 receptor agonist (i.e., semaglutide, dulaglutide, or liraglutide) may further improve liver health additionally reducing liver fat and improving noninvasive markers of liver injury, fibrosis, glucose, and lipid metabolism (NCT05039450) [140, 141]. However, clinical trials using combinatorial approaches have so far been disappointing despite promising preclinical data in preclinical models [10, 142].

## 4.4 Inflammation: Programmed Cell Death, Immune Cell Activation, and Fibrosis Progression

Metabolic injury results from a myriad of modifiable (e.g., lifestyle, diet, exercise, comorbidities) and non-modifiable (e.g., age, sex, ethnicity, genetics), intra- and extrahepatic factors, setting off cascades of pathogenic events such as ER stress, oxidative stress, and mitochondrial dysfunction in hepatocytes, prompting their cellular crosstalk with non-parenchymal and immune cells [143, 144]. Dysregulated lipid handling due to fatty acid overload and increased DNL leads to lipotoxicity, which in turn activates immune responses via cell death mechanisms and impairing autophagy indicating that overnutrition and insulin resistance can directly influence immune cell responses and composition in different organ systems. Hepatocyte stress and particularly cell death including apoptosis, necrosis, and necroptosis, triggers the release of signaling molecules like cytokines/chemokines, lipids, and extracellular vesicles, along with damage-associated molecular patterns (Fig. 4.1) [61]. Additionally, hepatocyte senescence contributes to inflammatory signals, which can be referred to as the senescence-associated secretory phenotype [61, 145]. Immune responses of sentinels to tissue perturbation exacerbate hepatocyte damage, fostering a vicious cycle of necroinflammation. In individuals with MASH, fibrosis exhibits varying rates of progression [7]. For most MASLD patients as well as those at risk, the quantity of hepatic fat accumulation can serve as a prognostic indicator for cardiovascular and cerebrovascular risks. Concurrently, inflammation and cellular damage fuel the progression of MASH and fibrosis, whereas fibrosis stage correlates with liver-specific morbidity and mortality including complications such as portal hypertension, end-stage cirrhosis or hepatocellular carcinoma (HCC), which significantly worsen prognosis [5, 8, 9, 14, 15].

Pharmacological strategies aim at metabolic dysregulation and hepatocyte injury, along with suppressing extrahepatic signals to reduce inflammatory cascades [10]. These approaches may involve modification of genetic risk factors or dampening immune actions associated with inflammation. By targeting metabolic pathways and modifying injury and inflammation, interventions may subsequently exhibit anti-inflammatory effects. Nevertheless, the extent to which targeting various pathways to diminish fat accumulation will affect the production of lipotoxic mediators remains uncertain—thus, representing a key question to identify the crucial metabolic vulnerabilities that need to be targeted to reach anti-inflammatory and antifibrotic efficacy. Despite identification of multiple promising drug targets, developing effective compounds for the treatment of MASH and fibrosis has been notably challenging over the last decades.

The US and European regulatory agencies, the FDA and the EMA, have concurred that achieving substantial histological improvement (i.e., resolution of MASH and/or decrease in fibrosis stage) in consecutive liver biopsies serve as relevant endpoints to warrant drug approval, given the correlation of inflammation and fibrosis with disease progression and clinical outcomes [89, 97]. As mentioned above, resmetirom is now the first drug specifically approved by the FDA for the treatment of MASH and liver fibrosis [72]. Nonetheless, available data indicate that THRβ-mediated antifibrotic efficacy is most likely a result of improved metabolic disturbance, while preclinical evidence elucidated direct antifibrotic effects via THRα signaling on hepatic stellate cells (HSCs) [146]. Similarly, the pan-PPAR agonist lanifibranor has demonstrated antifibrotic efficacy in MASH patients [88], most likely via PPARγ-mediated deactivation of HSCs and stimulating differentiation towards a quiescent phenotype [85]. Moreover, liver macrophages can be skewed towards an anti-inflammatory phenotype particularly via PPARβ/δ stimulation suggesting PPAR agonists as promising anti-inflammatory/antifibrotic candidates [85]. In line, FXR expression levels are relatively low on HSCs, while LXR expression is high. Nonetheless, FXR agonists such as cilofexor reported compelling improvement in portal hypertension [147], and especially obeticholic acid demonstrated significant antifibrotic potential in non-cirrhotic MASH patients, but will not be further evaluated in this indication [82]. On the contrary, LRXs agonism has in fact demonstrated protective effects regarding lipid metabolism and inflammatory immune responses in MASLD, potentially through stimulating a restorative phenotype in macrophages [67]. Yet, LXR-targeted approaches entering the clinical stage are still lacking [10].

Cellular stress signals such as excessive fatty acids, oxidative stress or endoplasmic reticulum stress trigger cell death mechanisms such as apoptosis, necrosis or necroptosis, subsequently stimulating secretion of reactive oxygen species and damage associated molecular patterns (DAMPs). Multiple inflammatory signaling pathways such as NF-kB, Apoptosis signal-regulating kinase 1 (ASK1), or c-Jun N-terminal kinase (JNK) have been identified in parenchymal liver cells, mainly hepatocytes, as well as immune cells such as liver macrophages and therefore represent attractive pharmacologic targets to modulate inflammation and fibrosis [10, 61]. Promising data of pharmacological ASK1 inhibition employing selonsertib reducing hepatic steatosis as well as inflammation and liver fibrosis corroborated evaluation in clinical trials [148]. However, despite demonstrating beneficial antisteatotic and antifibrotic signals at early stages, selonsertib could neither reach the primary endpoints of improving fibrosis by at least one stage in MASH patients (STELLAR-3, NCT03053050) nor in MASH-cirrhosis (STELLAR-4, NCT03053063) [149]. Moreover, insufficient efficacy of selonsertib was confirmed in a phase 2 trial (NCT02781584) evaluating a combinational approach of selonsertib with the ACC inhibitor firsocostat and the FXR agonist cilofexor in subjects with MASH [150].

Pathogen-associated molecular patterns (PAMPs) as well as DAMPs can induce formation and activation of inflammasomes via NF-κB signaling subsequently leading to secretion of inflammatory cytokines such as interleukin 1β (IL-1β) or interleukin 18 (IL-18) and cleavage of gasdermin D (GSDMD) causing pyroptosis, which in turn stimulates activation of hepatic macrophages in different entities of acute and chronic liver disease including MASLD [151, 152]. While no pharmacologic compound is approved as inflammasome-targeted therapy for liver disease [153], various preclinical and clinical studies have explored targeting downstream effectors such as IL-1β (e.g., anakinra, canakinumab or rilonacept, which are clinically approved) or IL-18 (e.g., the recombinant human IL-18 binding protein tadekinig alfa and the recombinant human IL-18-neutralizing antibody GSK1070806) in other inflammasome-associated diseases [154–156]. The NLRP3 inflammasome, which is triggered by pathogen-associated as well as sterile liver injury like MASLD, is characteristic for innate immunity [157, 158]. However, specific inhibitors of NLRP3 inflammasome have not entered advanced clinical stages with the indication of MASH and liver fibrosis, despite promising results in preclinical use [155, 159, 160]. Beneficially modulating the gut microbiota composition may limit release of inflammatory signals such as PAMPs. PAMPs display highly conserved molecules such as lipopolysaccharides (LPS) or endotoxins, which are frequently located on the cell membrane of gram-negative bacteria, potentially activating toll-like receptor 4 (TLR4) or TLR9-dependent signaling in immune cells [94]. Available data indicate that direct inhibition of TLR-mediated pathways hold the potential to suppress inflammasome formation or proinflammatory downstream signals, thereby highlighting major relevance of TLR4 signaling in other disease entities such as acute-on-chronic liver failure [161]. For instance, administering broad-spectrum antibiotics has been shown to mitigate steatohepatitis and liver fibrosis by attenuating TLR4-dependent activation of hepatic macrophages in experimental chronic liver injury [162–164]. In line, Eritoran tetrasodium (E5564), which is a synthetic lipid A analogue acting as a competitive TLR4 antagonist significantly attenuated inflammation and liver fibrosis in MASH and fibrosis models [165]. Interestingly the specific TLR4 inhibitor serelaxin amplified antifibrotic efficacy of PPARγ agonism. Nonetheless, despite of Eritoran currently being under evaluation in patients with obesity and type 2 diabetes (NCT02267317), TLR4 is not yet under clinical investigation for metabolic liver disease.

Various cell types within the liver serve as immune sentinels, including non-parenchymal populations like sinusoidal endothelial cells or HSCs, along with liver-resident immune cells such as macrophages or lymphocyte cells [5]. Upon detection of hepatocyte stress or injury signals from intra- or extrahepatic sources, liver-resident macrophages, referred to as Kupffer cells, respond by releasing inflammatory signals like chemokines recruiting further inflammatory cell types such as neutrophils or monocytes to the site of injury. Hepatic macrophages, i.e., Kupffer cells and infiltrating/accumulating monocyte-derived macrophages, encompass distinct subsets with notable context-dependent functional plasticity and play a pivotal role perpetuating inflammatory processes during the progression of MASLD as well as tissue-repair processes [93, 166–168]. In turn, anti-inflammatory approaches aim to mitigate the activation of immune sentinels, the recruitment of immune cells, and the intricate intercellular communication between parenchymal and non-parenchymal cell populations [10]. The chemokine (C-C motif) ligand 2 (CCL2), also known as monocyte chemoattractant protein 1 (MCP1) plays key role recruiting C–C motif chemokine receptor (CCR)2+ monocytes to the site of liver injury driving inflammation and MASH progression [94, 169]. In turn, pharmacologic inhibition of monocyte infiltration has shown anti-inflammatory and antifibrotic capacity in preclinical models [10]. Cenicriviroc, which works as a dual CCR2/CCR5 inhibitor, has been investigated extensively in preclinical models and demonstrated anti-MASH activity. However, despite favorable antifibrotic data after 1 year of treatment in MASH patients [170], clinical evaluation has been terminated early after interim analysis in the large phase 3 AURORA trial reporting insufficient efficacy to treat fibrosis in the long-term (NCT03028740) [171]. Compounds modulating chemokine receptor-mediated activities are currently approved for very specific applications but not metabolic liver disease. Similarly, directly targeting soluble effector molecules such as the cytokine galectin-3 represents an alternative approach. Galectin-3 is secreted by liver macrophages and has demonstrated inflammatory actions [172]. In turn, pharmacologic inhibition by belapectin ameliorated MASH and fibrosis in rodent models but lacked antifibrotic efficacy in a phase 2b clinical trial (NCT02462967) [173]. Nonetheless, positive data from a subanalysis on portal hypertension prompted further investigation in patients testing the potential to prevent oesophageal varices. Insufficient efficacy of promising agents like cenicriviroc might be explained by heterogeneity of MASLD and the redundancy within the chemokine system with overlapping targets, functions and the specific context-dependent plasticity of immune cells [10]. Moreover approaches evaluating other immune cells such as platelets, neutrophils and lymphocytes as well as their intercellular crosstalk in the course of MASLD as potential drug targets are less advanced but have demonstrated beneficial potential in metabolic liver disease in preclinical studies suggesting further investigation in that direction [10, 61].

Liver fibrogenesis can be described as an aberrant wound-healing process, characterized by excessive extracellular matrix deposition as well as depletion of functional hepatocytes, alongside persistent inflammation [5, 174]. During fibrogenesis, quiescent HSCs become activated via soluble signals (e.g., platelet-derived growth factor [PDGF] or transforming growth factor [TGF]-β) or cellular crosstalk with parenchymal or immune cells. Subsequently, HSCs transdifferentiate into myofibroblasts, which are the main source of scar tissue production and therefore represent an interesting target for direct antifibrotic agents. As this wound-healing process is highly dynamic and in principle reversible, current pharmacologic strategies aim at pathways leading to inhibition of HSC activation/transdifferentiation or to deactivation/elimination of myofibroblasts to a "quiescent"-like HSC phenotype or metabolic reprogramming particularly in the course of MASLD [10, 175]. However, directly targeting HSCs remained challenging. Especially systemic targeting of soluble mediators such as TGFβ has been terminated due to negative side effects such as immunosuppression or carcinogenesis [176]. Nonetheless, recent advances and promising results from experimental studies targeting cell surface integrins (e.g., integrins αvβ1 or αvβ3) promoted evaluation in clinical trials [177, 178]. As activation of HSCs and transdifferentiation towards myofibroblasts displays a highly energy-dependent process requiring complex metabolic reprogramming including intrinsic activation of glycolysis, glutaminolysis or lipogenesis [179], recent evidence supports direct antifibrotic efficacy of some compounds (e.g., inhibitor of ACC or FAS) modulating metabolic pathways such as DNL highlighting the importance of lipid metabolism as an energy source for HSC differentiation [10]. Moreover, despite clinical data are still lacking, preclinical evidence elucidated induction of glucose transporters and inhibition of gluconeogenesis in HSCs, suggesting a potential role for compounds influencing glucose metabolism (e.g., hexokinase or sodium glucose linked transporter [SGLT]2 inhibitors) [179, 180]. In turn, future studies need to address direct antifibrotic potential of metabolic compounds beyond indirect effects through reduction of liver fat [24, 31, 139]. Intriguingly, unmodifiable genetic risk factors such as PNPLA3 or MBOAT7 can also directly influence fibrogenic signaling in HSCs, suggesting that targeting the genetic mechanisms of lipid handling in hepatocytes may additionally exert immune cell-mediated antifibrotic effects [181, 182]. This observation may corroborate genetic risk prediction by PNPLA3 of liver fibrosis independent of the disease etiology beyond MASLD [183]. Alternatively, therapeutic strategies might augment scar-free tissue regeneration via attenuating metabolic injury, which stimulates release of proresolving factors, anti-inflammatory reprogramming of various immune cells as well as deactivation/elimination of HSCs [184–186]. However, the scar tissue formation especially in advanced liver fibrosis stages might be relatively resistant and pharmacologic agents such as simtuzumab, which potentially inhibits collagen cross-linking actions of lysyl oxidase-like (LOXL)2, lacked antifibrotic efficacy in clinical trials [187, 188]. Moreover, cell-based therapies emerge and are currently being explored to augment anti-inflammatory and antifibrotic potential [189, 190].

The high adaptability of various cellular components involved in liver fibrogenesis particularly in cases of ongoing tissue injury poses a tremendous challenge for effective treatment. This complexity underscores the potential benefit (e.g., amplifying efficacy, overcome signaling redundancy) of combining anti-inflammatory/antifibrotic compounds with one or more metabolic agents in the treatment of MASH [191]. However, despite promising results in preclinical studies, first results from clinical trials employing several combination therapies remained below expectations [139, 142]. One might speculate that counteracting the initial stages of the inflammatory activation cascades could bear advantages by mitigating pathogenic processes before highly conserved and complex inflammation/fibrosis downstream signals are stimulated. Moreover, one has to consider that improvement of liver fibrosis may correlate with better clinical outcomes but antifibrotic agents may not mitigate extrahepatic comorbidities such as cardiovascular events [192].

**Conflict of Interest** TP declares no conflict of interest.

FT's lab has received research funding from AstraZeneca, MSD, Gilead. FT has received honoraria for consulting or lectures from Astra Zeneca, Gilead, AbbVie, BMS, Boehringer, Madrigal, Intercept, Falk, Orphalan, Inventiva, Merz, Pfizer, Alnylam, CSL Behring, Novo Nordisk, Novartis, Sanofi, GSK, MSD.

## References

1. Estes C, Razavi H, Loomba R, Younossi Z, Sanyal AJ. Modeling the epidemic of nonalcoholic fatty liver disease demonstrates an exponential increase in burden of disease. Hepatology. 2018;67(1):123–33.
2. Estes C, Anstee QM, Arias-Loste MT, Bantel H, Bellentani S, Caballeria J, et al. Modeling NAFLD disease burden in China, France, Germany, Italy, Japan, Spain, United Kingdom, and United States for the period 2016-2030. J Hepatol. 2018;69(4):896–904.
3. Sanyal AJ. Past, present and future perspectives in nonalcoholic fatty liver disease. Nat Rev Gastroenterol Hepatol. 2019;16(6):377–86.
4. Rinella ME, Lazarus JV, Ratziu V, Francque SM, Sanyal AJ, Kanwal F, et al. A multisociety Delphi consensus statement on new fatty liver disease nomenclature. J Hepatol. 2023;79(6):1542–56.
5. Hammerich L, Tacke F. Hepatic inflammatory responses in liver fibrosis. Nat Rev Gastroenterol Hepatol. 2023;20(10):633–46.
6. Rinella ME, Lazarus JV, Ratziu V, Francque SM, Sanyal AJ, Kanwal F, et al. A multisociety Delphi consensus statement on new fatty liver disease nomenclature. Hepatology. 2023;78(6):1966–86.
7. Singh S, Allen AM, Wang Z, Prokop LJ, Murad MH, Loomba R. Fibrosis progression in nonalcoholic fatty liver vs nonalcoholic steatohepatitis: a systematic review and meta-analysis of paired-biopsy studies. Clin Gastroenterol Hepatol. 2015;13(4):643–54 e1–9.
8. Sanyal AJ, Van Natta ML, Clark J, Neuschwander-Tetri BA, Diehl A, Dasarathy S, et al. Prospective Study of Outcomes in Adults with Nonalcoholic Fatty Liver Disease. N Engl J Med. 2021;385(17):1559–69.
9. Simon TG, Roelstraete B, Khalili H, Hagstrom H, Ludvigsson JF. Mortality in biopsy-confirmed nonalcoholic fatty liver disease: results from a nationwide cohort. Gut. 2021;70(7):1375–82.
10. Tacke F, Puengel T, Loomba R, Friedman SL. An integrated view of anti-inflammatory and antifibrotic targets for the treatment of NASH. J Hepatol. 2023;79(2):552–66.
11. Esler WP, Cohen DE. Pharmacologic inhibition of lipogenesis for the treatment of NAFLD. J Hepatol. 2024;80(2):362–77.
12. Kawano Y, Cohen DE. Mechanisms of hepatic triglyceride accumulation in non-alcoholic fatty liver disease. J Gastroenterol. 2013;48(4):434–41.
13. Jacome-Sosa MM, Parks EJ. Fatty acid sources and their fluxes as they contribute to plasma triglyceride concentrations and fatty liver in humans. Curr Opin Lipidol. 2014;25(3):213–20.
14. Vilar-Gomez E, Calzadilla-Bertot L, Wai-Sun Wong V, Castellanos M, Aller-de la Fuente R, Metwally M, et al. Fibrosis Severity as a Determinant of Cause-Specific Mortality in Patients With Advanced Nonalcoholic Fatty Liver Disease: A Multi-National Cohort Study. Gastroenterology. 2018;155(2):443–57 e17.
15. Dulai PS, Singh S, Patel J, Soni M, Prokop LJ, Younossi Z, et al. Increased risk of mortality by fibrosis stage in nonalcoholic fatty liver disease: Systematic review and meta-analysis. Hepatology. 2017;65(5):1557–65.
16. Smith GI, Shankaran M, Yoshino M, Schweitzer GG, Chondronikola M, Beals JW, et al. Insulin resistance drives hepatic de novo lipogenesis in nonalcoholic fatty liver disease. J Clin Invest. 2020;130(3):1453–60.
17. Belew GD, Jones JG. De novo lipogenesis in non-alcoholic fatty liver disease: Quantification with stable isotope tracers. Eur J Clin Investig. 2022;52(3):e13733.
18. Jeyakumar SM, Vajreswari A. Stearoyl-CoA desaturase 1: A potential target for non-alcoholic fatty liver disease?-perspective on emerging experimental evidence. World J Hepatol. 2022;14(1):168–79.
19. ALJohani AM, Syed DN, Ntambi JM. Insights into stearoyl-CoA desaturase-1 regulation of systemic metabolism. Trends Endocrinol Metab. 2017;28(12):831–42.
20. Narce M, Bellenger J, Rialland M, Bellenger S. Recent advances on stearoyl-Coa desaturase regulation in fatty liver diseases. Curr Drug Metab. 2012;13(10):1454–63.
21. Goldiner I, van der Velde AE, Vandenberghe KE, van Wijland MA, Halpern Z, Gilat T, et al. ABCA1-dependent but apoA-I-independent cholesterol efflux mediated by fatty acid-bile acid conjugates (FABACs). Biochem J. 2006;396(3):529–36.
22. Brown JM, Rudel LL. Stearoyl-coenzyme A desaturase 1 inhibition and the metabolic syndrome: considerations for future drug discovery. Curr Opin Lipidol. 2010;21(3):192–7.
23. Safadi R, Konikoff FM, Mahamid M, Zelber-Sagi S, Halpern M, Gilat T, et al. The fatty acid-bile acid

conjugate Aramchol reduces liver fat content in patients with nonalcoholic fatty liver disease. Clin Gastroenterol Hepatol. 2014;12(12):2085–91 e1.
24. Ratziu V, de Guevara L, Safadi R, Poordad F, Fuster F, Flores-Figueroa J, et al. Aramchol in patients with nonalcoholic steatohepatitis: a randomized, double-blind, placebo-controlled phase 2b trial. Nat Med. 2021;27(10):1825–35.
25. Savage DB, Choi CS, Samuel VT, Liu ZX, Zhang D, Wang A, et al. Reversal of diet-induced hepatic steatosis and hepatic insulin resistance by antisense oligonucleotide inhibitors of acetyl-CoA carboxylases 1 and 2. J Clin Invest. 2006;116(3):817–24.
26. Ross TT, Crowley C, Kelly KL, Rinaldi A, Beebe DA, Lech MP, et al. Acetyl-CoA Carboxylase Inhibition Improves Multiple Dimensions of NASH Pathogenesis in Model Systems. Cell Mol Gastroenterol Hepatol. 2020;10(4):829–51.
27. Kelly KL, Reagan WJ, Sonnenberg GE, Clasquin M, Hales K, Asano S, et al. De novo lipogenesis is essential for platelet production in humans. Nat Metab. 2020;2(10):1163–78.
28. Kim CW, Addy C, Kusunoki J, Anderson NN, Deja S, Fu X, et al. Acetyl CoA Carboxylase Inhibition Reduces Hepatic Steatosis but Elevates Plasma Triglycerides in Mice and Humans: A Bedside to Bench Investigation. Cell Metab. 2017;26(2):394–406 e6.
29. Stiede K, Miao W, Blanchette HS, Beysen C, Harriman G, Harwood HJ Jr, et al. Acetyl-coenzyme A carboxylase inhibition reduces de novo lipogenesis in overweight male subjects: A randomized, double-blind, crossover study. Hepatology. 2017;66(2):324–34.
30. Loomba R, Kayali Z, Noureddin M, Ruane P, Lawitz EJ, Bennett M, et al. GS-0976 Reduces Hepatic Steatosis and Fibrosis Markers in Patients With Nonalcoholic Fatty Liver Disease. Gastroenterology. 2018;155(5):1463–73 e6.
31. Calle RA, Amin NB, Carvajal-Gonzalez S, Ross TT, Bergman A, Aggarwal S, et al. ACC inhibitor alone or co-administered with a DGAT2 inhibitor in patients with non-alcoholic fatty liver disease: two parallel, placebo-controlled, randomized phase 2a trials. Nat Med. 2021;27(10):1836–48.
32. Bergman A, Carvajal-Gonzalez S, Tarabar S, Saxena AR, Esler WP, Amin NB. Safety, Tolerability, Pharmacokinetics, and Pharmacodynamics of a Liver-Targeting Acetyl-CoA Carboxylase Inhibitor (PF-05221304): A Three-Part Randomized Phase 1 Study. Clin Pharmacol Drug Dev. 2020;9(4):514–26.
33. Amin NB, Darekar A, Anstee QM, Wong VW, Tacke F, Vourvahis M, et al. Efficacy and safety of an orally administered DGAT2 inhibitor alone or coadministered with a liver-targeted ACC inhibitor in adults with non-alcoholic steatohepatitis (NASH): rationale and design of the phase II, dose-ranging, dose-finding, randomised, placebo-controlled MIRNA (Metabolic Interventions to Resolve NASH with fibrosis) study. BMJ Open. 2022;12(3):e056159.
34. Fhu CW, Ali A. Fatty acid synthase: an emerging target in cancer. Molecules. 2020;25(17):3935.
35. Wu M, Singh SB, Wang J, Chung CC, Salituro G, Karanam BV, et al. Antidiabetic and antisteatotic effects of the selective fatty acid synthase (FAS) inhibitor platensimycin in mouse models of diabetes. Proc Natl Acad Sci USA. 2011;108(13):5378–83.
36. O'Farrell M, Duke G, Crowley R, Buckley D, Martins EB, Bhattacharya D, et al. FASN inhibition targets multiple drivers of NASH by reducing steatosis, inflammation and fibrosis in preclinical models. Sci Rep. 2022;12(1):15661.
37. Buhman KK, Smith SJ, Stone SJ, Repa JJ, Wong JS, Knapp FF Jr, et al. DGAT1 is not essential for intestinal triacylglycerol absorption or chylomicron synthesis. J Biol Chem. 2002;277(28):25474–9.
38. Cases S, Stone SJ, Zhou P, Yen E, Tow B, Lardizabal KD, et al. Cloning of DGAT2, a second mammalian diacylglycerol acyltransferase, and related family members. J Biol Chem. 2001;276(42):38870–6.
39. Qi J, Lang W, Geisler JG, Wang P, Petrounia I, Mai S, et al. The use of stable isotope-labeled glycerol and oleic acid to differentiate the hepatic functions of DGAT1 and −2. J Lipid Res. 2012;53(6):1106–16.
40. Choi CS, Savage DB, Abu-Elheiga L, Liu ZX, Kim S, Kulkarni A, et al. Continuous fat oxidation in acetyl-CoA carboxylase 2 knockout mice increases total energy expenditure, reduces fat mass, and improves insulin sensitivity. Proc Natl Acad Sci USA. 2007;104(42):16480–5.
41. Yu XX, Murray SF, Pandey SK, Booten SL, Bao D, Song XZ, et al. Antisense oligonucleotide reduction of DGAT2 expression improves hepatic steatosis and hyperlipidemia in obese mice. Hepatology. 2005;42(2):362–71.
42. Amin NB, Carvajal-Gonzalez S, Purkal J, Zhu T, Crowley C, Perez S, et al. Targeting diacylglycerol acyltransferase 2 for the treatment of nonalcoholic steatohepatitis. Sci Transl Med. 2019;11(520):eaav9701.
43. Sawant-Basak A, Bergman AJ, Mancuso J, Tripathy S, Gosset JR, Mendes da Costa L, et al. Investigation of pharmacokinetic drug interaction between clesacostat and DGAT2 inhibitor ervogastat in healthy adult participants. Clin Transl Sci. 2024;17(2):e13687.
44. Futatsugi K, Cabral S, Kung DW, Huard K, Lee E, Boehm M, et al. Discovery of Ervogastat (PF-06865571): A Potent and Selective Inhibitor of Diacylglycerol Acyltransferase 2 for the Treatment of Non-alcoholic Steatohepatitis. J Med Chem. 2022;65(22):15000–13.
45. Amin NB, Saxena AR, Somayaji V, Dullea R. Inhibition of Diacylglycerol Acyltransferase 2 Versus Diacylglycerol Acyltransferase 1: Potential Therapeutic Implications of Pharmacology. Clin Ther. 2023;45(1):55–70.
46. Loomba R, Morgan E, Watts L, Xia S, Hannan LA, Geary RS, et al. Novel antisense inhibition of diacylglycerol O-acyltransferase 2 for treatment

of non-alcoholic fatty liver disease: a multicentre, double-blind, randomised, placebo-controlled phase 2 trial. Lancet Gastroenterol Hepatol. 2020;5(9):829–38.
47. Herman MA, Birnbaum MJ. Molecular aspects of fructose metabolism and metabolic disease. Cell Metab. 2021;33(12):2329–54.
48. Yu S, Li C, Ji G, Zhang L. The Contribution of Dietary Fructose to Non-alcoholic Fatty Liver Disease. Front Pharmacol. 2021;12:783393.
49. Ferraris RP, Choe JY, Patel CR. Intestinal Absorption of Fructose. Annu Rev Nutr. 2018;38:41–67.
50. Staltner R, Burger K, Baumann A, Bergheim I. Fructose: a modulator of intestinal barrier function and hepatic health? Eur J Nutr. 2023;62(8):3113–24.
51. Zhao L, Zhang X, Coday M, Garcia DO, Li X, Mossavar-Rahmani Y, et al. Sugar-Sweetened and Artificially Sweetened Beverages and Risk of Liver Cancer and Chronic Liver Disease Mortality. JAMA. 2023;330(6):537–46.
52. Geidl-Flueck B, Gerber PA. Fructose drives de novo lipogenesis affecting metabolic health. J Endocrinol. 2023;257(2):e220270.
53. Gutierrez JA, Liu W, Perez S, Xing G, Sonnenberg G, Kou K, et al. Pharmacologic inhibition of ketohexokinase prevents fructose-induced metabolic dysfunction. Mol Metab. 2021;48:101196.
54. Kazierad DJ, Chidsey K, Somayaji VR, Bergman AJ, Birnbaum MJ, Calle RA. Inhibition of ketohexokinase in adults with NAFLD reduces liver fat and inflammatory markers: A randomized phase 2 trial. Med. 2021;2(7):800–13 e3.
55. Saxena AR, Lyle SA, Khavandi K, Qiu R, Whitlock M, Esler WP, et al. A phase 2a, randomized, double-blind, placebo-controlled, three-arm, parallel-group study to assess the efficacy, safety, tolerability and pharmacodynamics of PF-06835919 in patients with non-alcoholic fatty liver disease and type 2 diabetes. Diabetes Obes Metab. 2023;25(4):992–1001.
56. Luukkonen PK, Qadri S, Ahlholm N, Porthan K, Mannisto V, Sammalkorpi H, et al. Distinct contributions of metabolic dysfunction and genetic risk factors in the pathogenesis of non-alcoholic fatty liver disease. J Hepatol. 2022;76(3):526–35.
57. Trepo E, Valenti L. Update on NAFLD genetics: From new variants to the clinic. J Hepatol. 2020;72(6):1196–209.
58. Carlsson B, Linden D, Brolen G, Liljeblad M, Bjursell M, Romeo S, et al. Review article: the emerging role of genetics in precision medicine for patients with non-alcoholic steatohepatitis. Aliment Pharmacol Ther. 2020;51(12):1305–20.
59. Cherubini A, Casirati E, Tomasi M, Valenti L. PNPLA3 as a therapeutic target for fatty liver disease: the evidence to date. Expert Opin Ther Targets. 2021;25(12):1033–43.
60. Loomba R, Friedman SL, Shulman GI. Mechanisms and disease consequences of nonalcoholic fatty liver disease. Cell. 2021;184(10):2537–64.
61. Peiseler M, Schwabe R, Hampe J, Kubes P, Heikenwalder M, Tacke F. Immune mechanisms linking metabolic injury to inflammation and fibrosis in fatty liver disease - novel insights into cellular communication circuits. J Hepatol. 2022;77(4):1136–60.
62. Sunny NE, Bril F, Cusi K. Mitochondrial Adaptation in Nonalcoholic Fatty Liver Disease: Novel Mechanisms and Treatment Strategies. Trends Endocrinol Metab. 2017;28(4):250–60.
63. Rada P, Gonzalez-Rodriguez A, Garcia-Monzon C, Valverde AM. Understanding lipotoxicity in NAFLD pathogenesis: is CD36 a key driver? Cell Death Dis. 2020;11(9):802.
64. Fraser DA, Wang X, Lund J, Nikolic N, Iruarrizaga-Lejarreta M, Skjaeret T, et al. A structurally engineered fatty acid, icosabutate, suppresses liver inflammation and fibrosis in NASH. J Hepatol. 2022;76(4):800–11.
65. Samuel VT, Shulman GI. Nonalcoholic Fatty Liver Disease as a Nexus of Metabolic and Hepatic Diseases. Cell Metab. 2018;27(1):22–41.
66. Fuchs CD, Trauner M. Role of bile acids and their receptors in gastrointestinal and hepatic pathophysiology. Nat Rev Gastroenterol Hepatol. 2022;19(7):432–50.
67. Puengel T, Liu H, Guillot A, Heymann F, Tacke F, Peiseler M. Nuclear receptors linking metabolism, inflammation, and fibrosis in nonalcoholic fatty liver disease. Int J Mol Sci. 2022;23(5):2668.
68. Wirth EK, Puengel T, Spranger J, Tacke F. Thyroid hormones as a disease modifier and therapeutic target in nonalcoholic steatohepatitis. Expert Rev Endocrinol Metab. 2022;17(5):425–34.
69. Hones GS, Geist D, Moeller LC. Noncanonical Action of Thyroid Hormone Receptors alpha and beta. Exp Clin Endocrinol Diabetes. 2020;128(6–07):383–7.
70. Sinha RA, Bruinstroop E, Singh BK, Yen PM. Nonalcoholic Fatty Liver Disease and Hypercholesterolemia: Roles of Thyroid Hormones, Metabolites, and Agonists. Thyroid. 2019;29(9):1173–91.
71. Harrison SA, Bedossa P, Guy CD, Schattenberg JM, Loomba R, Taub R, et al. A Phase 3, Randomized, Controlled Trial of Resmetirom in NASH with Liver Fibrosis. N Engl J Med. 2024;390(6):497–509.
72. Pharmaceuticals M. Madrigal Pharmaceuticals Announces FDA Approval of Rezdiffra™ (resmetirom) for the Treatment of Patients with Noncirrhotic Nonalcoholic Steatohepatitis (NASH) with Moderate to Advanced Liver Fibrosis. 2024.
73. Pharmaceuticals M. Madrigal Pharmaceuticals Announces EMA Validation of its Marketing Authorization Application for Resmetirom for the Treatment of NASH/MASH with Liver Fibrosis. 2024.
74. Moskovich D, Finkelshtein Y, Alfandari A, Rosemarin A, Lifschytz T, Weisz A, et al. Targeting the DIO3 enzyme using first-in-class inhibitors effectively suppresses tumor growth: a new

paradigm in ovarian cancer treatment. Oncogene. 2021;40(44):6248–57.
75. Olker JH, Korte JJ, Denny JS, Hartig PC, Cardon MC, Knutsen CN, et al. Screening the ToxCast Phase 1, Phase 2, and e1k Chemical Libraries for Inhibitors of Iodothyronine Deiodinases. Toxicol Sci. 2019;168(2):430–42.
76. Tilg H, Adolph TE, Trauner M. Gut-liver axis: Pathophysiological concepts and clinical implications. Cell Metab. 2022;34(11):1700–18.
77. Evangelakos I, Heeren J, Verkade E, Kuipers F. Role of bile acids in inflammatory liver diseases. Semin Immunopathol. 2021;43(4):577–90.
78. Zhang S, Wang J, Liu Q, Harnish DC. Farnesoid X receptor agonist WAY-362450 attenuates liver inflammation and fibrosis in murine model of non-alcoholic steatohepatitis. J Hepatol. 2009;51(2):380–8.
79. Neuschwander-Tetri BA, Loomba R, Sanyal AJ, Lavine JE, Van Natta ML, Abdelmalek MF, et al. Farnesoid X nuclear receptor ligand obeticholic acid for non-cirrhotic, non-alcoholic steatohepatitis (FLINT): a multicentre, randomised, placebo-controlled trial. Lancet. 2015;385(9972):956–65.
80. Rinella ME, Dufour JF, Anstee QM, Goodman Z, Younossi Z, Harrison SA, et al. Non-invasive evaluation of response to obeticholic acid in patients with NASH: Results from the REGENERATE study. J Hepatol. 2022;76(3):536–48.
81. Pockros PJ, Fuchs M, Freilich B, Schiff E, Kohli A, Lawitz EJ, et al. CONTROL: A randomized phase 2 study of obeticholic acid and atorvastatin on lipoproteins in nonalcoholic steatohepatitis patients. Liver Int. 2019;39(11):2082–93.
82. Younossi ZM, Ratziu V, Loomba R, Rinella M, Anstee QM, Goodman Z, et al. Obeticholic acid for the treatment of non-alcoholic steatohepatitis: interim analysis from a multicentre, randomised, placebo-controlled phase 3 trial. Lancet. 2019;394(10215):2184–96.
83. Sanyal AJ, Ratziu V, Loomba R, Anstee QM, Kowdley KV, Rinella ME, et al. Results from a new efficacy and safety analysis of the REGENERATE trial of obeticholic acid for treatment of pre-cirrhotic fibrosis due to non-alcoholic steatohepatitis. J Hepatol. 2023;79(5):1110–20.
84. Staels B, Butruille L, Francque S. Treating NASH by targeting peroxisome proliferator-activated receptors. J Hepatol. 2023;79(5):1302–16.
85. Lefere S, Puengel T, Hundertmark J, Penners C, Frank AK, Guillot A, et al. Differential effects of selective- and pan-PPAR agonists on experimental steatohepatitis and hepatic macrophages(☆). J Hepatol. 2020;73(4):757–70.
86. Ratziu V, Harrison SA, Francque S, Bedossa P, Lehert P, Serfaty L, et al. Elafibranor, an Agonist of the Peroxisome Proliferator-Activated Receptor-alpha and -delta, Induces Resolution of Nonalcoholic Steatohepatitis Without Fibrosis Worsening. Gastroenterology. 2016;150(5):1147–59 e5.
87. Gawrieh S, Noureddin M, Loo N, Mohseni R, Awasty V, Cusi K, et al. Saroglitazar, a PPAR-alpha/gamma Agonist, for Treatment of NAFLD: A Randomized Controlled Double-Blind Phase 2 Trial. Hepatology. 2021;74(4):1809–24.
88. Francque SM, Bedossa P, Ratziu V, Anstee QM, Bugianesi E, Sanyal AJ, et al. A Randomized, Controlled Trial of the Pan-PPAR Agonist Lanifibranor in NASH. N Engl J Med. 2021;385(17):1547–58.
89. Rinella ME, Tacke F, Sanyal AJ, Anstee QM, participants of the AEW. Report on the AASLD/EASL joint workshop on clinical trial endpoints in NAFLD. J Hepatol. 2019;71(4):823–33.
90. Ahn SB, Jang K, Jun DW, Lee BH, Shin KJ. Expression of liver X receptor correlates with intrahepatic inflammation and fibrosis in patients with nonalcoholic fatty liver disease. Dig Dis Sci. 2014;59(12):2975–82.
91. Azzu V, Vacca M, Virtue S, Allison M, Vidal-Puig A. Adipose Tissue-Liver Cross Talk in the Control of Whole-Body Metabolism: Implications in Nonalcoholic Fatty Liver Disease. Gastroenterology. 2020;158(7):1899–912.
92. Nachit M, Kwanten WJ, Thissen JP, Op De Beeck B, Van Gaal L, Vonghia L, et al. Muscle fat content is strongly associated with NASH: A longitudinal study in patients with morbid obesity. J Hepatol. 2021;75(2):292–301.
93. Hundertmark J, Krenkel O, Tacke F. Adapted Immune Responses of Myeloid-Derived Cells in Fatty Liver Disease. Front Immunol. 2018;9:2418.
94. Heymann F, Tacke F. Immunology in the liver--from homeostasis to disease. Nat Rev Gastroenterol Hepatol. 2016;13(2):88–110.
95. Albillos A, de Gottardi A, Rescigno M. The gut-liver axis in liver disease: Pathophysiological basis for therapy. J Hepatol. 2020;72(3):558–77.
96. Bajaj JS, Ng SC, Schnabl B. Promises of microbiome-based therapies. J Hepatol. 2022;76(6):1379–91.
97. Ratziu V, Francque S, Sanyal A. Breakthroughs in therapies for NASH and remaining challenges. J Hepatol. 2022;76(6):1263–78.
98. Newsome PN, Ambery P. Incretins (GLP-1 receptor agonists and dual/triple agonists) and the liver. J Hepatol. 2023;79(6):1557–65.
99. Daniele G, Iozzo P, Molina-Carrion M, Lancaster J, Ciociaro D, Cersosimo E, et al. Exenatide Regulates Cerebral Glucose Metabolism in Brain Areas Associated With Glucose Homeostasis and Reward System. Diabetes. 2015;64(10):3406–12.
100. van Bloemendaal L, Veltman DJ, Ten Kulve JS, Groot PF, Ruhe HG, Barkhof F, et al. Brain reward-system activation in response to anticipation and consumption of palatable food is altered by glucagon-like peptide-1 receptor activation in humans. Diabetes Obes Metab. 2015;17(9):878–86.
101. Armstrong MJ, Houlihan DD, Rowe IA, Clausen WH, Elbrond B, Gough SC, et al. Safety and efficacy of liraglutide in patients with type 2 diabetes and

elevated liver enzymes: individual patient data meta-analysis of the LEAD program. Aliment Pharmacol Ther. 2013;37(2):234–42.
102. Armstrong MJ, Gaunt P, Aithal GP, Barton D, Hull D, Parker R, et al. Liraglutide safety and efficacy in patients with non-alcoholic steatohepatitis (LEAN): a multicentre, double-blind, randomised, placebo-controlled phase 2 study. Lancet. 2016;387(10019):679–90.
103. Armstrong MJ, Hull D, Guo K, Barton D, Hazlehurst JM, Gathercole LL, et al. Glucagon-like peptide 1 decreases lipotoxicity in non-alcoholic steatohepatitis. J Hepatol. 2016;64(2):399–408.
104. Newsome PN, Buchholtz K, Cusi K, Linder M, Okanoue T, Ratziu V, et al. A Placebo-Controlled Trial of Subcutaneous Semaglutide in Nonalcoholic Steatohepatitis. N Engl J Med. 2021;384(12):1113–24.
105. Thethi TK, Pratley R, Meier JJ. Efficacy, safety and cardiovascular outcomes of once-daily oral semaglutide in patients with type 2 diabetes: The PIONEER programme. Diabetes Obes Metab. 2020;22(8):1263–77.
106. Loomba R, Abdelmalek MF, Armstrong MJ, Jara M, Kjaer MS, Krarup N, et al. Semaglutide 2.4 mg once weekly in patients with non-alcoholic steatohepatitis-related cirrhosis: a randomised, placebo-controlled phase 2 trial. Lancet. Gastroenterol Hepatol. 2023;8(6):511–22.
107. Bosch R, Petrone M, Arends R, Vicini P, Sijbrands EJG, Hoefman S, et al. Characterisation of cotadutide's dual GLP-1/glucagon receptor agonistic effects on glycaemic control using an in vivo human glucose regulation quantitative systems pharmacology model. Br J Pharmacol. 2024;181:1874.
108. Kim T, Holleman CL, Nason S, Arble DM, Ottaway N, Chabenne J, et al. Hepatic Glucagon Receptor Signaling Enhances Insulin-Stimulated Glucose Disposal in Rodents. Diabetes. 2018;67(11):2157–66.
109. Parker VER, Hoang T, Schlichthaar H, Gibb FW, Wenzel B, Posch MG, et al. Efficacy and safety of cotadutide, a dual glucagon-like peptide-1 and glucagon receptor agonist, in a randomized phase 2a study of patients with type 2 diabetes and chronic kidney disease. Diabetes Obes Metab. 2022;24(7):1360–9.
110. Nahra R, Wang T, Gadde KM, Oscarsson J, Stumvoll M, Jermutus L, et al. Effects of Cotadutide on Metabolic and Hepatic Parameters in Adults With Overweight or Obesity and Type 2 Diabetes: A 54-Week Randomized Phase 2b Study. Diabetes Care. 2021;44(6):1433–42.
111. Bluher M, Rosenstock J, Hoefler J, Manuel R, Hennige AM. Dose-response effects on HbA(1c) and bodyweight reduction of survodutide, a dual glucagon/GLP-1 receptor agonist, compared with placebo and open-label semaglutide in people with type 2 diabetes: a randomised clinical trial. Diabetologia. 2024;67(3):470–82.
112. Romero-Gomez M, Lawitz E, Shankar RR, Chaudhri E, Liu J, Lam RLH, et al. A phase IIa active-comparator-controlled study to evaluate the efficacy and safety of efinopegdutide in patients with non-alcoholic fatty liver disease. J Hepatol. 2023;79(4):888–97.
113. El K, Campbell JE. The role of GIP in alpha-cells and glucagon secretion. Peptides. 2020;125:170213.
114. Ludwig MQ, Cheng W, Gordian D, Lee J, Paulsen SJ, Hansen SN, et al. A genetic map of the mouse dorsal vagal complex and its role in obesity. Nat Metab. 2021;3(4):530–45.
115. Thondam SK, Cuthbertson DJ, Wilding JPH. The influence of Glucose-dependent Insulinotropic Polypeptide (GIP) on human adipose tissue and fat metabolism: Implications for obesity, type 2 diabetes and Non-Alcoholic Fatty Liver Disease (NAFLD). Peptides. 2020;125:170208.
116. Jastreboff AM, Aronne LJ, Ahmad NN, Wharton S, Connery L, Alves B, et al. Tirzepatide Once Weekly for the Treatment of Obesity. N Engl J Med. 2022;387(3):205–16.
117. Gastaldelli A, Cusi K, Fernandez Lando L, Bray R, Brouwers B, Rodriguez A. Effect of tirzepatide versus insulin degludec on liver fat content and abdominal adipose tissue in people with type 2 diabetes (SURPASS-3 MRI): a substudy of the randomised, open-label, parallel-group, phase 3 SURPASS-3 trial. Lancet Diabetes Endocrinol. 2022;10(6):393–406.
118. Coskun T, Urva S, Roell WC, Qu H, Loghin C, Moyers JS, et al. LY3437943, a novel triple glucagon, GIP, and GLP-1 receptor agonist for glycemic control and weight loss: From discovery to clinical proof of concept. Cell Metab. 2022;34(9):1234–47 e9.
119. Jastreboff AM, Kaplan LM, Frias JP, Wu Q, Du Y, Gurbuz S, et al. Triple-Hormone-Receptor Agonist Retatrutide for Obesity - A Phase 2 Trial. N Engl J Med. 2023;389(6):514–26.
120. Rosenstock J, Frias J, Jastreboff AM, Du Y, Lou J, Gurbuz S, et al. Retatrutide, a GIP, GLP-1 and glucagon receptor agonist, for people with type 2 diabetes: a randomised, double-blind, placebo and active-controlled, parallel-group, phase 2 trial conducted in the USA. Lancet. 2023;402(10401):529–44.
121. Arab JP, Karpen SJ, Dawson PA, Arrese M, Trauner M. Bile acids and nonalcoholic fatty liver disease: Molecular insights and therapeutic perspectives. Hepatology. 2017;65(1):350–62.
122. Potthoff MJ, Boney-Montoya J, Choi M, He T, Sunny NE, Satapati S, et al. FGF15/19 regulates hepatic glucose metabolism by inhibiting the CREB-PGC-1alpha pathway. Cell Metab. 2011;13(6):729–38.
123. Harrison SA, Rossi SJ, Paredes AH, Trotter JF, Bashir MR, Guy CD, et al. NGM282 Improves Liver Fibrosis and Histology in 12 Weeks in Patients With Nonalcoholic Steatohepatitis. Hepatology. 2020;71(4):1198–212.

124. Harrison SA, Neff G, Guy CD, Bashir MR, Paredes AH, Frias JP, et al. Efficacy and Safety of Aldafermin, an Engineered FGF19 Analog, in a Randomized, Double-Blind, Placebo-Controlled Trial of Patients With Nonalcoholic Steatohepatitis. Gastroenterology. 2021;160(1):219–31. e1
125. Harrison SA, Abdelmalek MF, Neff G, Gunn N, Guy CD, Alkhouri N, et al. Aldafermin in patients with non-alcoholic steatohepatitis (ALPINE 2/3): a randomised, double-blind, placebo-controlled, phase 2b trial. Lancet Gastroenterol Hepatol. 2022;7(7):603–16.
126. Rinella ME, Lieu HD, Kowdley KV, Goodman ZD, Alkhouri N, Lawitz E, et al. A randomized, double-blind, placebo-controlled trial of aldafermin in patients with NASH and compensated cirrhosis. Hepatology. 2024;79(3):674–89.
127. Friedman SL, Neuschwander-Tetri BA, Rinella M, Sanyal AJ. Mechanisms of NAFLD development and therapeutic strategies. Nat Med. 2018;24(7):908–22.
128. Chen Z, Tian R, She Z, Cai J, Li H. Role of oxidative stress in the pathogenesis of nonalcoholic fatty liver disease. Free Radic Biol Med. 2020;152:116–41.
129. Puengel T, Tacke F. Efruxifermin, an investigational treatment for fibrotic or cirrhotic nonalcoholic steatohepatitis (NASH). Expert Opin Investig Drugs. 2023;32(6):451–61.
130. Lin R, Zhou J, Sun Q, Xin X, Hu Y, Zheng M, et al. Meta-analysis: Efficacy and safety of fibroblast growth factor 21 analogues for the treatment of non-alcoholic steatohepatitis and non-alcoholic steatohepatitis-related fibrosis. Aliment Pharmacol Ther. 2024;59(7):802–11.
131. Abdelmalek MF, Charles ED, Sanyal AJ, Harrison SA, Neuschwander-Tetri BA, Goodman Z, et al. The FALCON program: Two phase 2b randomized, double-blind, placebo-controlled studies to assess the efficacy and safety of pegbelfermin in the treatment of patients with nonalcoholic steatohepatitis and bridging fibrosis or compensated cirrhosis. Contemp Clin Trials. 2021;104:106335.
132. Abdelmalek MF, Sanyal AJ, Nakajima A, Neuschwander-Tetri BA, Goodman ZD, Lawitz EJ, et al. Pegbelfermin in Patients With Nonalcoholic Steatohepatitis and Compensated Cirrhosis (FALCON 2): A Randomized Phase 2b Study. Clin Gastroenterol Hepatol. 2024;22(1):113–23 e9.
133. Loomba R, Sanyal AJ, Nakajima A, Neuschwander-Tetri BA, Goodman ZD, Harrison SA, et al. Pegbelfermin in Patients With Nonalcoholic Steatohepatitis and Stage 3 Fibrosis (FALCON 1): A Randomized Phase 2b Study. Clin Gastroenterol Hepatol. 2024;22(1):102–12 e9.
134. Brown EA, Minnich A, Sanyal AJ, Loomba R, Du S, Schwarz J, et al. Effect of pegbelfermin on NASH and fibrosis-related biomarkers and correlation with histological response in the FALCON 1 trial. JHEP Rep. 2023;5(4):100661.
135. Harrison SA, Frias JP, Neff G, Abrams GA, Lucas KJ, Sanchez W, et al. Safety and efficacy of once-weekly efruxifermin versus placebo in non-alcoholic steatohepatitis (HARMONY): a multicentre, randomised, double-blind, placebo-controlled, phase 2b trial. Lancet Gastroenterol Hepatol. 2023;8(12):1080–93.
136. Mahgoub S, Newsome PN. Efruxifermin in non-alcoholic steatohepatitis. Lancet Gastroenterol Hepatol. 2023;8(12):1058–9.
137. Bhatt DL, Bays HE, Miller M, Cain JE 3rd, Wasilewska K, Andrawis NS, et al. The FGF21 analog pegozafermin in severe hypertriglyceridemia: a randomized phase 2 trial. Nat Med. 2023;29(7):1782–92.
138. Loomba R, Sanyal AJ, Kowdley KV, Bhatt DL, Alkhouri N, Frias JP, et al. Randomized, Controlled Trial of the FGF21 Analogue Pegozafermin in NASH. N Engl J Med. 2023;389(11):998–1008.
139. Alkhouri N, Herring R, Kabler H, Kayali Z, Hassanein T, Kohli A, et al. Safety and efficacy of combination therapy with semaglutide, cilofexor and firsocostat in patients with non-alcoholic steatohepatitis: A randomised, open-label phase II trial. J Hepatol. 2022;77(3):607–18.
140. Harrison SA, Frias JP, Lucas KJ, Reiss G, Neff G, Bollepalli S, et al. Safety and efficacy of efruxifermin in combination with a GLP-1 receptor agonist in patients with NASH/MASH and type 2 diabetes in a randomized phase 2 study. Clin Gastroenterol Hepatol. 2024;
141. Carvalho T. Efruxifermin combined with a GLP-1 receptor agonist reduces liver fat in NASH. Nat Med. 2023;29(8):1881.
142. Puengel T, Lefere S, Hundertmark J, Kohlhepp M, Penners C, Van de Velde F, et al. Combined therapy with a CCR2/CCR5 antagonist and FGF21 analogue synergizes in ameliorating steatohepatitis and fibrosis. Int J Mol Sci. 2022;23(12):6696.
143. Wallace SJ, Tacke F, Schwabe RF, Henderson NC. Understanding the cellular interactome of non-alcoholic fatty liver disease. JHEP Rep. 2022;4(8):100524.
144. Carvalho-Gontijo R, Han C, Zhang L, Zhang V, Hosseini M, Mekeel K, et al. Metabolic injury of hepatocytes promotes progression of NAFLD and AALD. Semin Liver Dis. 2022;42(3):233–49.
145. Engelmann C, Tacke F. The potential role of cellular senescence in non-alcoholic fatty liver disease. Int J Mol Sci. 2022;23(2):652.
146. Puengel T, Tacke F. Cell type-specific actions of thyroid hormones in nonalcoholic steatohepatitis and liver fibrosis. Liver Int. 2024;44(2):275–8.
147. Schwabl P, Hambruch E, Budas GR, Supper P, Burnet M, Liles JT, et al. The non-steroidal FXR agonist cilofexor improves portal hypertension and reduces hepatic fibrosis in a rat NASH model. Biomedicines. 2021;9(1):60.
148. Puengel T, De Vos S, Hundertmark J, Kohlhepp M, Guldiken N, Pujuguet P, et al. The medium-chain fatty acid receptor GPR84 mediates myeloid cell infiltration promoting steatohepatitis and fibrosis. J Clin Med. 2020;9(4):1140.

149. Harrison SA, Wong VW, Okanoue T, Bzowej N, Vuppalanchi R, Younes Z, et al. Selonsertib for patients with bridging fibrosis or compensated cirrhosis due to NASH: Results from randomized phase III STELLAR trials. J Hepatol. 2020;73(1):26–39.
150. Lawitz EJ, Bhandari BR, Ruane PJ, Kohli A, Harting E, Ding D, et al. Fenofibrate Mitigates Hypertriglyceridemia in Nonalcoholic Steatohepatitis Patients Treated With Cilofexor/Firsocostat. Clin Gastroenterol Hepatol. 2023;21(1):143–52 e3.
151. Triantafilou M, Hughes TR, Morgan BP, Triantafilou K. Complementing the inflammasome. Immunology. 2016;147(2):152–64.
152. Szabo G, Petrasek J. Inflammasome activation and function in liver disease. Nat Rev Gastroenterol Hepatol. 2015;12(7):387–400.
153. Tilg H, Adolph TE, Tacke F. Therapeutic modulation of the liver immune microenvironment. Hepatology. 2023;78(5):1581–601.
154. Abbate A, Toldo S, Marchetti C, Kron J, Van Tassell BW, Dinarello CA. Interleukin-1 and the Inflammasome as Therapeutic Targets in Cardiovascular Disease. Circ Res. 2020;126(9):1260–80.
155. Chauhan D, Vande Walle L, Lamkanfi M. Therapeutic modulation of inflammasome pathways. Immunol Rev. 2020;297(1):123–38.
156. Gorelik M, Lee Y, Abe M, Andrews T, Davis L, Patterson J, et al. IL-1 receptor antagonist, anakinra, prevents myocardial dysfunction in a mouse model of Kawasaki disease vasculitis and myocarditis. Clin Exp Immunol. 2019;198(1):101–10.
157. Knorr J, Wree A, Tacke F, Feldstein AE. The NLRP3 Inflammasome in Alcoholic and Nonalcoholic Steatohepatitis. Semin Liver Dis. 2020;40(3):298–306.
158. Wree A, Eguchi A, McGeough MD, Pena CA, Johnson CD, Canbay A, et al. NLRP3 inflammasome activation results in hepatocyte pyroptosis, liver inflammation, and fibrosis in mice. Hepatology. 2014;59(3):898–910.
159. Mridha AR, Wree A, Robertson AAB, Yeh MM, Johnson CD, Van Rooyen DM, et al. NLRP3 inflammasome blockade reduces liver inflammation and fibrosis in experimental NASH in mice. J Hepatol. 2017;66(5):1037–46.
160. Perera AP, Fernando R, Shinde T, Gundamaraju R, Southam B, Sohal SS, et al. MCC950, a specific small molecule inhibitor of NLRP3 inflammasome attenuates colonic inflammation in spontaneous colitis mice. Sci Rep. 2018;8(1):8618.
161. Engelmann C, Sheikh M, Sharma S, Kondo T, Loeffler-Wirth H, Zheng YB, et al. Toll-like receptor 4 is a therapeutic target for prevention and treatment of liver failure. J Hepatol. 2020;73(1):102–12.
162. Seki E, De Minicis S, Osterreicher CH, Kluwe J, Osawa Y, Brenner DA, et al. TLR4 enhances TGF-beta signaling and hepatic fibrosis. Nat Med. 2007;13(11):1324–32.
163. Dapito DH, Mencin A, Gwak GY, Pradere JP, Jang MK, Mederacke I, et al. Promotion of hepatocellular carcinoma by the intestinal microbiota and TLR4. Cancer Cell. 2012;21(4):504–16.
164. Schneider KM, Bieghs V, Heymann F, Hu W, Dreymueller D, Liao L, et al. CX3CR1 is a gatekeeper for intestinal barrier integrity in mice: Limiting steatohepatitis by maintaining intestinal homeostasis. Hepatology. 2015;62(5):1405–16.
165. Hsieh YC, Lee KC, Wu PS, Huo TI, Huang YH, Hou MC, et al. Eritoran Attenuates Hepatic Inflammation and Fibrosis in Mice with Chronic Liver Injury. Cells. 2021;10(6):1562.
166. Krenkel O, Hundertmark J, Abdallah AT, Kohlhepp M, Puengel T, Roth T, et al. Myeloid cells in liver and bone marrow acquire a functionally distinct inflammatory phenotype during obesity-related steatohepatitis. Gut. 2020;69(3):551–63.
167. Ramachandran P, Matchett KP, Dobie R, Wilson-Kanamori JR, Henderson NC. Single-cell technologies in hepatology: new insights into liver biology and disease pathogenesis. Nat Rev Gastroenterol Hepatol. 2020;17(8):457–72.
168. Wen Y, Lambrecht J, Ju C, Tacke F. Hepatic macrophages in liver homeostasis and diseases-diversity, plasticity and therapeutic opportunities. Cell Mol Immunol. 2021;18(1):45–56.
169. Krenkel O, Puengel T, Govaere O, Abdallah AT, Mossanen JC, Kohlhepp M, et al. Therapeutic inhibition of inflammatory monocyte recruitment reduces steatohepatitis and liver fibrosis. Hepatology. 2018;67(4):1270–83.
170. Ratziu V, Sanyal A, Harrison SA, Wong VW, Francque S, Goodman Z, et al. Cenicriviroc Treatment for Adults With Nonalcoholic Steatohepatitis and Fibrosis: Final Analysis of the Phase 2b CENTAUR Study. Hepatology. 2020;72(3):892–905.
171. Anstee QM, Neuschwander-Tetri BA, Wai-Sun Wong V, Abdelmalek MF, Rodriguez-Araujo G, Landgren H, et al. Cenicriviroc Lacked Efficacy to Treat Liver Fibrosis in Nonalcoholic Steatohepatitis: AURORA Phase III Randomized Study. Clin Gastroenterol Hepatol. 2024;22(1):124–34 e1.
172. Al Attar A, Antaramian A, Noureddin M. Review of galectin-3 inhibitors in the treatment of nonalcoholic steatohepatitis. Expert Rev Clin Pharmacol. 2021;14(4):457–64.
173. Chalasani N, Abdelmalek MF, Garcia-Tsao G, Vuppalanchi R, Alkhouri N, Rinella M, et al. Effects of Belapectin, an Inhibitor of Galectin-3, in Patients With Nonalcoholic Steatohepatitis With Cirrhosis and Portal Hypertension. Gastroenterology. 2020;158(5):1334–45. e5
174. Schwabe RF, Tabas I, Pajvani UB. Mechanisms of Fibrosis Development in Nonalcoholic Steatohepatitis. Gastroenterology. 2020;158(7):1913–28.
175. Kisseleva T, Brenner D. Molecular and cellular mechanisms of liver fibrosis and its regression. Nat Rev Gastroenterol Hepatol. 2021;18(3):151–66.

176. Henderson NC, Rieder F, Wynn TA. Fibrosis: from mechanisms to medicines. Nature. 2020;587(7835):555–66.
177. Henderson NC, Arnold TD, Katamura Y, Giacomini MM, Rodriguez JD, McCarty JH, et al. Targeting of alphav integrin identifies a core molecular pathway that regulates fibrosis in several organs. Nat Med. 2013;19(12):1617–24.
178. Rahman SR, Roper JA, Grove JI, Aithal GP, Pun KT, Bennett AJ. Integrins as a drug target in liver fibrosis. Liver Int. 2022;42(3):507–21.
179. Gilgenkrantz H, Mallat A, Moreau R, Lotersztajn S. Targeting cell-intrinsic metabolism for antifibrotic therapy. J Hepatol. 2021;74(6):1442–54.
180. Harrison SA, Manghi FP, Smith WB, Alpenidze D, Aizenberg D, Klarenbeek N, et al. Licogliflozin for nonalcoholic steatohepatitis: a randomized, double-blind, placebo-controlled, phase 2a study. Nat Med. 2022;28(7):1432–8.
181. Bruschi FV, Claudel T, Tardelli M, Starlinger P, Marra F, Trauner M. PNPLA3 I148M Variant Impairs Liver X Receptor Signaling and Cholesterol Homeostasis in Human Hepatic Stellate Cells. Hepatol Commun. 2019;3(9):1191–204.
182. Thangapandi VR, Knittelfelder O, Brosch M, Patsenker E, Vvedenskaya O, Buch S, et al. Loss of hepatic Mboat7 leads to liver fibrosis. Gut. 2021;70(5):940–50.
183. Buch S, Stickel F, Trepo E, Way M, Herrmann A, Nischalke HD, et al. A genome-wide association study confirms PNPLA3 and identifies TM6SF2 and MBOAT7 as risk loci for alcohol-related cirrhosis. Nat Genet. 2015;47(12):1443–8.
184. Tacke F, Trautwein C. Mechanisms of liver fibrosis resolution. J Hepatol. 2015;63(4):1038–9.
185. Serhan CN, Levy BD. Resolvins in inflammation: emergence of the pro-resolving superfamily of mediators. J Clin Invest. 2018;128(7):2657–69.
186. Calvente CJ, Tameda M, Johnson CD, Del Pilar H, Lin YC, Adronikou N, et al. Neutrophils contribute to spontaneous resolution of liver inflammation and fibrosis via microRNA-223. J Clin Invest. 2019;129(10):4091–109.
187. Caligiuri A, Gentilini A, Pastore M, Gitto S, Marra F. Cellular and molecular mechanisms underlying liver fibrosis regression. Cells. 2021;10(10):2759.
188. Harrison SA, Abdelmalek MF, Caldwell S, Shiffman ML, Diehl AM, Ghalib R, et al. Simtuzumab Is Ineffective for Patients With Bridging Fibrosis or Compensated Cirrhosis Caused by Nonalcoholic Steatohepatitis. Gastroenterology. 2018;155(4):1140–53.
189. Friedman SL. Fighting Cardiac Fibrosis with CAR T Cells. N Engl J Med. 2022;386(16):1576–8.
190. Amor C, Feucht J, Leibold J, Ho YJ, Zhu C, Alonso-Curbelo D, et al. Senolytic CAR T cells reverse senescence-associated pathologies. Nature. 2020;583(7814):127–32.
191. Ratziu V, Charlton M. Rational combination therapy for NASH: Insights from clinical trials and error. J Hepatol. 2023;78(5):1073–9.
192. Sanyal AJ, Anstee QM, Trauner M, Lawitz EJ, Abdelmalek MF, Ding D, et al. Cirrhosis regression is associated with improved clinical outcomes in patients with nonalcoholic steatohepatitis. Hepatology. 2022;75(5):1235–46.

# 5 Diagnostic Advances in MASLD

Paulina Vidal-Cevallos, Norberto Chávez-Tapia, and Emmanuel Tsochatzis

## 5.1 Introduction

In 2020, an update on the definition of nonalcoholic fatty liver disease (NAFLD) to metabolic-associated fatty liver disease (MAFLD) was proposed. It was suggested that the definition should be based on the presence of metabolic dysfunction, and emphasize the coexistence of MAFLD with other liver diseases [1].

The proposed criteria for the diagnosis of MAFLD requires the histological (biopsy), imaging (ultrasound, measurement of controlled attenuation parameter, magnetic resonance spectroscopy, or magnetic resonance-derived proton density fact fraction), or serum biomarker (fatty liver index) evidence of hepatic steatosis in addition to one of the three criteria presented in Table 5.1 [2].

The new definition also suggests that the activity grade and stage of fibrosis of MAFLD should be a continuum, eliminating the stratification into nonalcoholic steatohepatitis (NASH) and non-steatohepatitis. MAFLD-related cirrhosis is also addressed in the proposition, they suggest that it should be diagnosed in the absence of histological signs suggestive of steatohepatitis in patients with past or present evidence of metabolic risk factors, as described in the above criteria, and meet at least one of the following: (1) documentation of MAFLD on a previous liver biopsy, or (2) historical documentation of steatosis by hepatic imaging [2].

In June 2023, another consensus [3] proposed a change in nomenclature to metabolic dysfunction-associated steatotic liver disease (MASLD), the criterion of diagnosis is very similar to MAFLD. It can be diagnosed in any patient with steatosis identified by imaging of biopsy with at least 1 of 5 cardiometabolic criteria (Table 5.2).

This new definition added a new category named metabolic- and alcohol-related/associated liver disease (MetALD) to describe those with MAFLD who consume 140–350 g/week of alcohol for females and 210–420 g/week for males, and considers other causes of liver steatosis as a combination etiology.

From here onwards the terms NAFLD, MAFLD, and MASLD will be used as originally published by the authors.

P. Vidal-Cevallos · N. Chávez-Tapia (✉)
Obesity and Digestive Disease Unit, Medica Sur Clinic and Foundation, Mexico City, Mexico
e-mail: nchavezt@medicasur.org.mx

E. Tsochatzis
Royal Free Sheila Sherlock Liver Centre, Royal Free Hospital and UCL Institute of Liver and Digestive Health, London, UK
e-mail: e.tsochatzis@ucl.ac.uk


N. Méndez-Sánchez, X. Qi (eds.), *Metabolic Dysfunction-Associated Steatotic Liver Disease*,
https://doi.org/10.1007/978-981-97-9519-2_5

**Table 5.1** Diagnostic criteria for MAFLD

| Criteria 1 | Criteria 2 | Criteria 3 |
|---|---|---|
| **Overweight or obesity** | **Type 2 diabetes mellitus** | **The presence of at least 2 metabolic risk abnormalities** |
| BMI ≥25 kg/m² in Caucasians or BMI ≥23 kg/m² in Asians | According to the international criteria | Waist circumference ≥102/88 cm in Caucasian men/women, or ≥90/80 cm in Asian men/women |
| | | Blood pressure ≥130/85 mmHg or specific drug treatment |
| | | Plasma triglycerides ≥150 mg/dl (≥1.70 mmol/l) or specific drug treatment |
| | | Plasma HDL-cholesterol <40 mg/dl (<1.0 mmol/L) for men and <50 mg/dl (<1.3 mmol/L) for women or specific drug treatment |
| | | Prediabetes (i.e., fasting glucose levels 100–125 mg/dl (5.6–6.9 mmol/L), or 2-h post-load glucose levels 140–199 mg/dl (7.8–11 mmol) or HbA1c 5.7–6.4% (39–47 mmol/mol) |
| | | Plasma high-sensitivity C-reactive protein level >2 mg/l |

Modified from Ref. [2] *BMI* body mass index

**Table 5.2** Diagnostic criteria for MASLD

| |
|---|
| BMI ≥ 25 kg/m² in Caucasians or waist circumference >94 cm (male) 80 cm (female) or ethnicity adjusted equivalent. |
| Fasting serum glucose ≥5.6 mmol/L (100 mg/dl) or 2-h post-load glucose levels ≥7.8 mmol/L (140 mg/dl) or HbA1c ≥ 5.7% (39 mmol/L) or type 2 diabetes or treatment for type 2 diabetes. |
| Blood pressure ≥130/85 mmHg or specific antihypertensive drug treatment. |
| Plasma triglycerides ≥1.70 mmol/L (150 mg/dl) or lipid lowering treatment. |
| Plasma HDL-cholesterol ≤1.0 mmol/L (40 mg/dl) (male) and ≤1.3 mmol/L (50 mg/dl) (female) or lipid lowering treatment. |

Modified from Ref. [3] *BMI* body mass index, HbA1c glycosylated hemoglobin. HDL

## 5.2 Noninvasive Methods for Diagnosing MASLD

The gold standard for the diagnosis of NAFLD is the liver biopsy, with the limitations of cost, invasiveness, interobserver variability, sampling errors as it only represents 1/50,000 of the liver and complications [4]. For this reason, it is important to develop noninvasive methods for the diagnosis of MASLD.

### 5.2.1 Blood Biomarkers for the Diagnosis of Steatosis

Different scores have been developed for the noninvasive diagnosis of hepatic steatosis, with many advantages, such as high applicability, reproducibility, and availability; however, none are liver-specific and the results can be influenced by comorbidities, which should be taken into account for interpretation [5] (Table 5.3). It is difficult to compare these scores with each other because for the development they were compared to biopsy, ultrasound, and magnetic resonance.

The SteatoTest was one of the first panel of biomarkers developed for the diagnosis of steatosis, it uses FibroTest-ActiTest (Gamma-glutamyl transferase GGT, total bilirubin, alpha-2-macroglobulin, apolipoprotein A1, haptoglogin, and alanine aminotransferase ALT), body mass index (BMI), cholesterol, triglycerides (TG), and glucose adjusted for age and gender, it has an AUROC of 0.80 for the diagnosis of grade 2–4 steatosis [6].

The Fibrosis Liver Index (FLI) was a score developed in Northern Italy by selecting a population with elevated ALT or GGT and excluding patients infected with hepatitis B virus (HBV) or

**Table 5.3** Blood biomarker-based scores for the diagnosis of liver steatosis

| Score | Diagnostic yield | Interpretation |
|---|---|---|
| SteatoTest [6] | AUROC = 0.80 (0.02) | Cutoff of 0.72 NPV 93% for steatosis with a prevalence of 30% |
| Fibrosis liver index (FLI) [7] | AUROC = 0.85 (95%CI 0.81–0.88) | An FLI < 30 rules out fatty liver and an FLI ≥ 60 rules in fatty liver |
| Liver accumulation product (LAP) [8] | N/A | More severe vs. less severe steatosis increased for increasing values OR = 4.28 (95% CI 3.28–5.58) |
| Hepatic steatosis index (HSI) [9] | AUROC = 0.812 (95% CI 0.801–0.824) | <30.0 rules out NAFLD >36.0 detects NAFLD |
| Index of NASH (ION) [10] | AUROC = 0.77 (95% CI 0.75–0.79) | <11 rules out NAFLD >22 detects NAFLD |
| NAFLD liver fat score (NAFLD-FSL) [11] | AUROC = 0.87 (95% CI 0.84–0.92) | >−0.640 detects NAFLD |

*AUROC* area under the receiver operating characteristic curve, *NPV* negative predictive value, *OR* odds ratio, *NAFLD* nonalcoholic fatty liver disease

hepatitis C virus (HCV), all patients were compared with paired healthy subjects, the algorithm is based on BMI, waist circumference (WC), TG, and GGT, resulting in an AUROC of 0.85 (95%CI 0.81–0.88) for the detection of fatty liver. A recent meta-analysis found that the score has a good discriminatory performance excluding the disorder (negative predictive value 84%), but is not good for the diagnosis of NAFLD (sensitivity 81%, specificity 65%) [7].

Other formulas developed include the Liver Accumulation Product (LAP) that uses WC, fasting TG and sex, they found that the odds of more severe vs. less severe steatosis increased for increasing values OR = 4.28 (95% CI 3.28–5.58) for each log-unit increment [8]; the Hepatic Steatosis Index (HSI) that includes ALT, AST, BMI, sex, and the presence of type 2 diabetes mellitus [9]; the index of NASH (ION) that uses sex, waist-to-heap ratio, TG, ALT, homeostasis model assessment (HOMA), and a constant to determine the presence of steatosis, the score was compared with FLI and NFS [10]; the NAFLD liver fat score (NAFLD-LFS) was developed for the prediction of NAFLD and liver fat content using the presence of metabolic syndrome, type 2 diabetes, fasting insulin, AST, and ALT, noteworthy the addition of the presence of PNPLA3 gene variant did not improve accuracy [11].

More recently, a study assessed the triglyceride-glucose index (TyG) combined with different evaluations to predict MAFLD, TyC x waist circumference had an AUROC of 0.832 (95% CI 0.814–0.850), TyC x waist-to-height ratio 0.826 (95% CI 0.808–0.844), and TyC x body mass index 0.822 (95% CI 0.803–0.840); in the subgroup analysis the predictive values of TyG-WC were higher in the following subgroups of patients, nondiabetic ($p$ < 0.05), non-overweight ($p$ < 0.05), and people aged ≤53 years ($p$ < 0.05) [12]. This index has been proposed to use as an early screening for MAFLD.

### 5.2.2 Blood Biomarkers for the Diagnosis of Fibrosis

The development of a noninvasive test for diagnosis of liver fibrosis is of the utmost importance since fibrosis is the single most important predictor of mobility and mortality in these population (Table 5.4).

One of the first models developed to predict fibrosis was the AST/Platelet index (APRI) in patients with chronic HCV infection, this simple test has an AUROC of 0.80 for predicting significant fibrosis [13]; however, a recent meta-analysis in patients with MAFLD found it does not perform well in patients with NAFLD with an AUROC of 0.76 for significant fibrosis and of 0.77 for advanced fibrosis [14].

Another score was developed for the detection of fibrosis in patients with a BMI ≥ 25 kg/m$^2$, BAAT combines age, BMI, TG, and ALT with a

**Table 5.4** Blood biomarker-based scores for the diagnosis of liver fibrosis

| Score | AUROC | Interpretation |
|---|---|---|
| AST/platelet index (APRI) [13, 14] | Significant fibrosis 0.76<br>Advanced fibrosis 0.77 | >1.50 predicts significant fibrosis |
| Fibrosis-4 (FIB-4) [14, 23] | Advanced fibrosis 0.84 | <1.45 rules out advanced fibrosis<br>>3.25 detects advanced fibrosis |
| BAAT [15] | 0.84 | 0–1 rules out septal fibrosis |
| BARD [16] | 0.86 (95% CI 0.79–0.92) | ≥2 detects advanced fibrosis |
| NAFLD fibrosis score (NFS) [17] | 0.82 (95% CI 0.76–0.88) | <−1.455 rules out advanced fibrosis<br>>0.676 detects advanced fibrosis |
| Hepamet fibrosis score (HFS) [19] | 0.84 (95% CI 0.82–0.86) | <0.12 rules out advanced fibrosis<br>>0.47 detects advanced fibrosis |
| ADAPT [18] | 0.87 (95% CI 0.83–0.91) | >6.31 to rule in advanced fibrosis (≥F3) |
| Proprietary algorithms | | |
| FibroTest [20] | 0.870 (0.340) | <0.1 rules out fibrosis ≥F2<br>>0.6 detects fibrosis ≥F2 |
| Enhanced liver fibrosis (ELF) [21] | 0.87 (95% CI 0.66–1.00) | 0.375 detects fibrosis stage 3–4 (NPV 98%) |
| FibroMeter [22] | 0.911 | >0.256 detects significant fibrosis (≥F2) |

100% NPV for septal fibrosis when scoring 0–1 [15]. The BARD score was developed in patients with NAFLD diagnosed with biopsy in Poland, it includes AST/ALT ratio, BMI, and the presence of diabetes, the score has NPV of 96% for advanced fibrosis [16].

The NAFLD Fibrosis Score (NFS) predicts advance fibrosis in patients with biopsy-proven NAFLD, it includes age, hyperglycemia, BMI, platelet count, albumin, and AST/ALT ratio, with an NPV of 88% to rule out advanced fibrosis [17].

The Fibrosis-4 (FIB-4) was a model developed in patients with coinfection of HIV and HCV, it considers the platelet count, age, AST, and ALT, with an AUROC of 0.76 to detect advanced fibrosis, a meta-analysis in patients with NAFLD showed a very good AUROC for the detection of advanced fibrosis (AUROC 0.84) [14].

An algorithm including PRO-C3, a marker of type III collagen formation that elevates in the presence of fibrosis, along with age, presence of diabetes, and platelet count was recently developed for the identification of advanced fibrosis (≥F3) in patients with NAFLD, demonstrating superiority to APRI, FIB-4, and NFS [18].

More recently the Hepamet Fibrosis score was developed as a noninvasive method to detect advanced fibrosis in patients with NAFLD, including variables as sex, age, HOMA, presence of diabetes, AST, albumin, and platelet counts to discriminate between patients with and without fibrosis with an NPV of 92% [19].

Some proprietary algorithms have also been developed. The FibroTest was developed in patients with HCV infection, it contains 11 surrogate serological markers for the assessment of liver fibrosis, with a negative predictive value of 100% to rule out F2–F4 [20].

A group in Europe developed a panel of immunoassays to detect matrix constituents and mediators of matrix remodeling in serum for the detection of liver fibrosis containing nine markers (ELF), they used a multinational cohort including patients with liver disease due to different etiologies, in the subgroup of patients with NAFLD a score of 0.375 had a sensitivity of 89% and a negative predictive value (NPV) of 98% for detecting fibrosis stage 3–4 [21].

FibroMeter is a tool including age, sex, platelets, alpha-2-macroglobulin, ALT, urea, prothrombin index, GGT, and AST, developed for the evaluation of significant or advanced fibrosis in patients with chronic viral hepatitis, a group in Greece assessed its accuracy in patients with MASLD with and AUROC of 0.911 for predicting $F \geq 2$ [22].

Recently a test was developed for the early diagnosis of NAFLD; the NAFLD test uses elevated C-reactive protein, cholesterol, BMI, and ALT levels to discriminated patients with NAFLD from healthy subjects with an AUROC of 0.94 (95% CI 0.88–0.93) and an NPV of 86% [24].

## 5.3 Imaging Techniques: Beyond Ultrasound and Biopsy

**Steatosis Assessment**

Imaging techniques are the most commonly used methods to diagnose steatosis. The most accessible method is an abdominal ultrasound with a specificity of 93.6% (95% CI 87.2–97.0) and an AUC of 0.93 (0.91–0.95) for the detection of moderate-severe fatty liver [25], unfortunately, when steatosis is <30% the sensitivity is significantly reduced [26]. The computed tomography (CT) also has a limited capability of detecting mild steatosis, and the radiation exposure limits is used as a screening method [26].

### 5.3.1 Transient Elastography

The transient elastography is performed with an ultrasound and uses the controlled attenuation parameter (CAP) to assess the quantity of steatosis [26] by detecting the velocity of the shear waves induced in the liver tissue [5]. The CAP is an estimate of the total ultrasonic attenuation at 3.5 MHz, values range from 100 to 400 dB/m, steatosis grade 1 (S1) indicates 10–32% of hepatocytes with fat, grade 2 indicates 33–65%, and grade 3 indicates ≥66% of hepatocytes with fat [27].

A meta-analysis including 20% of patients with NAFLD, 37% hepatitis B, and 36% hepatitis C found a cutoff value of 248 dB/m (95% CI 237–261) for the detection of S1, noteworthy, it suggested deducting 10 dB/m for NAFLD and/or diabetes patients, and deducting/adding 4.4 dB/m for each unit of BMI above/below 25 kg/m$^2$ over the range of 20–30 kg/m$^2$. [28] Another individual patient data meta-analysis found that the AUROC for the use of the XL probe in patients with NAFLD 0.819 (95% CI 0.769–0.869) for S0 versus S1–S3 and 0.754 (0.72–0.787) for S0–S1 versus S2–S3 [29].

An observational study including patients diagnosed with MAFLD found that a CAP value >353 dB/m was associated with the presence of chronic kidney disease, and more strongly associated than the presence of fibrosis [30]. Another study in patients with NAFLD found that a CAP >295 dB/m value was associated with an increased risk of cardiovascular events (OR 8.661, CI 95% 1.11–6702; $p = 0.039$) [31].

### 5.3.2 Magnetic Resonance Imaging (MRI)

Multiple MRI-based techniques that have emerged for quantifying liver fat, however, widespread use is limited due to cost and availability [32].

The use of magnetic resonance spectroscopy (MRS) is technically difficult and it only measures a small volume of the tissue, conventional MRI is limited by eddy frequencies and the effects of protons in fat that interfere with singling, giving an inaccurate quantification of liver fat; the magnetic resonance imaging proton density fat fraction (MRI-PDFF) correlates well with MRS-PDFF, additionally it allows measurement of the entire liver and can be applied in any MRI platform [33].

The accuracy of the MRI-PDFF was assessed in a meta-analysis including patients with NAFLD, the AUROC value for classifying steatosis grades 0 vs. 1–3 was 0.98, for 0–1 vs. 2–3 was 0.91, and for 0–2 vs. 3 was 0.90, this technique can accurately detect 5% steatosis [34].

A cross-sectional study comparing MRI-DFF with liver biopsy in patients with NAFLD found that it identified patients with grade 2 steatosis with an AUROC of 0.90 (95% CI 0.820; $p < 0.001$), and performed better when compared to transient elastography [35]. The MRI-PDFF is currently the gold standard for the assessment of liver steatosis, used in phase II and III clinical trials.

**Fibrosis Assessment**

Fibrosis is the most important predictor of liver-related morbidity and mortality in patients with fatty liver, the gold standard for the diagnosis is the liver biopsy with all the above-mentioned limitations. Imaging methods have been developed for the noninvasive assessment of fibrosis.

### 5.3.3 Transient Elastography

The transient elastography measures liver stiffness by measuring the propagation velocity of a low-frequency wave (50 Hz) through the liver by pulse-echo ultrasound [36]. The values can range from 2.5 to 75 kPa and are inversely proportional to the liver elasticity, ten measurements are required for reliable evaluations [37].

A meta-analysis performed with the M probe in patients with NAFLD found that the pooled sensitivities and specificities to diagnose $F \geq 2$ were 79% and 75% (cutoff 6.7–7.7 kPa), $F \geq 3$ 85% and 85% (cutoff 8–10.4 kPa), and F4 92% and 92% (cutoff 10.3–17.5 kPa), respectively. They also found that liver stiffness measurement often failed in patients with obesity [38].

A more recent meta-analysis in patients with NAFLD found that the M and the XL probe have an AUROC of 0.88 and 0.85 for diagnosis advanced fibrosis ($F \geq 3$), respectively. A prospective cohort study including patients with biopsy-proven NAFLD found that the optimal cutoff value for advanced fibrosis was 9.9 kPa, with a sensitivity of 95%, and specificity of 75%, with an AUROC of 0.93 (95% CI 0.86–0.96) [39].

The use of transient elastography is currently recommended as a diagnostic method for NAFLD by the EASL guidelines [40]. A real-world multicenter study found that the cutoff of <7 kPa for excluding and >12 kPa for diagnosing compensated advanced chronic liver disease has a 91% sensitivity and 92% specificity (AUROC 0.87; 95% CI 0.86–0.88; $p < 0.001$), and should be used as an optimal cutoff [41].

Recently the AGILE 3+ score was developed to combine liver stiffness measurement (LSM) with AST/ALT ratio, platelet count, presence of diabetes, sex, and age for the diagnosis of advanced fibrosis (AUROC 0.88) and the prediction of liver-related events (AUROC 0.95) in patients with NAFLD [42].

### 5.3.4 Magnetic Resonance Elastography (MRE)

MRE is a noninvasive method that uses propagating waves with a phase contrast to quantify liver stiffness. It holds the additional value that it can be performed in patients with ascites, anatomical variants and transplant recipients, with the caveat of the cost, the practicality, and the availability [27].

A meta-analysis comparing laboratory markers, transient elastography, and MRI for diagnosing liver fibrosis in patients with NAFLD found that the MRE had a sensitivity of 77% for detecting significant fibrosis (F2–F4) with a specificity of 91.5%, with and AUROC of 0.92, and an AUROC of 0.96 for the detection of advanced fibrosis ($F \geq 3$) [14].

A recent meta-analysis found that the MRE had a sAUC of 0.92 (sensitivity 78%, specificity 89%) for $F \geq 2$, sAUC of 0.92 (sensitivity 83%, specificity 89%) for $F \geq 3$, and sAUC of 0.90 (sensitivity 81%, specificity 90%) for F4 [43].

A more advanced version of the MRE, the three-dimensional MRE has been assessed for diagnostic accuracy compared with 2D-MRE in a cross-sectional study in patients with biopsy-proven NAFLD and found an AUROC for diagnosing advanced fibrosis of 0.981 at 40 Hz and 0.927 for 60 Hz, compared with 0.921 for 2D-MRE at 60 Hz; with a cutoff point of 2.43 kPa the 3D-MRE at 40 Hz had a sensitivity of 1.0 and specificity of 0.94 [44].

The interobserver agreement of the MRE is very good, a study performed in patients with chronic viral hepatitis and biopsy-proven fibrosis reported an intraclass correlation coefficient of 0.99 (95% CI 0.98–1.00) [45]. An individual patient meta-analysis including international cohorts found the following cutoff values for MRE: 3.14 kPa for significant fibrosis (F2), 3.53 kPa for advanced fibrosis (F3), and 4.45 kPa for cirrhosis (F4) [46].

## 5.4 Other Imaging Techniques

The acoustic radiation force impulse (ARFI) is an elastography method included in the conventional ultrasound machine using short-duration acoustic pulses with a frequency of 2.67 MHz that result in localized tissue displacements, the propagation velocity is then measured and the results are expressed in meters per second in a range of 0.5–4.4 m/s [47].

A meta-analysis including patients with biopsy-proven liver fibrosis found that the AUROC for the diagnosis of $F \geq 2$ was 0.84 (DOR, 11.54), for $F \geq 3$ was 0.89 (DOR, 33.54) and for the diagnosis of F4 0.91 (DOR, 45.35) [47]. However, this method is not standardized and is not currently recommended for the diagnosis of fibrosis.

The two-dimensional shear wave elastography (2D-SWE) is another wave-based elastography method based on supersonic shear imaging integrated into the conventional ultrasound machine, it localizes the exact region during the B-mode ultrasound and is not limited by ascites [48]. An individual patient-data meta-analysis assessed the diagnostic accuracy in patients with multiple etiology biopsy-proven liver fibrosis and found an AUROC of 85.5% in patients with NAFLD for the diagnosis of significant fibrosis [48].

However, there is no data on the follow-up of patients with this method and it is not currently recommended for the diagnosis of fibrosis.

## 5.5 Novel Imaging Techniques

A novel technique using the MRI is the multiparametric MRI, which includes T1 mapping for fibrosis/inflammation, T2 mapping for liver iron quantification, and spectroscopy for liver fat quantification; it is completed in 23 min and does not require special hardware or the injection of contrast [27].

A study conducted in patients with multiple etiology liver fibrosis, comparing the multiparametric MRI with the liver biopsy found a strong correlation for fibrosis ($r_s = 0.68$, $p < 0.0001$; AUROC 0.94), steatosis ($r_s = 0.89$, $p < 0.001$; AUROC 0.93). More studies are needed to standardize the use of this method [49].

## 5.6 Early Identification of at-Risk Population

There is an unmet need for noninvasive tests for the screening of patients at higher risk of nonalcoholic steatohepatitis (NASH), disease progression, and/or developing liver-related events. Over the last few years, several panels and algorithms have been developed for this purpose.

A multicenter study assessed the ability of the FibroScan-AST (FAST) score to identify patients with NASH at higher risk of progression to cirrhosis, it combined liver stiffness measurement and CAP measured by FibroScan with the AST/ALT ratio, the rule-out cutoff of 0.2 and the rule-in cutoff of 5 had a negative predictive value of 0.73–1.0. [50]

The NIS2+™ score was developed later for the same purpose using 2 biomarkers (miR-34a-5p, YKL-40) and corrected by sex with and AURCO of 0.81 (95% CI 0.79–0.83) to rule-in/rule-out individuals at-risk of NASH, with a low cutoff of 0.45 to rule-out NASH and a high cutoff of 0.68 to rule-in NASH [51].

The metabolomics-advanced steatohepatitis fibrosis score (MASEF) was developed for the early identifications of patients with NAFLD activity score ≥ 4 and significant fibrosis ($F \geq 2$) in patients with MASLD to prioritize patients with increased risk of disease progression, it included 12 lipids, BMI, AST, and ALT, it had an AUROC of 0.79 (95% CI 0.75–0.83), with a negative predictive value of 0.88 [52].

The LiverRisk score was developed to identify patients at risk of cirrhosis, it included individuals from six countries, variables included were age, sex, fasting glucose, cholesterol, AST, ALT, GGT, and platelet count; the AUROC for the diagnosis of liver fibrosis at 10 kPa measured by FibroScan was 0.83 (95% CI 0.78–0.89). Four groups were created according to selected cutoff values, minimal-, low-, medium-, and high-risk, the score is very specific for predicting liver-related mortality, with an HR of 471 (95% CI 347–641) for liver-related mortality when comparing the high-risk group with the minimal-risk group, with an AUROC of 0.90 (95% CI 0.88–0.91) to predict 10-year liver-related mortality [53].

## 5.7 The Role of Artificial Intelligence and Machine Learning in Diagnosis

Artificial intelligence (AI) has been rapidly developing and has entered the field of medicine. Logic, statistics, cognitive psychology, decision theory, neuroscience, linguistics, cybernetics, and computer engineering are the disciplines underlying AI, the subdiscipline of AI that enables computers to learn from data is called Machine Learning (ML) [54].

In medicine, ML has emerged as a tool to make predictions and to support decision making, it can be categorized into (1) Supervised learning, where the machine generates results by learning from both input and output data; (2) Unsupervised learning, where it produces results without training of labeled data; and (3) Deep learning, where it learns from a training dataset and uses this to predict outcomes for new data [54].

The different developed models can be divided according to their purpose into diagnostic models, therapeutic models, and prognostic models [55].

### 5.7.1 Artificial Intelligence Based on Imaging

A study in China developed an ML model to classify MRE-derived liver stiffness using clinical and non-elastographic MRI radiomic features by using support vector machine models in pediatric patients, and found that the combination of clinical and radiomic (handcrafted image analysis) features has an AUC of 0.84, with a 72.2% sensitivity and 87% specificity in the internal validation; in the external validation it achieved an AUC of 0.80 [56].

Another group assessed the diagnostic accuracy of texture analysis-derived parameters combined with ML of non-contrast-enhanced T1w and T2w fat-saturated images with MRE for liver fibrosis quantification, categorized in low-grade (0–2) and high-grade (3, 4) fibrosis, and found an AU for T1w of 0.82 (95% CI 0.59–0.95) and 0.57 (95% CI 0.34–0.78) on T2w for classification into low-grade and high-grade fibrosis [57].

A study using inception-ResNet-v2 deep convolutional neural network (CNN) pretrained on the ImageNet dataset to extract high-level features in liver B-mode ultrasound image sequences compared with wedge biopsy found an AUROC of 0.977 [58]. An automated framework using CNN with ultrasound shear wave elastography images for the staging of fibrosis was developed yielding an AUROC of 0.89 compared to 0.74 of conventional stiffness for the diagnosis of fibrosis ≥2 [59].

Another study assessed the fully automated liver segmentation algorithm in non-contrast abdominal CT scans from asymptomatic adults by using convolutional neuronal networks, with excellent agreement between automated and manual measurements ($r^2 = 0.92$) [60].

A prospective study compared the accuracy of a deep learning tool using data from ultrasounds with MRI-PDFF for the diagnosis of NAFLD and found a correlation of Pearson $r = 0.85$, with an accuracy of 96% (95% CI 90–99%) [61]. Another retrospective study compared using deep convolutional neural network for staging fibrosis using gadoxetic acid-enhanced hepatobiliary phase MR images compared with liver biopsies, irrespective of etiology and showed an AUROC of 0.84 for F4, 0.84 for F3, and 0.85 for F2 [62].

### 5.7.2 Artificial Intelligence on Histology

One of the first published studies using automated assessment of histological features of NAFLD to reduce interobserver variability used hematoxylin and eosin-stained liver biopsies to quantify steatosis using supervised machine learning created from annotations by two expert pathologists with an overall accuracy of 89% [63].

A Chinese group developed qFIBS a system that uses second harmonic generation/two photon excitation fluorescence imaging-based tool to provide and automated quantitative assessment of the histological features of nonalcoholic steatohepatitis using the Clinical Research Network score to reduce interobserver variability and found a strong correlation for fibrosis ($r = 0.776$, $p < 0.001$) and a high AUROC value (0.87, 95% CI 0.787–1.000; $p < 0.001$) [64].

Another study assessed a computer-aided diagnosis system to predict NAFLD activity using the NAFLD activity score from histopathology slides with a good fibrosis stage prediction (AUC 83.8%) [65].

A further one study analyzed the ability of an integrated AI-based automated tool to quantify hepatic fibrosis and assess its architectural pattern in NAFLD biopsies compared with two expert pathologist and showed an AUROC of 78.6% for detection of periportal fibrosis, 83.3% for pericellular fibrosis, 86.4% for portal fibrosis, and >90% for detection of normal fibrosis, bridging fibrosis, and cirrhosis [66].

## 5.8 Novel Biomarkers and Their Role in Early Detection

The extracellular vesicles (EVs) are derived from the cellular membranes of living cells with lipid bilayer membranes; proteins, lipids, DNA, RNA, and metabolic products that regulated gene expression and signaling pathways in cells function as cargo for EVs [67]. There are three types of EVs—exosomes (40–120 nm) formed by exocytosis, microvesicles (50–1000 nm) derived from cellular budding, and apoptotic bodies (500–2000 nm) derived from dead cells [67].

EVs carry inflammatory molecules which lead to the progression of NAFLD, EV levels can induce activation of hepatic stellate cells and influence liver fibrosis [68]. The EV levels change from the early stage of NAFLD and throughout the different stages of progression and may be useful for the early diagnosis of NAFLD and for monitoring disease progression [69, 70]. A recent study found that the differences in protein expression of the extracellular vesicles can be useful differentiating patients with alcoholic liver disease from patients with NAFLD [71].

## 5.9 Conclusion

Significant advancements have been made in the noninvasive diagnostics of MASLD. A holistic approach should integrate various biomarkers, imaging techniques, and AI technologies. These innovations offer a promising future for accurately assessing liver steatosis and fibrosis, potentially transforming the clinical management of MASLD. Further research is needed to validate and standardize the diagnostic track and provide more precise, accessible, and patient-friendly diagnostic approaches in the evolving landscape of liver disease management.

## References


1. Eslam M, Sanyal AJ, George J. International consensus panel. MAFLD: a consensus-driven proposed nomenclature for metabolic associated fatty liver disease. Gastroenterology. 2020;158:1999–2014.e1.
2. Eslam M, Newsome PN, Sarin SK, Anstee QM, Targher G, Romero-Gomez M, et al. A new definition for metabolic dysfunction-associated fatty liver disease: an international expert consensus statement. J Hepatol. 2020;73:202–9.
3. Rinella ME, Lazarus JV, Ratziu V, Francque SM, Sanyal AJ, Kanwal F, et al. A multi-society delphi consensus statement on new fatty liver disease nomenclature. Ann Hepatol. 2023;62:101133.
4. Sumida Y, Nakajima A, Itoh Y. Limitations of liver biopsy and non-invasive diagnostic tests for the diagnosis of nonalcoholic fatty liver disease/nonalcoholic steatohepatitis. World J Gastroenterol. 2014;20:475–85.
5. Castera L, Friedrich-Rust M, Loomba R. Noninvasive assessment of liver disease in patients with nonalcoholic fatty liver disease. Gastroenterology. 2019;156:1264–1281.e4.
6. Poynard T, Ratziu V, Naveau S, Thabut D, Charlotte F, Messous D, et al. The diagnostic value of biomarkers (SteatoTest) for the prediction of liver steatosis. Comp Hepatol. 2005;4:10.
7. Castellana M, Donghia R, Guerra V, Procino F, Lampignano L, Castellana F, et al. Performance of fatty liver index in identifying non-alcoholic fatty liver disease in population studies. A meta-analysis. J Clin Med. 2021;10(9):1877. https://doi.org/10.3390/jcm10091877.
8. Bedogni G, Bellentani S, Miglioli L, Masutti F, Passalacqua M, Castiglione A, et al. The fatty liver index: a simple and accurate predictor of hepatic steatosis in the general population. BMC Gastroenterol. 2006;6:33.

9. Lee J-H, Kim D, Kim HJ, Lee C-H, Yang JI, Kim W, et al. Hepatic steatosis index: a simple screening tool reflecting nonalcoholic fatty liver disease. Dig Liver Dis. 2010;42:503–8.
10. Otgonsuren M, Estep MJ, Hossain N, Younossi E, Frost S, Henry L, et al. Single non-invasive model to diagnose non-alcoholic fatty liver disease (NAFLD) and non-alcoholic steatohepatitis (NASH). J Gastroenterol Hepatol. 2014;29:2006–13.
11. Kotronen A, Peltonen M, Hakkarainen A, Sevastianova K, Bergholm R, Johansson LM, et al. Prediction of non-alcoholic fatty liver disease and liver fat using metabolic and genetic factors. Gastroenterology. 2009;137:865–72.
12. Xue Y, Xu J, Li M, Gao Y. Potential screening indicators for early diagnosis of NAFLD/MAFLD and liver fibrosis: triglyceride glucose index-related parameters. Front Endocrinol (Lausanne). 2022;13:951689.
13. Wai C-T, Greenson JK, Fontana RJ, Kalbfleisch JD, Marrero JA, Conjeevaram HS, et al. A simple noninvasive index can predict both significant fibrosis and cirrhosis in patients with chronic hepatitis C. Hepatology. 2003;38:518–26.
14. Xiao G, Zhu S, Xiao X, Yan L, Yang J, Wu G. Comparison of laboratory tests, ultrasound, or magnetic resonance elastography to detect fibrosis in patients with nonalcoholic fatty liver disease: a meta-analysis. Hepatology. 2017;66:1486–501.
15. Ratziu V, Giral P, Charlotte F, Bruckert E, Thibault V, Theodorou I, et al. Liver fibrosis in overweight patients. Gastroenterology. 2000;118:1117–23.
16. Cichoż-Lach H, Celiński K, Prozorow-Król B, Swatek J, Słomka M, Lach T. The BARD score and the NAFLD fibrosis score in the assessment of advanced liver fibrosis in nonalcoholic fatty liver disease. Med Sci Monit. 2012;18:CR735-40.
17. Angulo P, Hui JM, Marchesini G, Bugianesi E, George J, Farrell GC, et al. The NAFLD fibrosis score: a noninvasive system that identifies liver fibrosis in patients with NAFLD. Hepatology. 2007;45:846–54.
18. Daniels SJ, Leeming DJ, Eslam M, Hashem AM, Nielsen MJ, Krag A, et al. ADAPT: an algorithm incorporating PRO-C3 accurately identifies patients with NAFLD and advanced fibrosis. Hepatology. 2019;69:1075–86.
19. Ampuero J, Pais R, Aller R, Gallego-Durán R, Crespo J, García-Monzón C, et al. Development and validation of hepamet fibrosis scoring system-a simple, noninvasive test to identify patients with nonalcoholic fatty liver disease with advanced fibrosis. Clin Gastroenterol Hepatol. 2020;18:216–225.e5.
20. Imbert-Bismut F, Ratziu V, Pieroni L, Charlotte F, Benhamou Y, Poynard T, et al. Biochemical markers of liver fibrosis in patients with hepatitis C virus infection: a prospective study. Lancet (London, England). 2001;357:1069–75.
21. Rosenberg WMC, Voelker M, Thiel R, Becka M, Burt A, Schuppan D, et al. Serum markers detect the presence of liver fibrosis: a cohort study. Gastroenterology. 2004;127:1704–13.
22. Arvaniti P, Giannoulis G, Lygoura V, Gatselis NK, Gabeta S, Rigopoulou E, et al. FibroMeter scores are predictive noninvasive markers of advanced and significant liver fibrosis in patients with chronic viral hepatitis or metabolic dysfunction-associated steatotic liver disease. Ann Gastroenterol. 2023;36:661–9.
23. Sterling RK, Lissen E, Clumeck N, Sola R, Correa MC, Montaner J, et al. Development of a simple noninvasive index to predict significant fibrosis in patients with HIV/HCV coinfection. Hepatology. 2006;43:1317–25.
24. Omran M, Omr M, Mohamed AA, Abdelghafour RA, Muharram NM, Hassan MB, et al. Development and validation of nonalcoholic fatty liver disease test: a simple sensitive and specific marker for early diagnosis of nonalcoholic fatty liver disease. Eur J Gastroenterol Hepatol. 2023;35:874–80.
25. Hernaez R, Lazo M, Bonekamp S, Kamel I, Brancati FL, Guallar E, et al. Diagnostic accuracy and reliability of ultrasonography for the detection of fatty liver: a meta-analysis. Hepatology. 2011;54:1082–90.
26. Xian Y-X, Weng J-P, Xu F. MAFLD vs. NAFLD: shared features and potential changes in epidemiology, pathophysiology, diagnosis, and pharmacotherapy. Chin Med J. 2020;134:8–19.
27. Han MAT, Saouaf R, Ayoub W, Todo T, Mena E, Noureddin M. Magnetic resonance imaging and transient elastography in the management of Nonalcoholic Fatty Liver Disease (NAFLD). Expert Rev Clin Pharmacol. 2017;10:379–90.
28. Karlas T, Petroff D, Sasso M, Fan J-G, Mi Y-Q, de Lédinghen V, et al. Individual patient data meta-analysis of controlled attenuation parameter (CAP) technology for assessing steatosis. J Hepatol. 2017;66:1022–30.
29. Petroff D, Blank V, Newsome PN, Shalimar VCS, Thiele M, et al. Assessment of hepatic steatosis by controlled attenuation parameter using the M and XL probes: an individual patient data meta-analysis. Lancet Gastroenterol Hepatol. 2021;6:185–98.
30. Marc L, Mihaescu A, Lupusoru R, Grosu I, Gadalean F, Bob F, et al. Liver steatosis: better predictor of CKD in MAFLD than liver fibrosis as determined by transient elastography with controlled attenuation parameter. Front Med. 2021;8:788881.
31. de Sousa MR, Xavier S, Magalhães J, Rosa B, Marinho C, Cotter J. Transient elastography through controlled attenuated parameter assisting the stratification of cardiovascular disease risk in NAFLD patients. Clin Res Hepatol Gastroenterol. 2021;45:101580.
32. Chandra Kumar CV, Skantha R, Chan W-K. Non-invasive assessment of metabolic dysfunction-associated fatty liver disease. Ther Adv Endocrinol Metab. 2022;13:20420188221139616.
33. Noureddin M, Lam J, Peterson MR, Middleton M, Hamilton G, Le T-A, et al. Utility of magnetic resonance imaging versus histology for quantifying changes in liver fat in nonalcoholic fatty liver disease trials. Hepatology. 2013;58:1930–40.

34. Gu J, Liu S, Du S, Zhang Q, Xiao J, Dong Q, et al. Diagnostic value of MRI-PDFF for hepatic steatosis in patients with non-alcoholic fatty liver disease: a meta-analysis. Eur Radiol. 2019;29:3564–73.
35. Imajo K, Kessoku T, Honda Y, Tomeno W, Ogawa Y, Mawatari H, et al. Magnetic resonance imaging more accurately classifies steatosis and fibrosis in patients with nonalcoholic fatty liver disease than transient elastography. Gastroenterology. 2016;150:626–637.e7.
36. Andersen ES, Christensen PB, Weis N. Transient elastography for liver fibrosis diagnosis. Eur J Intern Med. 2009;20:339–42.
37. Jin M, Yu Q, Liu Y, Xu W, Fu X, Ji B. Safety and efficacy of physical thermal ablation combined sorafenib for hepatocellular carcinoma: a meta-analysis. J Clin Transl Hepatol. 2021;9(2):149–59.
38. Kwok R, Tse Y-K, Wong GL-H, Ha Y, Lee AU, Ngu MC, et al. Systematic review with meta-analysis: non-invasive assessment of non-alcoholic fatty liver disease--the role of transient elastography and plasma cytokeratin-18 fragments. Aliment Pharmacol Ther. 2014;39:254–69.
39. Tapper EB, Challies T, Nasser I, Afdhal NH, Lai M. The performance of vibration controlled transient elastography in a US cohort of patients with nonalcoholic fatty liver disease. Am J Gastroenterol. 2016;111:677–84.
40. European Association for the Study of the Liver (EASL), European Association for the Study of Diabetes (EASD), European Association for the Study of Obesity (EASO). EASL-EASD-EASO clinical practice guidelines for the management of non-alcoholic fatty liver disease. J Hepatol. 2016;64:1388–402.
41. Papatheodoridi M, Hiriart JB, Lupsor-Platon M, Bronte F, Boursier J, Elshaarawy O, et al. Refining the Baveno VI elastography criteria for the definition of compensated advanced chronic liver disease. J Hepatol. 2021;74:1109–16.
42. Pennisi G, Enea M, Pandolfo A, Celsa C, Antonucci M, Ciccioli C, et al. AGILE 3+ score for the diagnosis of advanced fibrosis and for predicting liver-related events in NAFLD. Clin Gastroenterol Hepatol. 2023;21:1293–1302.e5.
43. Selvaraj EA, Mózes FE, Jayaswal ANA, Zafarmand MH, Vali Y, Lee JA, et al. Diagnostic accuracy of elastography and magnetic resonance imaging in patients with NAFLD: a systematic review and meta-analysis. J Hepatol. 2021;75:770–85.
44. Loomba R, Cui J, Wolfson T, Haufe W, Hooker J, Szeverenyi N, et al. Novel 3D magnetic resonance Elastography for the noninvasive diagnosis of advanced fibrosis in NAFLD: a prospective study. Am J Gastroenterol. 2016;111:986–94.
45. Runge JH, Bohte AE, Verheij J, Terpstra V, Nederveen AJ, van Nieuwkerk KMJ, et al. Comparison of interobserver agreement of magnetic resonance elastography with histopathological staging of liver fibrosis. Abdom Imaging. 2014;39:283–90.
46. Liang J-X, Ampuero J, Niu H, Imajo K, Noureddin M, Behari J, et al. An individual patient data meta-analysis to determine cut-offs for and confounders of NAFLD-fibrosis staging with magnetic resonance elastography. J Hepatol. 2023;79:592–604.
47. Nierhoff J, Chávez Ortiz AA, Herrmann E, Zeuzem S, Friedrich-Rust M. The efficiency of acoustic radiation force impulse imaging for the staging of liver fibrosis: a meta-analysis. Eur Radiol. 2013;23:3040–53.
48. Herrmann E, de Lédinghen V, Cassinotto C, Chu WC-W, Leung VY-F, Ferraioli G, et al. Assessment of biopsy-proven liver fibrosis by two-dimensional shear wave elastography: an individual patient data-based meta-analysis. Hepatology. 2018;67:260–72.
49. Banerjee R, Pavlides M, Tunnicliffe EM, Piechnik SK, Sarania N, Philips R, et al. Multiparametric magnetic resonance for the non-invasive diagnosis of liver disease. J Hepatol. 2014;60:69–77.
50. Newsome PN, Sasso M, Deeks JJ, Paredes A, Boursier J, Chan W-K, et al. FibroScan-AST (FAST) score for the non-invasive identification of patients with non-alcoholic steatohepatitis with significant activity and fibrosis: a prospective derivation and global validation study. Lancet. Gastroenterol Hepatol. 2020;5:362–73.
51. Harrison SA, Ratziu V, Magnanensi J, Hajji Y, Deledicque S, Majd Z, et al. NIS2+™, an optimisation of the blood-based biomarker NIS4® technology for the detection of at-risk NASH: a prospective derivation and validation study. J Hepatol. 2023;79:758–67.
52. Noureddin M, Truong E, Mayo R, Martínez-Arranz I, Mincholé I, Banales JM, et al. Serum identification of at-risk MASH: the metabolomics-advanced steatohepatitis fibrosis score (MASEF). Hepatology. 2024;79:135–48.
53. Serra-Burriel M, Juanola A, Serra-Burriel F, Thiele M, Graupera I, Pose E, et al. Development, validation, and prognostic evaluation of a risk score for long-term liver-related outcomes in the general population: a multicohort study. Lancet (London, England). 2023;402:988–96.
54. Zhang L, Mao Y. Artificial intelligence in NAFLD: will liver biopsy still be necessary in the future? Healthcare (Basel). 2022;11(1):117. https://doi.org/10.3390/healthcare11010117.
55. Li Y, Wang X, Zhang J, Zhang S, Jiao J. Applications of artificial intelligence (AI) in researches on non-alcoholic fatty liver disease(NAFLD): A systematic review. Rev Endocr Metab Disord. 2022;23:387–400.
56. He L, Li H, Dudley JA, Maloney TC, Brady SL, Somasundaram E, et al. Machine learning prediction of liver stiffness using clinical and T2-weighted MRI Radiomic data. AJR Am J Roentgenol. 2019;213:592–601.
57. Schawkat K, Ciritsis A, von Ulmenstein S, Honcharova-Biletska H, Jüngst C, Weber A, et al. Diagnostic accuracy of texture analysis and machine learning for quantification of liver fibrosis in MRI: correlation with MR elastography and histopathology. Eur Radiol. 2020;30:4675–85.

58. Byra M, Styczynski G, Szmigielski C, Kalinowski P, Michałowski Ł, Paluszkiewicz R, et al. Transfer learning with deep convolutional neural network for liver steatosis assessment in ultrasound images. Int J Comput Assist Radiol Surg. 2018;13:1895–903.
59. Brattain LJ, Telfer BA, Dhyani M, Grajo JR, Samir AE. Objective liver fibrosis estimation from shear wave elastography. Annu Int Conf IEEE Eng Med Biol Soc IEEE Eng Med Biol Soc Annu Int Conf. 2018;2018:1–5.
60. Graffy PM, Sandfort V, Summers RM, Pickhardt PJ. Automated liver fat quantification at nonenhanced abdominal CT for population-based steatosis assessment. Radiology. 2019;293:334–42.
61. Han A, Byra M, Heba E, Andre MP, Erdman JW, Loomba R, et al. Noninvasive diagnosis of nonalcoholic fatty liver disease and quantification of liver fat with radiofrequency ultrasound data using one-dimensional convolutional neural networks. Radiology. 2020;295:342–50.
62. Yasaka K, Akai H, Kunimatsu A, Abe O, Kiryu S. Liver fibrosis: deep convolutional neural network for staging by using gadoxetic acid-enhanced hepatobiliary phase MR images. Radiology. 2018;287:146–55.
63. Vanderbeck S, Bockhorst J, Komorowski R, Kleiner DE, Gawrieh S. Automatic classification of white regions in liver biopsies by supervised machine learning. Hum Pathol. 2014;45:785–92.
64. Liu F, Goh GB-B, Tiniakos D, Wee A, Leow W-Q, Zhao J-M, et al. qFIBS: an automated technique for quantitative evaluation of fibrosis, inflammation, ballooning, and steatosis in patients with nonalcoholic steatohepatitis. Hepatology. 2020;71:1953–66.
65. Qu H, Minacapelli CD, Tait C, Gupta K, Bhurwal A, Catalano C, et al. Training of computational algorithms to predict NAFLD activity score and fibrosis stage from liver histopathology slides. Comput Methods Prog Biomed. 2021;207:106153.
66. Gawrieh S, Sethunath D, Cummings OW, Kleiner DE, Vuppalanchi R, Chalasani N, et al. Automated quantification and architectural pattern detection of hepatic fibrosis in NAFLD. Ann Diagn Pathol. 2020;47:151518.
67. Jiang W, Xu Y, Chen J-C, Lee Y-H, Hu Y, Liu C-H, et al. Role of extracellular vesicles in nonalcoholic fatty liver disease. Front Endocrinol (Lausanne). 2023;14:1196831. https://doi.org/10.3389/fendo.2023.1196831.
68. Kostallari E, Valainathan S, Biquard L, Shah VH, Rautou P-E. Role of extracellular vesicles in liver diseases and their therapeutic potential. Adv Drug Deliv Rev. 2021;175:113816.
69. Tryndyak VP, Latendresse JR, Montgomery B, Ross SA, Beland FA, Rusyn I, et al. Plasma microRNAs are sensitive indicators of inter-strain differences in the severity of liver injury induced in mice by a choline- and folate-deficient diet. Toxicol Appl Pharmacol. 2012;262:52–9.
70. Ban LA, Shackel NA, McLennan SV. Extracellular vesicles: a new frontier in biomarker discovery for non-alcoholic fatty liver disease. Int J Mol Sci. 2016;17:376.
71. Nguyen H-Q, Lee D, Kim Y, Bang G, Cho K, Lee Y-S, et al. Label-free quantitative proteomic analysis of serum extracellular vesicles differentiating patients of alcoholic and nonalcoholic fatty liver diseases. J Proteome. 2021;245:104278.

# 6 Histopathology of MASLD: Insights into Liver Tissue Changes

Sven M. Francque and Ann Driessen

## 6.1 Introduction

The earliest descriptions of liver steatosis not attributable to what was then known as a common cause, namely alcohol consumption, date from the mid nineteenth century. Those first reports include descriptions of the macroscopic and microscopic appearance of "fatty livers" and hence imply that, as for several other diseases, the description of the disease was based on these pathology examinations. Also, the root cause of the disease, which would later be named Non-Alcoholic Fatty Liver Disease (NAFLD), was already recognised, being overnutrition, sedentarism and adiposity [1].

It was only in 1980 that the Mayo Clinic's pathologist Jurgen Ludwig described a series of 20 predominantly female patients with presence of striking fatty changes in the liver with evidence of lobular hepatitis, focal necrosis with mixed inflammatory infiltrates, and, in most instances, Mallory bodies [2]. Many patients also showed fibrosis, and cirrhosis was present in a few. He noted that the disease mimicked alcoholic hepatitis, but the patients were not drinking alcohol, so, despite the fact that he also observed that most patients were moderately obese and had obesity-associated diseases, e.g. diabetes, he called it non-alcoholic steatohepatitis, introducing NASH in the hepatology lexicon. Some years later, the broader term NAFLD was introduced, encompassing both those with NASH and those with fatty liver without features of steatohepatitis.

It became, however, clear over the last decades that this disease was indeed linked, in the vast majority of people, to what we currently know as the components of the metabolic syndrome, in particular overweight/obesity, insulin resistance, (pre)diabetes and dyslipidaemia [3]. The problem that NAFLD did not reflect this root cause of the disease was rapidly acknowledged, as well as the fact that the exclusionary definition of NAFLD did not allow to accurately describe chronic liver disease in the context of

S. M. Francque (✉)
Department of Gastroenterology and Hepatology, Antwerp University Hospital, Edegem, Belgium

InflaMed Centre of Excellence, Laboratory for Experimental Medicine and Paediatrics, Translational Sciences in Inflammation and Immunology, Faculty of Medicine and Health Sciences, University of Antwerp, Wilrijk, Belgium
e-mail: sven.francque@uza.be; sven.francque@uantwerpen.be

A. Driessen
Department of Pathology, Antwerp University Hospital, Edegem, Belgium

Department of Molecular Imaging, Pathology, Radiotherapy, Oncology, Faculty of Medicine and Health Sciences, University of Antwerp, Wilrijk, Belgium
e-mail: ann.driessen@uza.be; ann.driessen@uantwerpen.be



N. Méndez-Sánchez, X. Qi (eds.), *Metabolic Dysfunction-Associated Steatotic Liver Disease*,
https://doi.org/10.1007/978-981-97-9519-2_6

combined metabolic and alcoholic risk factors, but nevertheless the nomenclature remained unchanged. Recently, a large consensus process involving a wide and comprehensive range of stakeholders and following a stringent methodology, issued a new framework of terminology and definitions to settle the issue [4]. First, the term "fatty" was replaced by "steatotic" to avoid stigma. Second, the new nomenclature introduced the overarching concept of steatotic liver disease (SLD), hence with the starting point of diagnosis being the feature of steatosis, regardless of the aetiology. This concept deliberately favours a broad differential diagnosis, stressing the potential coexistence of multiple risk factors of liver steatosis and hence supporting a holistic care. Under this umbrella, you hence find all potential causes of liver steatosis, obviously with alcohol and metabolic dysfunction being the two leading aetiologies. The "old" NAFLD referring to liver steatosis in the context of cardiometabolic risk factors is now named metabolic dysfunction-associated steatotic liver disease (MASLD), requiring a diagnosis of steatosis and at least one cardiometabolic risk factor. People with liver steatosis in whom no cause can be identified, were previously also labelled NAFLD, which contributed to disease heterogeneity, and are now appropriately labelled cryptogenic SLD. The new framework did not change the concepts of steatohepatitis (only changing non-alcoholic steatohepatitis (NASH) to metabolic dysfunction-associated steatohepatitis (MASH)) nor the fibrosis staging. This, and the large overlap between NAFLD and MASLD also implies that the scientific data gathered so far with the "old" nomenclature are still valid [5].

Anyhow, the initial description of lipid accumulation in hepatocytes and the associated features of liver damage and inflammation in the context of metabolic dysfunction have been driven by pathology examination, and to date the histological characterisation of the disease and its features plays a pivotal role in the clinical management of these patients as well as in research.

The change in defining NAFLD as a diagnosis through exclusion to MASLD, a multisystemic disorder, could also significantly impact the histological understanding of the disease. While the histological features of NAFLD were considered similar to alcoholic liver disease, this comparison was inherently limited. The transition to MASLD acknowledges the multifactorial origin of the disease, leading to a more comprehensive pathology. MASLD is characterised by fluctuating phases of steatosis and steatohepatitis, influenced by lifestyle changes, therapeutic interventions, and concurrent liver diseases. Consequently, liver biopsy emerges even more as crucial for accurately diagnosing MASLD, as it offers insights into the dynamic nature of the disease and aids in tailored management strategies [6, 7].

## 6.2 The Role of the Liver Biopsy

The liver biopsy, an invasive technique, is still used as a reference standard for diagnosing liver diseases, evaluating necroinflammatory activity, assessing fibrosis and monitoring hepatic architecture alterations. Its diagnostic significance is underscored by its ability to alter preclinical diagnosis and treatment plans in 36% and 58% of patients, respectively, with liver diseases. Additionally, it exhibits high diagnostic specificity in 87% of patients with elevated liver tests [8–10]. Beyond diagnosis, liver biopsy plays a crucial role in assessing prognosis and evaluating treatment efficacy in clinical trials by examining activity grades and fibrosis stages. In SLD, it also helps excluding other causes of steatosis like alcoholic liver disease and evaluating concurrent chronic liver disorders such as viral hepatitis and autoimmune liver disease [11]. The role of the liver biopsy is summarised in Table 6.1.

To ensure accurate assessment, the American Association for the Study of Liver Diseases (AASLD) recommends a liver biopsy of at least 2 cm in length, containing no fewer than 11 portal tracts [12]. Adequate evaluation of the lobular architecture requires a biopsy with a diameter, ranging between 0.8 mm and 1 mm, corresponding to a 16-Gauge needle [13]. The importance of biopsy length and the number of portal tracts was underscored by Vuppalaini et al., demonstrating

**Table 6.1** Role of the liver biopsy

| | |
|---|---|
| 1. | Detection of steatosis |
| 2. | Differentiation between steatosis and steatohepatitis based on assessment of features of cell injury, namely ballooning, and inflammation |
| 3. | Assessment of the grade of activity based on the presence of ballooning and inflammation |
| 4. | Assessment of the stage of disease by evaluating the degree of fibrosis |
| 5. | Estimation of the severity of the disease by application of a histological scoring system, evaluating the grade and stage of MASLD |
| 6. | Estimation of the course of the disease by evaluation of paired-biopsies or follow-up biopsies at different moments in order to evaluate disease progression and prognosis |
| 7. | Exclusion of other causes of steatosis/ steatohepatitis |
| 8. | Assessment of an associated chronic liver disease |
| 9. | Exclusion of malignancy, such as a hepatocellular carcinoma |

significantly higher diagnostic accuracy in MASH patients with a 25 mm long biopsy and an average of 13 portal tracts compared to a 10 mm long biopsy with fewer portal tracts (65% vs 29%) [14]. Insufficiently sized biopsies with a limited number of portal tracts poses challenges in ascertaining the disease pattern and fibrosis stage [15]. Hence, it is recommended to use a sufficiently thick needle and collect two of more samples with adequate length. For transjugular biopsies, usually using a thinner needle, optimal tissue sampling requires four passes with a 19-gauge true-cut needle [16].

Sampling error is influenced not only by the size but also by the location of the biopsy. As the degree of fibrosis and inflammation may significantly vary between the two lobes, a standardised approach with sampling of the right lobe is advised [17]. Additionally, the expertise of the pathologist plays a crucial role in the quality of the histological examination of the liver. This expertise relies on the quality of the training of the hepatopathologist and the extent of exposure to liver diagnostics [18]. Inter- and intra-observer variability, particularly in the assessment of inflammation and ballooning, remains a challenge [19, 20]. Hence, in clinical trials the assessment of liver biopsies is usually done by a panel of pathologists in consensus [21, 22].

## 6.3 Histological Features

MASLD development is driven multiple hits, including factors as obesity, insulin resistance, genetic and epigenetic factors, and alterations in the intestinal microbiome. Insulin resistance plays a key role, leading to hepatic de novo lipogenesis and impaired lipolysis in the adipose tissue with changes in inflammatory cytokines and adipokines. In the liver, lipid accumulation results in mitochondrial dysfunction, producing free oxygen radicals and initiating hepatic cell injury [23]. Histologically, the disease ranges from steatosis due to hepatic lipid accumulation, to liver cell injury, inflammation and ballooning, and fibrosis.

### 6.3.1 Steatosis

Steatosis is the histologic hallmark feature of MASLD, which is found in different phases of the disease from the begin to the end stage. Steatosis in MASLD is defined as lipid accumulation in at least 5% of the hepatocytes. This threshold has been introduced to avoid clinically irrelevant diagnoses [24]. However, steatosis may also be inconspicuous in the final stage of the disease, cirrhosis. Diagnosis in these circumstances is based on other features, such as ballooning and Mallory-Denk bodies [25].

Lipid accumulation in hepatocytes is not diagnostic for MASLD, but is also found in other chronic liver diseases, such as chronic hepatitis C genotype 3, alcoholic liver disease, autoimmune disorder and primary biliary cholangitis (PBC) [26]. The lipids in the cytoplasm organise themselves into globules, which are distinguished by their size into macrovesicular or microvesicular or an intermediate form mediovesicular, which may be intermingled with macrovesicular steatosis, the so-called macro-mediovesicular steatosis. Whereas in macrovesicular steatosis a large globule of more than 3 μm is seen in the cytoplasm of the hepatocyte, resulting in enlargement of the cell with displacement of nucleus, in microvesicular steatosis the nucleus remains centred and surrounded by a cytoplasm with numerous small globules or droplets of less than 3 μm. Microvesicular steatosis, which gives a foamy appearance to the cytoplasm, occurs either in single cells or as a small patch. This uncommon type is observed in rare diseases such as acute fatty liver of pregnancy and Reye syndrome [27]. In MASH however, its presence in approximately 10% of the biopsies points towards a more severe liver disease [28, 29] (Fig. 6.1).

The distribution of macrovesicular steatosis in adults has a zonal pattern with centralisation in the centrilobular area or zone 3, but with progression of the disease, the steatosis extends towards the periportal area or zone 1 or becomes more irregularly distributed, giving an azonal pattern or a diffuse pattern in the acinus. Azonal steatosis is associated with a higher grade of ballooning, activity and an advanced fibrosis stage, hence a more severe liver disease with a higher risk of poor outcome [30]. In the paediatric liver biopsy the distribution is opposite to the adults, as it is more situated periportally [31, 32] (Fig. 6.2).

Whereas originally the degree of steatosis was scored from 0%, the threshold is nowadays, as mentioned, 5% to define clinically relevant lipid accumulation in the liver [24, 33]. The degree of steatosis is graded into three classes, namely grade 1 from 5% up to 33%, grade 2 from 33% to 66% and finally grade 3 from 66%. This grading system is applied in the NASH/MASH Clinical Research Network (CRN) as well as Steatosis-Activity-Fibrosis (SAF) histological scoring system [24, 34]. Steatosis or steatosis with some mild inflammation is a rather benign disease, but steatohepatitis, diagnosed on the concomitant presence of ballooned hepatocytes, may progress in severity [35] (Fig. 6.3).

### 6.3.2 Inflammation

In MASLD inflammation may be present in the liver. Numerous elements contribute to the onset of hepatic inflammation, namely intrahepatic,

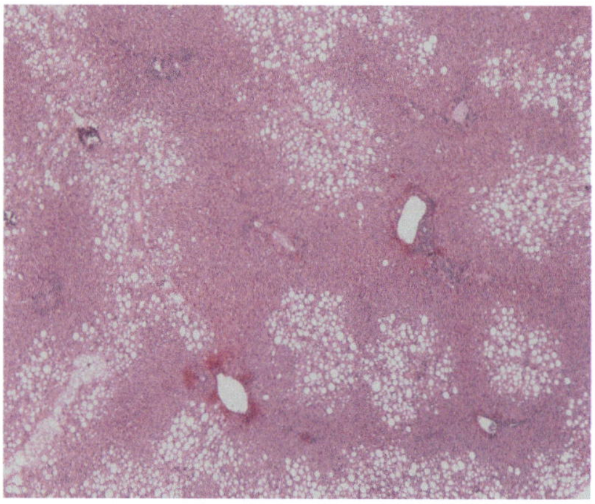

**Fig. 6.2** The liver shows a zonal pattern with steatosis around the central vein (HE, 2.5x)

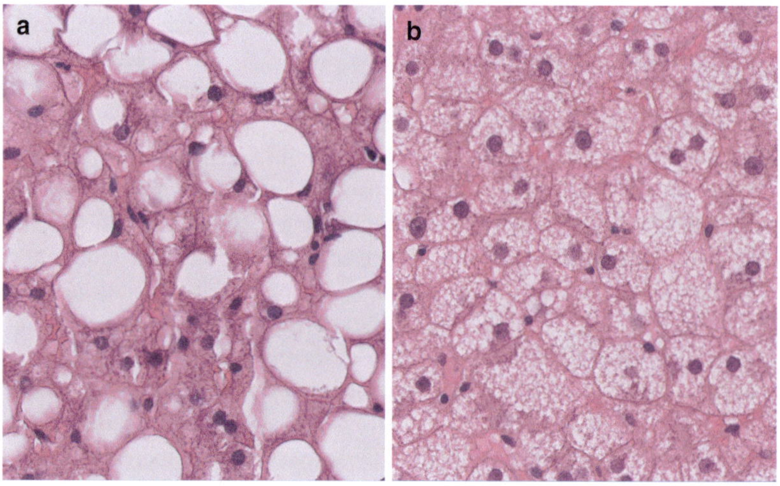


**Fig. 6.1** In macrovesicular steatosis, the nucleus relocates to the cell's periphery due to lipid accumulation (HE, 63x), whereas in microvesicular steatosis, cells display a foamy cytoplasm with the nucleus positioned centrally (HE, 63x)

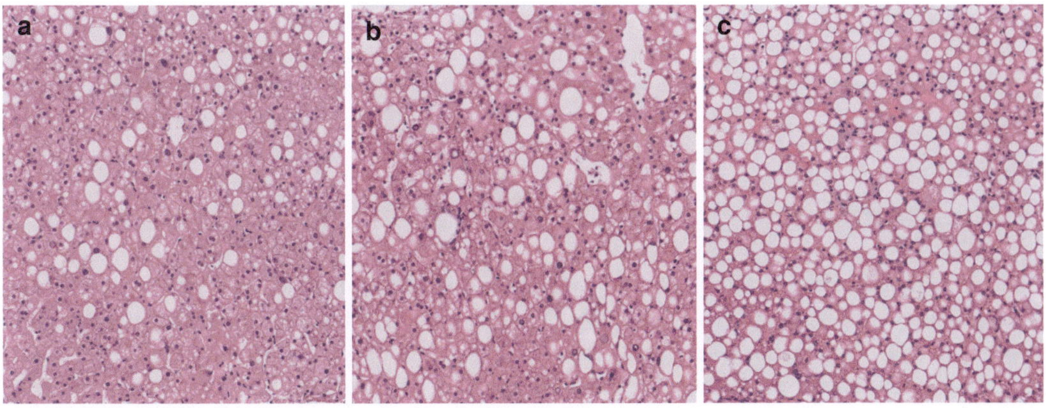


**Fig. 6.3** The steatosis grade is based on the percentage of hepatocytes, showing macrovesicular steatosis, namely: score 5–33% (A: HE, 63x), score 2 > 33–66% (B: HE, 63x) and score 3 > 67% (C: HE, 63x)

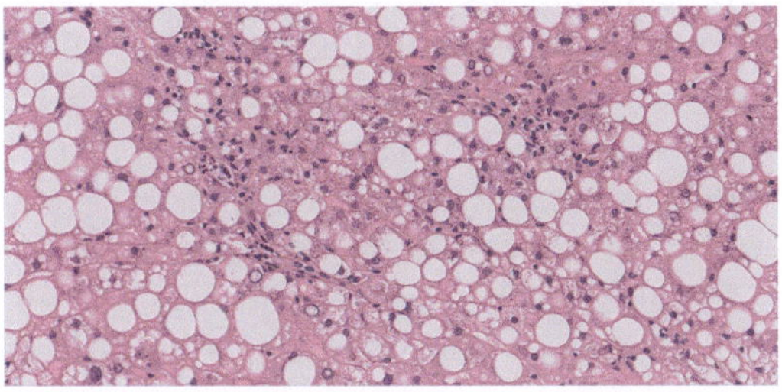

**Fig. 6.4** The steatohepatitis, observed in this liverbiopsy, is defined by the presence of steatotic hepatocytes alongside some ballooned cells interspersed with inflammatory cells (HE, 40x)

such as lipotoxicity, mitochrondrial dysfunction, endoplasmatic reticulum stress, activation of apoptotic mechanisms and autophagy, and extrahepatic, e.g. the microbiome and changes in the intestinal permeability. These factors induce a response of the innate immune system [36]. Besides activation of the resident Kupffer cells, the liver becomes infiltrated by different types of immune cells as neutrophils, lymphocytes and macrophages (Fig. 6.4).

The neutrophils, which are activated first by cell damage, are predominantly found in the portal tract. Their presence correlates with progression of the disease to MASH [37]. Likewise neutrophils, lymphocytes and macrophages are present in the portal tracts, but usually less significantly than in the liver parenchyma. An intense portal inflammation, however, is found in severe disease or in case of an associated chronic liver disease, such as viral hepatitis or autoimmune hepatitis. Although there is a relationship between the density of the portal inflammation and the severity of the disease, the infiltrate may also increase in intensity in case of therapy response, indicating resolution of the disease [38]. In contrast to biopsies of adults, portal inflammation is a characteristic inflammation pattern in the paediatric liver biopsy. In adults a more predominant lobular inflammation, situated thus in the liver parenchyma, is present.

The lobular inflammation consists mainly of mononuclear cells, T-lymphocytes, macrophages and a few plasma cells. This infiltrate is irregularly distributed either in the sinusoids or as small collections in the parenchyma. Macrophages can be organised as a microgranuloma, consisting of a small collection of histiocytic cells, or a lipogranuloma, which is composed of a histiocytic infiltrate with a lipid droplet in the centre. Neutrophils are uncommon except in case of satellitosis, in which they surround a ballooned hepatocyte, especially if the latter contains a Mallory-Denk body [39]. Satellitosis is, however, more commonly observed in alcohol-related steatohepatitis [40].

The intensity of the lobular inflammation is based on the number of collections in a microscopic field, defined by a 20x magnification. The NASH/MASH CRN network subdivides the intensity of the lobular inflammation in three grades and in the SAF scoring only two grades exist. The prevalence of lipogranulomas or microgranulomas does not influence the scoring of the intensity of the lobular inflammation [24, 34].

### 6.3.3 Ballooning

Ballooned hepatocytes are not diagnostic for MASH as they may be found in alcoholic steatohepatitis, cholestatic liver diseases, liver damage due to ischemia-reperfusion disturbances and as a feature of drug toxicity, e.g. amiodarone [41]. In MASH hepatocytic ballooning is a cardinal morphological feature in the distinction between steatosis and steatohepatitis. Ballooned hepatocytes are most commonly found in the centrilobular area or zone 3 of Rappaport in liver biopsies of adults. In a paediatric liver biopsy, however, the periportal (zone 1 of Rappaport) is mostly involved. Besides this, it is an essential feature in diagnosis of MASLD in cases of so-called cryptogenic cirrhosis (as steatosis itself is sometimes absent in these advanced stages), in the selection of patients at risk to develop fibrosis, in inclusion of these patients in trials and the evaluation of the efficacy of new drugs in clinical trials [42, 43].

However, it is an ill-defined term, on which several definitions, based on cell size, cell shape and appearance of the cytoplasm, are applied in the literature. Ballooned hepatocytes are swollen cells with an enlargement of 1.5 to 2x of the normal hepatocyte, resulting in a loss of the polygonal shape and giving a rounded appearance and a pale flocculent cytoplasm. All these morphological changes are due to an alteration of the cytoskeleton with a loss of intermediate filaments. Another cause of ballooning is hydropic swelling of endoplasmatic reticulum, as in viral hepatitis [44]. The water retention is the result of mitochondrial damage leading to dysfunction of the $Na^+/K^+$ pump [45]. Ballooned hepatocytes are frequently surrounded by tiny collagen fibres which are visualised using collagen stains such as Sirius Red or Masson trichrome [46]. Mimickers of ballooned hepatocytes are glycogen-containing hepatocytes or those with small lipid droplets, corresponding to microvesicular steatosis. In case of glycogenosis the hepatocyte has a pale cytoplasm, but in contrast to ballooned cells it retains its polygonal shape.

The detection of ballooned cells is a challenge in the routine Haematoxilin/Eosin-stain, which explains the significant inter-observer variability with a kappa-value between 0.43 and 0.66. This inter-observer variability does not only exist between general pathologists and hepatopathologists, but also between expert pathologists [45]. Hence immunohistochemistry with antibodies against CK 8 or CK18, p62, ubiquitin or sonic-hedgehog are used to highlight these cells [47, 48].

Ballooned hepatocytes may eventually contain Mallory-Denk bodies in their cytoplasm, which also stain with these previously described markers, as they are composed of cytokeratins CK8/CK18, ubiquitin and p62 (sequestosome 1). These cytoplasmic hyaline bodies were discovered by Mallory in 1911 in alcoholic liver disease and created by Denk by experimental research in mice fed with the antifungal product griseofulvin [49]. The morphology of these structures varies from cytoplasmic granules to large irregular eosinophilic structures. Mallory-bodies can be found in different conditions, where they are found in the centrilobular area as in MASLD and alcoholic liver disease, or in the periportal area as in cholestatic liver diseases such as PBC (Fig. 6.5).

Ballooned hepatocytes are evaluated to determine the grade of steatohepatitis. In the NASH/MASH CRN grading system, grading is based on the number of ballooned cells, varying between none, few and numerous, but in the SAF score is determined by the size of these cells: ballooned cells with a size comparable to a normal hepatocyte are grade 1, whereas in grade 2 these cells are twice as large as the normal hepatocyte [24, 34]. In 2022, the NASH CRN Pathology Committee introduced the "NASH extended hepatocyte ballooning score" (eB score), comprising five distinct scores. They differentiate based on their absence (0) or presence of ballooned hepatocytes, further categorised into non-classic [1] and classic [2–4] ballooned hepatocytes. A non-classic ballooned hepatocyte is a small hepatocyte with similar cytoplasmic features as the classic ballooned hepatocyte.

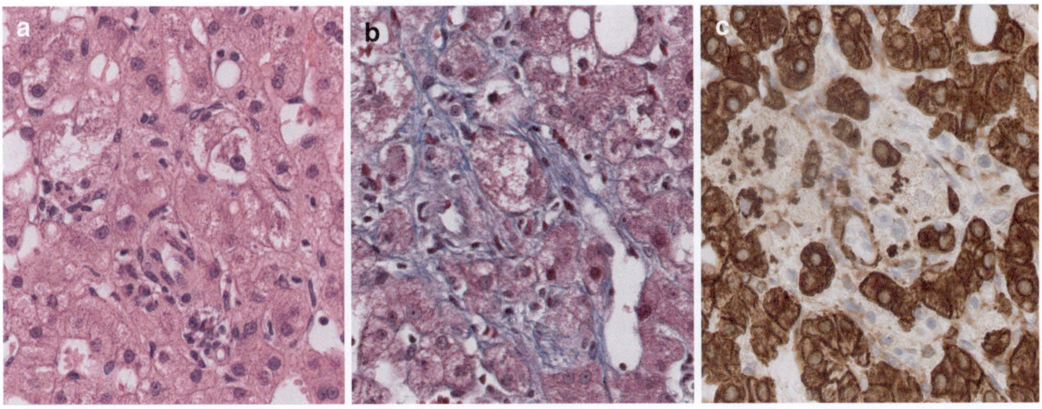


**Fig. 6.5** In the centre of the liver biopsy, one can observe some ballooned hepatocytes, distinguished by their enlarged size with a pale, flocculent cytoplasm, sometimes with the presence of a Mallory-Denk body. These cells are surrounded by some tiny collagen fibres and may be accentuated using a CK8/C18 immunohistochemical stain (A: HE, 63x; B: Masson, 63x, CK8/18 63x)

Scores 2 and 3 correspond to the previous scores 1 (few) and 2 (many, indicating foci of at least 4 classic hepatocytes). The highest score, 4, indicates visibly ballooned hepatocytes at low magnification. The eB score facilitates a more precise identification of the morphologically different ballooned hepatocytes and aligns with the stage of fibrosis [50].

### 6.3.4 Other Histological Features

In MASLD other histological features may be found in the liver, such as megamitochondria, apoptotic bodies and iron deposition.

**Megamitochondria** or giant mitochondria were for the first time described by R.V. Stewart in 1982 in association with MASLD on light microscopy: the structures, which are less common than in alcohol-related liver disease, are round or needle-shaped and randomly distributed in the hepatic lobule. Compared to normal mitochondria, giant mitochondria are ultrastructurally significant of size and are characterised by filamentous crystalline inclusions, enlarged matrix granules and irregularly arranged cristae. These ultrastructural abnormalities may be responsible for the mitochondrial dysfunction in MASLD, although the exact function of these structures remains unclear [51].

In MASH apoptotic pathways are involved, resulting in **apoptotic bodies** or Councilman bodies in the liver parenchyma [52]. The prevalence of these bodies, which are characterised by an irregular nucleus surrounded by an eosinophilic cytoplasm, correlates with the intensity of lobular inflammation and hepatic ballooning and may be used in the diagnosis of MASH [53]. Nevertheless, apoptotic bodies alone do no serve as a diagnostic marker for this condition, as they can also be present in other situations leading to cell injury, such as viral hepatitis or drug-induced liver disease [54].

Biliary epithelium cell injury and **ductular rection** can be observed in advanced MASLD with pronounced portal inflammation and interphase hepatitis, indicating an increased hepatic activity. Furthermore, in the context of MASH, ductular reaction manifests both in the periportal and centrilobular area, exhibiting a correlation with fibrosis in these areas. Research has indicated that the occurrence of ductular reaction, particularly in the centrilobular region, is associated with a more advanced stage of fibrosis [55, 56].

In MASLD **iron deposition**, which occurs in approximately a quarter of the liver biopsies, is irregularly distributed in the liver, namely hepatocytic, reticulo-endothelial or with a mixed pattern of both [57, 58]. Iron may be involved in the development of liver fibrosis through a process of ferroptosis, an iron-dependent non-apoptotic cell death related to lipid peroxidation and oxidative stress [45, 59]. Studies have shown that there is a relationship between the distribution pattern of iron deposition and liver fibrosis, in which deposition in the reticulo-endothelial cells is associated, besides fibrosis, with other histologic features such as portal inflammation and hepatocyte ballooning [58]. Moreover the study of Eder et al. has shown that not only the reticulo-endothelial pattern, but also the mixed pattern is associated with an adverse outcome of the disease [57].

### 6.3.5 Fibrosis

The necroinflammatory state in MASLD activates hepatic stellate cells, which become myofibroblasts. These cells induce hepatic fibrosis, characterised by the deposition of extracellular matrix, consisting of collagens (type I and III), glycoproteins (laminin, fibronectin) and proteoglycans (e.g. syndecan, glypican). The deposition causes disturbance of the microcirculation and alteration of the architecture of the liver parenchyma in time, with as end-stage cirrhosis.

Fibrosis occurs in different stages varying from delicate perisinusoidal fibrosis centrilobularly with a preserved angioarchitecture in steatosis, to centrilobular fibrosis eventually progressing to centro-central bridging fibrosis and portal fibrosis in steatohepatitis. In time the architecture of the liver acquires a nodular appearance, in which the noduli are surrounded by fibrous connective septa. The development of fibrosis is associated with vascular changes, such as early sinusoidal capillarisation and, later on, phlebosclerosis and neoangiogenesis [60–62]. Follow-up studies have indicated that fibrosis in MASLD may progress with at least one stage in around 40% of patients both with MASL and with MASH [63]. MASL-patients with fibrosis often manifest steatohepatitis in their second biopsy, in line with steatohepatitis being the driving force of disease progression [64]. The study of Pelusi et al. reveals similar results, in which the development of fibrosis correlates with the degree of steatosis in MASL, while in MASH ballooning and inflammation are identified as the primary determining factors [65]. Fibrosis progresses significantly slower in MASL, requiring 14 years per stage, whereas in MASH, each stage proceeds over 7 years [66]. In the final stage of cirrhosis the diagnosis of MASH is based on the presence of ballooning and Mallory bodies, as steatosis is limited or even absent. If these features are not found, a diagnosis of cryptogenic cirrhosis is made from a pathologist's perspective. This cryptogenic cirrhosis is frequently due to MASH [25, 67] and clinical criteria still allow for a presumable diagnosis of MASLD-related cirrhosis in that case [68] (Fig. 6.6).

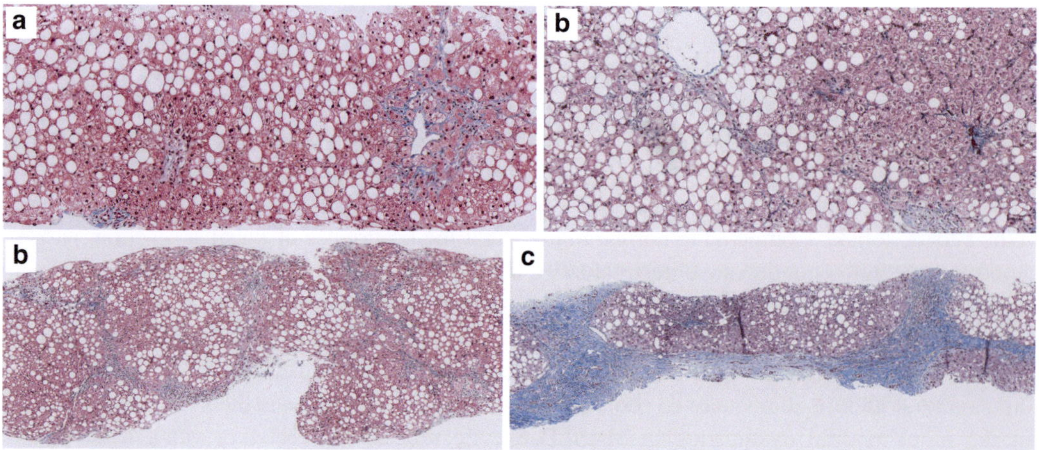


**Fig. 6.6** The stages of fibrosis is subclassified into stage 1 fibrosis restricted to the perivenular/centrilobular area, stage 2 periportal and perivenular fibrosis in periportal, stage 3 bridging fibrosis and stage 4 cirrhosis (Masson, A: 20x, B: 20x, C: 10x, D: 5x)

In contrast to the original thinking, MASLD is not a straight forward process of steatosis progressing to steatohepatitis causing fibrosis and ultimately cirrhosis. In this disease a continuous repetitive injury, in which periods of steatosis and steatohepatitis vary, may progress to different stages of fibrosis and the final stage of cirrhosis [69]. However, by changes in nutrition and diet, as well as by anti-inflammatory or antifibrogenic treatment, regression of hepatic fibrosis and even cirrhosis may occur [70, 71]. Gastric bypass surgery may induce resolution of MASH and decrease or disappearance of fibrosis even in advanced stage fibrosis [72]. The morphological features of regression of cirrhosis, a controversial issue in the past, have been for the first time described in a patient with hepatitis B by Wanless et al. in 2000. He introduced the term "human hepatic repair complex", a set of histopathological features pointing to regression of cirrhosis with decrease of fibrosis, parenchymal regeneration causing disappearance of the parenchymal nodular architecture, eventually associated with vascular changes. Regression of cirrhosis is characterised by a resorption of broad fibrous septa, which change into perforated septa. As a result the architecture of the liver changes from macronodular to micronodular to incomplete septal cirrhosis. The latter is easily missed on biopsy. The latter can also lead to clinical presentation with portal hypertension without cirrhosis on liver biopsy. The portal hypertension is in this case due to the persistence of vascular changes, such as portal tract remnants, characterised by the absence of portal veins [73, 74]. According to the Beijing classification, fibrous septa are subtyped into progressed, indefinite or regressed septa based on the degree and the cellularity of the fibrous scarring tissue. This distinction is important as progressed or indefinite septa points to active disease. The Beijing classification originally applied on biopsies of viral hepatitis patients, can also be used in other chronic liver diseases, such as MASLD [75, 76]. The exact mechanism of regression of cirrhosis in MASLD, however, is not yet exactly known.

## 6.4 Histological Scoring

Originally, MASLD was considered a disease with two distinct manifestations or histological phenotypes, in which steatosis evolved into steatohepatitis. Progressively, however, it has become clear that the disease is rather a continuum in which the severity of steatosis and steatohepatitis can vary with concomitant different degrees of activity and fibrosis, resulting during the disease course in a fluctuation and even regression of both conditions due to treatment. Therefore, the assessment of the grade of steatosis and activity as well the stage of fibrosis is an essential part of the histological examination of the liver biopsy. Various histological scoring systems are used for this purpose. The advantage of a histological scoring system is that it provides a standardised approach to assess histological features, such as steatosis, activity and fibrosis. This makes it possible to evaluate the severity of these histological abnormalities in an objective way, in addition to the more classical descriptive way. By methodological analysis of follow-up biopsies, using histological scoring systems, changes in the degree of activity and progression of fibrosis over time as well as the influence of the treatment can be evaluated [77].

Similar to the histological scoring systems, utilised in chronic liver disease, the initial histological scoring system, introduced by Brunt et al. in 1999, differentiates between "grade", indicating activity and "stage", representing fibrosis. The grade reflects the actual condition of the liver with features as steatosis, inflammation and ballooning, which are reversible due to diet and treatment. On the other hand, the stage results of the cumulative impact of the disease over time and necessitates prolonged treatment for reversal. The application of this scoring system is intended for the diagnosis of steatohepatitis in biopsies of adults [33]. Further details about this semiquantitative scoring of the features are elaborated in Table 6.2.

In 2005 a new histological scoring system, adapting some of the criteria of Brunt et al., was proposed by the pathology department of the NASH CRN [24]. This histologic scoring system

**Table 6.2** Grading and staging of the histological scoring system of Brunt, Kleiner and Bedossa, and the staging system of EPoS

| Feature | Brunt score | Kleiner score | Bedossa score | EPoS |
|---|---|---|---|---|
| **Grade** | | | | |
| Macrovesicular steatosis | 0: None | 0: < 5% | 0: < 5% | |
| | 1: < 33% | 1: 5–33% | 1: 5–33% | |
| | 2: > 33–66% | 2: > 33–66% | 2: > 33–66% | |
| | 3: > 67% | 3: > 67% | 3: > 67% | |
| Portal inflammation* | 0: No inflammation | 0: None–minimal | | |
| | 1: 0–1 | 1: Mild | | |
| | 2: 1–2 | | | |
| | 3: 1–2 | | | |
| Lobular inflammation | 0: No inflammation | 0: No inflammation | 0: No inflammation | |
| (foci number/20x) | 1: < 2 | 1: < 2 | 1: < 2 | |
| | 2: 2–4 | 2: 2–4 | 2: >2 | |
| | 3: > 4 | 3: > 4 | | |
| Ballooning | 0: Absent | 0: Absent | 0: Normal hepatocytes | |
| | 1: Mild, zone 3 | 1: Few | 1: Clusters of hepatocytes with round shape and reticulated cytoplasm | |
| | 2: Prominent, zone 3 | 2: Many | 2: Enlarged 2x size normal hepatocyte | |
| **Stage** | | | | |
| Fibrosis | 0: No fibrosis | 0: No fibrosis | 0: No fibrosis | 0: No fibrosis |
| | 1: Perivenular perisinusoidal fibrosis | 1a: Delicate perivenular fibrosis (connective tissue stain) | 1: Perivenular/ periportal perisinusoidal fibrosis | 1: Perivenular/ periportal perisinusoidal fibrosis |
| | | 1b: Dense perivenular fibrosis (H/E) | | |
| | | 1c: Portal perisinusoidal fibrosis | | |
| | 2: Perivenular and periportal fibrosis | 2: Perivenular and periportal fibrosis | 2: Perivenular and periportal fibrosis | 2: Perivenular and intralobular/ periportal fibrosis |
| | 3: Bridging fibrosis | 3: Bridging fibrosis | 3: Bridging fibrosis | 3: Bridging fibrosis with few septa (2/10 mm) |
| | | | | 4: Bridging fibrosis with many septa (> 2/10 mm) without nodules |
| | 4: Cirrhosis | 4: Cirrhosis | 4: Cirrhosis | 5: Incomplete cirrhosis with many septa with a few nodules |
| | | | | 6: Cirrhosis with numerous nodules |

*Portal inflammation not included in NAS-score or SAF-score

assesses the full spectrum of MASLD, varying from MASL to MASH. As also the portal fibrosis is analysed, this scoring system can be applied to biopsies of adults as well as children. The scoring system, which is developed to use in clinical trials, is a semiquantitative analysis of the same morphological features as in the previous scoring system. In contrast to the previous scoring system, steatosis is scored from 5% onwards in order to evaluate only clinically relevant features. The severity of the disease in this second classification is mirrored in the NAFLD/MASLD activity score (NAS, now MAS), an unweighted sum of the scores for steatosis, lobular inflammation and ballooning, varying between 0 and 8. Including steatosis in the NAS/MAS may, however, give an erroneous impression of the severity of the disease, e.g. in biopsies with mild steatohepatitis with severe steatosis or in those progressing towards cirrhosis, as in the latter the degree of steatosis may be less than 5% [39]. The study of Pai et al. found indeed that steatosis correlates poorly with disease activity [78].

Solving this issue of mixing steatosis with active disease is the main advantage of the third histological scoring system, SAF, developed by the Fatty Liver: Inhibition of Progression (FLIP) consortium [34, 79]. Similar features are assessed, namely steatosis, inflammation and ballooning, but in the SAF-score the activity is only determined by the degree of inflammation and cell injury. Despite the absence or limited occurrence of steatosis (<5%), patients with severe liver disease could still be classified as having MASH in the burned-out stage, based on the activity in their cirrhotic liver [25, 80]. More so, application of the FLIP algorithm, in which ballooning is the cardinal feature, improved the consensus between pathologists for the overall diagnosis of steatohepatitis [34, 79]. The clinical value of this scoring system has also been validated in the clinical trial of the pan-peroxisome proliferator-activated receptor (PPAR) agonist Lanifibrinor in MASH patients with as primary endpoint a two-point score decrease in the SAF-A-score and no increase of fibrosis stage [81].

In 2018 a refined fibrosis staging classification was introduced by Bedossa et al., known as the EPoS-staging (Elucidating (E) Pathways (P) of (o) Steatohepatitis (S) consortium). This reproducible 7-tiered system better represents the continuum of the fibrosis in MASH. In contrast to the situated CRN groups (F1a, b, c), mild fibrosis is one single group, in which the fibrosis may be either periportal, pericentral or perisinusoidal. The CRN stage 3, which may vary between only one septum or bridging fibrosis without nodularity in the liver biopsy, is subtyped into F3 or F4 in EPoS. Similarly, CRN F4 corresponds to EPoS F5 or F6 stage, in which the last stage is further categorised according to the Laennec system [82]. The primary objective of this new system is to enhance the accuracy and granularity of the fibrosis scoring. Notably, the EPoS system demonstrates a significant inter-observer agreement among pathologists, whether evaluating liver biopsies through a microscope (κ score 0.84) or digital pathology (κ score 0.80). However, widespread adoption among pathologists remains limited as the scoring system is currently available only as an abstract or via the atlas of histological images, published in collaboration with the European Society of Pathology [83].

## 6.5 Histopathology of Paediatric MASLD

Similar to adults there is a considerable burden of paediatric MASLD with a prevalence of nearly 35% in clinically obese children [84]. In the paediatric population three different patterns are described. Type 1 resembles the adult pattern with pericentral distribution of the macrovesicular steatosis, lobular inflammation and ballooning, and pericentral fibrosis. The type 2 pattern is opposite to the adult pattern. The macrovesicular steatosis has a zonal 1 pattern of distribution, with periportal lobular infiltration, however, without ballooning or presence of Mallory bodies. As the diagnostic feature of steatohepatitis, namely ballooning, is frequently missing for a definite diagnosis steatohepatitis, the CRN applies the term “bordeline pattern”. In parallel with the distribution of the steatosis and inflammation, fibrosis extends from the portal tracts into the liver parenchyma with sparing of the central veins. The uncommon type 3 pattern is characterised by a panacinar (diffuse) pattern of macrovesicular steatosis, and may progress from either a type 1 or 2 pattern. Paediatric MASH type 2, defined by its characteristic zonal 1 pattern, is more commonly found in young age and less mature children of Hispanic origin with a prevalence of 28%, which is in contrast to adults where only 1% of MASH patients may show this pattern. This suggests that type 2 MASH may either progress toward type 1 or disappear in time [39, 85, 86]. As in children portal inflammation is present in their liver biopsy, a new histologic score system, based on the Brunt's criteria was developed. This paediatric histologic score system, in which the degree of portal inflammation is scored along with other features, relates well with the presence of MASH in the paediatric setting [86].

## 6.6 Clinical Relevance of the Histological Features

The histological definition, grading and staging has undergone several adaptations since the terms NAFLD and NASH have been introduced. As mentioned, the concept of steatohepatitis reflects damage to hepatocytes, hepatocyte suffering and inflammation, triggering fibrogenesis. Although the dichotomy of steatohepatitis vs. no-steatohepatitis is an artificial construct not accurately reflecting the continuum of disease severity, it is a useful concept [87] to make a distinction between people who only show accumulation of lipid laden vacuoles in the hepatocytes, but little or no other lesions and with a very low likelihood of developing progressive liver disease (the vast majority of patients) vs. those with more active disease, at risk for more progressive disease and clinical outcomes (a limited number of patients).

The presence of fibrosis, currently mostly staged on a 0–4 scale as described above, implies that the mechanisms of liver damage are not completely counterbalanced by repair mechanisms [88]. Indeed, progressive liver disease is not only determined by the damage the liver suffers from, and by the forces that cause this damage, but also by the armamentarium of the liver to cope with the damaging mechanism. That concept of balance is also important to understand disease regression, as, upon resolving the cause of the disease, you do not only expect halting disease progression; by the repair mechanisms taking over and the balance being restored, you can expect regression of the lesions.

The concept is hence that steatohepatitis is the driving force of disease progression and the motor of fibrogenesis and evolution towards cirrhosis and decompensation [89]. Clinical outcome studies have shown, however, that fibrosis, and not the presence of steatohepatitis, is the strongest predictor of prognosis, not only in terms of liver-related morbidity and mortality, but also in terms of overall morbidity and mortality [90]. The latter is important, as indeed cardiovascular disease and non-hepatological malignancies are the most frequent cause of death in these patients, and several studies point towards an independent contribution of the liver disease to these extrahepatic diseases [91]. The extrahepatic complications are not driven by fibrogenesis as such, it rather indicates that fibrosis is the most accurate reflector of a longstanding active disease not adequately counterbalanced by repair mechanisms. The severity (or activity) of the steatohepatitis is probably fluctuating over time, and, in contrast to fibrosis which has a progressive staging from 0 to 4, has not that concept of progression along a scale, as was outlined before. The severity of the steatohepatitis on a liver biopsy is hence also more a snap shot observation, whereas fibrosis is more stable over time and a better reflection of the average disease activity over a certain time period. These considerations probably explain why the stage of fibrosis is a stronger predictor of prognosis than the steatohepatitis, despite the latter being the true disease driver. Nevertheless, the activity of the steatohepatitis and the fibrosis stage are correlated. As highlighted, fibrosis progression rate in patients with MASH is double the progression rate in patients with isolated steatosis [66]. And in terms of risks associated with MASLD, the odds ratios of cardiovascular events are higher in those with MASH compared to the broader group with MASLD [92]. These latter observations clearly illustrate the role of steatohepatitis in disease progression.

Accurate assessment of the fibrosis stage as well as the presence and severity of steatohepatitis is therefore an important step in disease management (Table 6.1). Given the aforementioned data, isolated steatosis is unlikely to lead to significant liver disease. Conversely, this is not considered an indication for a liver-targeted treatment [93, 94]. This does not imply that it is without meaning: it is a clear sign of whole-body metabolic dysfunction and should hence trigger an appropriate investigation and management of all metabolic syndrome features. A liver-targeted treatment, is, however, indicated in those who are clearly at risk of clinical outcomes associated to the liver disease. The current consensus is that this concerns people with steatohepatitis with some indication of the severity of the steatohepatitis and with already some fibrosis, as the latter better reflects longstanding steatohepatitis and the imbalance between tissue damage and repair.

As such, the current definition of steatohepatitis requires the presence of three cardinal features, being steatosis, lobular inflammation and ballooning [95, 96]. The people deemed at risk for clinical outcomes and hence the target population for liver-targeted therapies are those with steatohepatitis, a NAS/MAS of at least 4 (see above) and a fibrosis stage of at least 2 on the NASH/MASH and SAF 0–4 scale (Table 6.2). This population is currently considered to be "at risk" MASH [97].

It is important to repeat that when disease is in the cirrhotic stage and advances further, the features of steatosis and steatohepatitis tend to disappear [25], a condition in which the Liver Forum guidance to attribute MASH as an aetiology of cirrhosis in the absence of steatosis or steatohepatitis (one of the popular terms used is "burned-out MASH") is to be recommended [68].

Finally, the prognostic value of the individual cardinal features, as well as other features like Mallory bodies and portal inflammation are ill defined and have been discussed above. As mentioned, the latter has been linked in adults with a higher likelihood of progressive disease, but is nevertheless currently not included in the definition or severity assessment [98].

In summary, the histopathological features of MASLD have an important role, not just in diagnosis of the disease and its more severe subtype of steatohepatitis, but also in assessing disease severity. Furthermore, they harbour prognostic information and are therefore used in defining the target population for a liver-targeted treatment in people with MASH (Table 6.1).

## 6.7 Histological Endpoints of Therapy

Fibrosis is an important target for therapy. Despite MASH being the driver of disease progression, fibrosis has been shown to be the strongest predictor of adverse outcomes, both liver-related outcomes and overall mortality [90]. Liver-related events also drive morbidity and mortality in F3–4 patients [99]. These patients do not decompensate and die from the fibrosis per se, but fibrosis progression is intimately linked to the development and worsening of portal hypertension as well as the impairment of liver function, both closely associated drivers of liver-related complications. Fibrosis regression is therefore a desirable endpoint with biological plausibility in terms of efficacy of treatment, although whether it indeed translates in improved outcomes still needs to be unequivocally demonstrated.

Hence regression of fibrosis, defined as a ≥1 stage of fibrosis regression without worsening of MASH (for which several definitions exist, e.g. increase in NAS/MAS, increase in any score for the individual MASH features…) is an important endpoint and also a regulatory endpoint in Phase 3 clinical trials for non-cirrhotic MASH [70, 94]. This endpoint is used in the majority of both non-pharmacological and pharmacological intervention trials to assess their efficacy, although, as said, whether it truly translate into clinical benefit remains to be proven. It is therefore a reasonably likely but not a validated surrogate for clinical benefit. Only one study so far could link regression of fibrosis of 1 stage (in this case, as it was studied in patients with cirrhosis) with a reduced risk of liver-related events [70]. This hence requires much more study.

The definition of this endpoint only considers patients who show improvement in their fibrosis stage. However, halting disease progression might be as valuable, and absence of progression should even so be considered to capture the whole effect on fibrosis. For example, the placebo-subtracted effect size of obeticholic acid (OCA) was 15% (per protocol) for the 20 mg dose in terms of fibrosis regression, but there were also 8% less patients who progressed compared to placebo [100]. The pan-PPAR agonist lanifibranor showed a comparable picture, with 14% and 5% placebo-subtracted effect size for regression and reduced progression of fibrosis respectively [81]. A secondary analysis of the F1–2 population (so, not the F2–3 population that is used for the primary analysis) of the phase III data of the thyroid hormone receptor beta agonist resmetirom showed 33% vs. 15% fibrosis regression comparing 100 mg resmetirom vs. placebo (so, an effect size of 18% in this case), but also only 19% progressors vs. 34%, meaning a total effect size of 33% in terms of fibrosis benefit [101]. The ≥1 stage improvement in fibrosis is a high barrier endpoint. Despite numerical differences, semaglutide, a glucagon-like peptide receptor 1 agonist, although drastically reducing steatohepatitis, did not reach this endpoint, but here too, the rate of fibrosis progressors was lower on the drug compared to placebo, suggesting overall also a beneficial impact on fibrosis, albeit not powerful enough to hit the endpoint of fibrosis regression [102].

The latter brings back the concept of MASH as the driver of disease progression. Paired biopsy studies have shown that evolution in fibrosis over time correlates with evolution in disease activity over time [64]. NASH/MASH resolution was also the strongest predictor of fibrosis regression in a recent post-hoc analysis of NASH/MASH CRN trials [103] and a subanalysis of the elafibranor phase II showed changes in disease activity and changes in fibrosis evolution to be correlated [104]. Therefore, MASH resolution without worsening of fibrosis is another histology-based endpoint and a regulatory endpoint in non-cirrhotic MASH trials. The definition of resolution of MASH has also evolved over time, and is currently defined as no longer having the diagnosis of MASH, requiring the absence of ballooning but allowing for a minor degree of lobular inflammation to be present.

Lanifibranor not only regressed fibrosis but highly significantly induced MASH resolution. Also, the combined endpoint of MASH resolution and fibrosis regression, which makes sense given the intimate link between activity of the disease and the evolution of fibrosis, was tested for the first time in this phase II trial and was met [81]. Later on, this endpoint was also used for other trials. Resmetirom has shown efficacy also on both resolution of MASH and fibrosis regression in a phase III trial and is the first drug to be approved by the FDA as an anti-MASH drug. It also met the combined endpoint of MASH resolution and fibrosis regression [101].

OCA, although not significant on the MASH resolution endpoint, significantly improved the three cardinal features of MASH [81, 100]. As mentioned, the strong effect of semaglutide on MASH resolution also was accompanied by a signal of beneficially impacting fibrosis evolution over time [81]. By contrast, the dual C–C motif chemokine receptor 2 and 5 antagonist cenicriviroc showed no effect on steatohepatitis [105] and did also not add to the effect of tropifexor in a combined therapy regimen [106]. Also, other compounds without effect on MASH (e.g. simtuzumab [107] and selonsertib [108]) failed to show effect on fibrosis. All these results illustrate again the tight relationship between histological activity and fibrosis.

In summary, histological resolution of MASH and regression of fibrosis are widely used histological endpoints in the assessment of efficacy of interventions in MASH patients. These endpoints have regulatory value, but their value as surrogates for improved clinical outcomes still requires validation. They are high barrier endpoints, and a clinically meaningful benefit of more subtle improvements, e.g. absence of progression of disease, cannot be excluded.

## 6.8 Limitations of the Histological Assessment in MASLD

The liver biopsy comes with an inherent cost and risk. Performance of the liver biopsy as well as its analysis requires expertise, which has an impact on feasibility. The liver biopsy is hence not suitable as a screening tool or first-line diagnostic tool, and should be appropriately positioned in the diagnostic algorithm of patients at risk of or with a suspicion of MASH. Several algorithms are currently available and beyond the scope of this chapter.

Another issue is the inter-observer variability. Although as we discussed before, the latter is undeniably real in cross-sectional diagnosis [20], it is less relevant when it comes to comparing biopsies before and after treatment to detect a treatment effect. What matters in the latter case, is that biopsies before and after are read in the same way, which is the case in most of the recent trials. A recent re-analysis of the OCA trial confirmed previous results [109], and a re-analysis by a machine learning and artificial intelligence approach of the phase IIb study of semaglutide yielded the same conclusions and numerically roughly the same effect sizes as the primary analysis [110]. Sampling variability is also an inherent limitation of the liver biopsy, but a study with left and right lobe per-operative biopsy also showed that, regarding fibrosis, a two or more stages difference is rare [111]. Obviously, in an individual patient, this is still relevant, in intervention trials this can be overcome by appropriate sample sizes. Liver histology hence remains a crucial tool in the accurate diagnosis and staging of MASLD, as well as in the assessment of the efficacy of treatment intervention (Table 6.1). Although the place of the liver biopsy in diagnostic assessment in routine clinical practice is rather well-defined based on algorithms, its place in follow-up outside the setting of interventional trails is ill-defined and depending on local expertise and protocols.

Can the liver biopsy be replaced by non-invasive tests (NIT)? Liver steatosis can be diagnosed and quantified adequately by magnetic resonance-based imaging techniques. Diagnosis of moderate and severe steatosis is also quite accurate, but not mild steatosis. Liver stiffness measurements correlate cross-sectionally with the fibrosis stage, but with large overlap [112]. The same holds true for blood-based fibrosis tests and scores. All these tests can be used to rule-in or rule-out a certain stage of fibrosis, but not as an accurate predictor of the actual fibrosis stage. There is still no reliable test to diagnose MASH, although a few tests seem to have acceptable accuracy to diagnose at risk MASH [113, 114]. As well as the biopsy comes with the issue of sampling variability, NITs come with a non-neglectable coefficient of variability, hampering the interpretation of pre-post treatment differences (e.g. 31% of the patients on placebo in the pegbelfermin trial of patients with NASH and F3 had ≥15% relative reduction in liver stiffness measured by MRE despite the absence of significant metabolic improvement) [115]. Also, we need to better understand how changes in NIT over time correlate with changes in histology or long-term outcomes (there is a paucity of data on this highly relevant question [116]), and what magnitude of change is clinically meaningful and can be defined as a surrogate endpoint. For all these items, we refer to the appropriate chapters.

## 6.9 Differential Diagnosis of Steatohepatitis

### 6.9.1 Alcohol-Related Liver Disease

Steatohepatitis is not diagnostic for MASLD. One major differential diagnosis is alcohol-related liver disease (ALD), which is a major global health problem. Its risk depends on the amount of alcohol consumption: drinking more than five glasses a day increases the risk of liver cirrhosis in men (5–6 drinks: RR 3.80, 95% CI: 0.85–17.02, ≥7 drinks RR 6.93, 95% CI: 1.07–44.99) and even more in women (5–6 drinks: RR 12.44, 95% CI: 6.65–23.27, ≥7 drinks: RR 24.58, 95% CI: 14.77–40.90) [117]. ALD encompasses a range of conditions, including steatosis, steatohepatitis, steatotic liver with cholestasis, and cirrhosis. Within 5–10 years, around 30% advance to alcohol-related hepatitis, while approximately 15% develop cirrhosis [118]. ALD disease resembles MASLD histologically but there are some clues that are more characteristic for ALD (Table 6.3), e.g. the preponderance of the degree of macrovesicular steatosis, the degree of ballooning and the number of Mallory-Denk bodies, the neutrophilic inflammation in the portal as well as lobular area, where they often encircle the ballooned hepatocytes in large numbers (known as "neutrophilic satellitosis"). Characteristically there is pronounced pericellular fibrosis, resulting in the typical chicken-wire pattern as well as the perivenular fibrosis and phlebosclerosis, occasionally accompanied by sclerosing hyaline necrosis and obliterative fibrosis. Foamy degeneration is diagnostically significant but is infrequently observed in ALD [40, 119–121].

For patients vulnerable to liver decompensation secondary to alcohol, a liver biopsy may be performed. Its purpose is not primarily to confirm the diagnosis, but rather to assess the severity of the activity of the alcohol-related hepatitis. This evaluation is particularly important as corticosteroid treatment may be applied in case of significant activity. The activity can be assessed using histological scoring systems, as the validated alcohol-related hepatitis scoring system and the Salve grade, both having a prognostic significance [122, 123] (Fig. 6.7).

**Table 6.3** Characteristic histologic features of NASH versus ASH

| | NASH | ASH |
|---|---|---|
| Macrovesicular steatosis | ++ | + |
| Microvesicular steatosis | –/+ | +/– |
| Foamy degeneration | – | + |
| Ballooning | + | ++ |
| Mallory-bodies | +/– | ++ |
| Lobular inflammation | + | ++ |
| Portal neutrophilic inflammation | –/+ | ++ |
| Ductular reaction | –/+ | + |
| Neutrophilic infiltration | + | ++ |
| Neutrophilic satellitosis | – | ++ |
| Perivenular hyaline sclerosis | –/+ | + |
| Phlebosclerosis | –/+ | + |
| Pericellular fibrosis | – | ++ |
| Periportal fibrosis | +/– | +/++ |
| Cholestasis | +/– | + |
| Giant mitochondria | + | ++ |
| Glycogen nuclei | ++ | + |
| Lipogranuloma | + | +/– |
| Iron deposition | –/+ | +/– |

– Absent; –/+ Uncommon; +/– Variable; + Common; ++ Frequent

### 6.9.2 Wilson's Disease and Other Genetic Diseases

Wilson's disease, initially described by the British neurologist Samuel Alexander Kinnier Wilson in 1912, is an autosomal recessive disorder with genetic mutations within the ATP7B gene. This gene encodes a transmembrane copper transporting ATPase, resulting in copper accumulation in organs as the liver and the brain. Although relatively rare, with a prevalence of 1 in 30,000 individuals, certain regions exhibit higher incidence, often linked to familial occurrences due to consanguinity, as in Sardinia [124].

The histological spectrum varies significantly from minimal changes, chronic hepatitis (resembling viral hepatitis or autoimmune hepatitis), to steatosis or steatohepatitis. Hence Wilson's disease is a mimicker of MASLD as it presents with macrovesicular steatosis with a variable portal/lobular lymphocytic infiltrate, lipogranulomas and ballooning. Glycogenated nuclei, characterised by their pale appearance, are focally seen. However, while rhodanine stain or rubeanic acid stains may reveal copper deposits in the liver cells, such findings lack specificity for Wilson's disease, as they are also observed in cholestatic liver diseases, ALD and PBC. Disease progression may lead to fibrotic changes and eventual development of liver cirrhosis [125, 126].

In addition to Wilson's disease there exists other genetic conditions, where the liver manifests steatohepatitis, such as α1-antitrypsin deficiency (A1AT). This uncommon disorder, originating from mutations in the Serpina1 gene (chromosome 14), exhibits with different variants, the Pi*ZZ variant being the most severe. Patients often develop emphysema and severe liver disease,

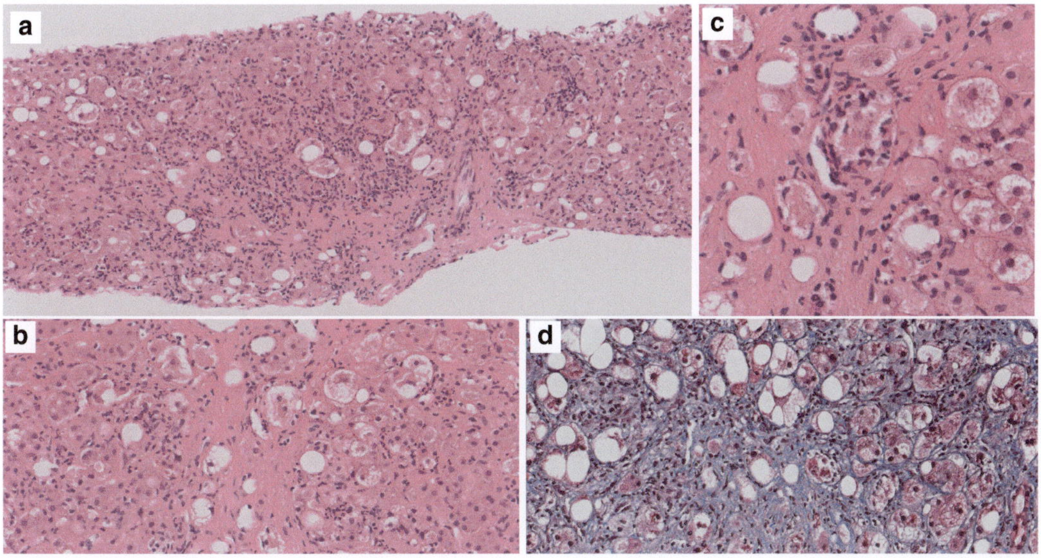


**Fig. 6.7** Acute alcoholic hepatitis in a fibrotic liver, characterised by a polymorphonuclear infiltrate, interspersed between the ballooned hepatocytes containing Mallory-Denk bodies (MB) (A: HE, 20x). Higher magnification of numerous MB containing ballooned hepatocytes and neutrophils (B: HE, 40x). In neutrophilic sattelitosis a ballooned hepatocyte with an MB is encircled by several neutrophils (C: HE, 63x). Alcoholic liver disease exhibits pericellular fibrosis as a predominant pattern of fibrosis (D: HE, 40x)

which may progress to cirrhosis. A distinguishing feature is the zone 1 localisation of the steatosis, unlike in adult MASLD, and the presence of eosinophilic globules in the periportal hepatocytes. These globules, which represent dilated endoplasmatic reticulum membranes engorged with polymerised AAT mutant Z protein, can be identified on a Periodic Acid-Schiff stain and with immunohistochemistry [127–129] (Fig. 6.8).

The cholesterol ester storage disease is a rare genetic disorder, with a prevalence ranging from 1/40,000 to 1/300,000, caused by mutation in the Lysosomal Acid Lipase Gene (LIPA Gene). This gene encodes the enzyme lysosomal acid lipase (LAL), which plays a vital role in the breakdown of cholesterol esters and triglycerides within lysosomes. The disease, caused by a reduced enzyme activity, manifests itself usually at an age of 5 years, but rarely also only in adulthood. These children develop liver disease with diffuse microvesicular steatosis, due to accumulation of lipids in the hepatocytes. As mimicker of MASLD it has some distinctive features: pigmented macrophages are dispersed in the portal tracts and in between the steatotic hepatocytes. Additionally fibrosis exhibits a portal-portal distribution, eventually progressing to cirrhosis. Patients are treated with enzyme substitution. In Wolman's disease, a variant of cholesterol ester storage disease, there is a complete absence of the enzyme. The disease presents at neonatal age and is fatal due to multi-organ failure [130–132].

### 6.9.3 Drug-Related Steatosis and Steatohepatitis

Diagnosis of drug-induced liver injury (DILI) through biopsy poses a significant challenge for pathologists due to its diverse histological presentations, often necessitating a nuanced differential diagnosis from other hepatic diseases. One such manifestation is steatosis or steatohepatitis, mimicking MASLD. These hepatic histological alterations arise from a dual impact: the toxic effects of drugs inducing a mitochondrial dysfunction and the secondary metabolic dysfunction occurring in obese patients [133, 134]. A study of Kleiner et al. showed that steatosis is a prevalent feature of DILI patients with an unfavourable outcome

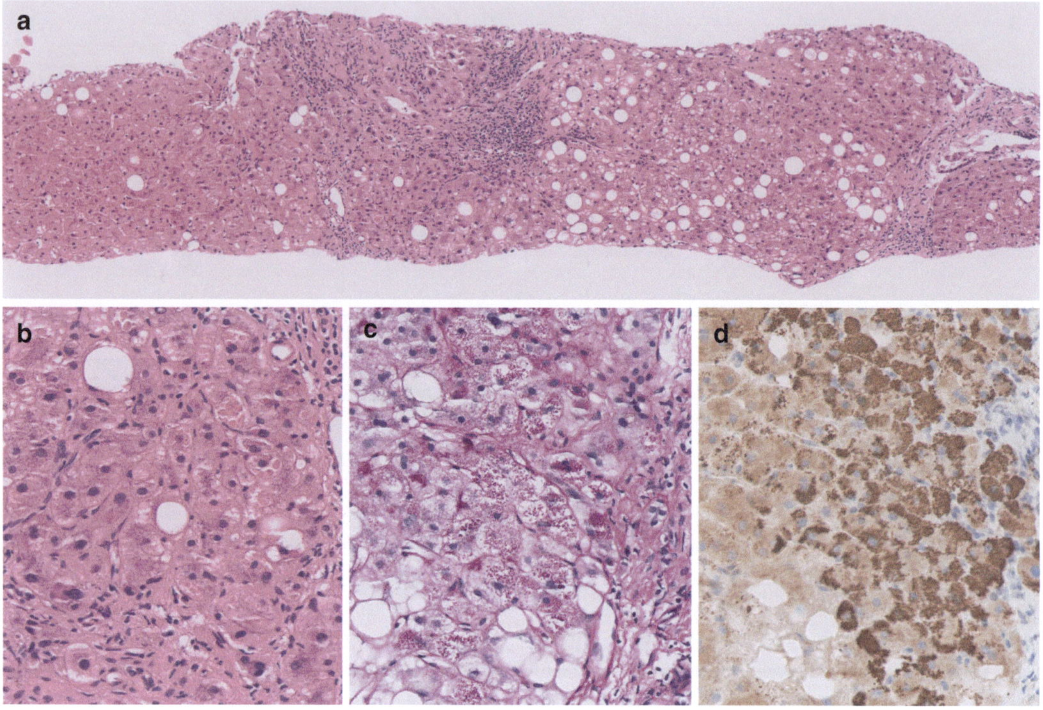


**Fig. 6.8** Fibrotic liver with a steatohepatitis in a patient with an α1-antitrypsin deficiency. Within the cytoplasm of the periportal hepatocytes are eosinophilic globules present, which can be highlighted using a PAS-diastase and immunohistochemical staining techniques (A: HE 5x, B: HE 40x, C: PAS-diastase 40x, D: immunohistochemistry 40x)

accounting for 64% ($n$ = 134/208) of cases, exhibiting different patterns: macrovesicular (72%, $n$ = 96/134), microvesicular (14%, $n$ = 19) and mixed pattern of steatosis (14%, $n$ = 19). Microvesicular steatosis is frequently linked with severe or fatal liver injury, often resulting in fatal outcomes [135]. Despite sharing similarities with MASH, certain DILI display distinctive features: for instance amiodarone is associated with microvesicular steatosis and prominently ballooned hepatocytes containing numerous Mallory bodies. Allende et al. have provided a comprehensive table delineating the relationship between drugs and their histological presentations [136].

## 6.10 Artificial Intelligence in MASLD Histopathology

Artificial intelligence (AI), utilising numerical algorithms, aims to replicate human intelligence. Machine learning, a subset of AI, enables computers to discern patterns from datasets and make decisions autonomously. Tasks in machine learning are categorised into supervised, unsupervised, and reinforcement learning, each serving distinct purposes. AI in medicine is on the rise, including in pathology. Application of artificial intelligence is of paramount interest in MASLD. Whole Slide Imaging (WSI) and supervised machine learning with annotations by expert pathologists are utilised to better identify and quantify histological features such as steatosis, inflammation, hepatocyte ballooning and fibrosis [137, 138]. The utilisation of a training atlas to identify ballooned hepatocytes could enhance the quality of annotations made by pathologists, especially considering the lack of consensus even among expert pathologists [20]. This helps to address the issue of inter-observer variation among pathologists by accurately grading and staging of liver biopsies and contributes to early detection of disease. Moreover they can also provide ongoing metrics to monitor therapy-related changes [139, 140]. As a result, artificial-assisted digital pathology tools are increasingly utilised in clinical trials to assess the impact of drug therapy on histological endpoints like regression of liver fibrosis. These tools can even reveal effects that conventional histology may fail to detect emphasising their importance in clinical trials [106, 110, 141].

## 6.11 New Technologies

Efforts to go beyond standard reading of the biopsy by the pathologist have focused on unique imaging methodologies on the one hand, and machine-learning approaches to enhance the precision and reproducibility of results on the other hand.

Machine-learning-approaches, starting from a large number of annotated histological sections, have been used to identify key features such as steatosis, ballooning, inflammation and fibrosis and are used for quantification or to produce an equivalent of the conventional scoring systems [142]. This approach was first of all able to diagnose steatohepatitis comparably to pathologists, and fibrosis scores also correlated well with conventional staging. This is, as mentioned, a way that can help standardising diagnosis and avoid inter-observer variability (although it obviously doesn't chance the issue of sampling variability). It also allows reading large numbers of slides in a short time frame. Also, re-analysis of trials with machine learning approaches, although revealing differences in cross-sectional read between the trial pathologist (1–3 pathologists with different approaches in terms of consensus reaching vs. the machine learning approach), the effect sizes (active treatment vs. placebo) by both approaches are almost identical [106, 140]. This illustrates that in that setting the most important point is that pre- and post-treatment biopsies are read in exactly the same way, and hence previous results are valid and solid.

Innovative imaging approaches include second-harmonic generated images from unstained paraffin-embedded sections to measure several aspects of fibrosis, resulting in quantifiable collagen fibrillar parameters (qFP) or in a continuous fibrosis staging system [143]. Meanwhile this has been commercialised. A qFP-based score for fibrosis, with zone-specific differentiation, has been applied to various independent cohorts of MASH patients with interesting results [144]. Additional parameters include septal areas, septal width and septal cellularity. Such a granular approach assessing various features of fibrosis beyond conventional scoring allows to detect subtle changes that otherwise remain unnoticed, as we could demonstrate in the trial with the non-steroidal FXR agonist tropifexor [145].

**Disclosures** SF holds a senior clinical investigator fellowship from the Research Foundation Flanders (FWO) (1,802,154 N). His institution has received grants from Astellas, Falk Pharma, Genfit, Gilead Sciences, GlympsBio, Janssens Pharmaceutica, Inventiva, Merck Sharp & Dome, Pfizer, Roche. He has acted as consultant for Abbvie, Actelion, Aelin Therapeutics, AgomAb, Aligos Therapeutics, Allergan, Alnylam, Astellas, Astra Zeneca, Bayer, Boehringer Ingelheim, Bristoll-Meyers Squibb, CSL Behring, Coherus, Echosens, Dr. Falk Pharma, Eisai, Enyo, Galapagos, Galmed, Genetech, Genfit, Genflow Biosciences, Gilead Sciences, Intercept, Inventiva, Janssens Pharmaceutica, PRO.MED.CS Praha, Julius Clinical, Madrigal, Medimmune, Merck Sharp & Dome, Mursla Bio, NGM Bio, Novartis, Novo Nordisk, Promethera, Roche, Siemens Healthineers. SF has been lecturer for Abbvie, Allergan, Bayer, Eisai, Genfit, Gilead Sciences, Janssens Cilag, Intercept, Inventiva, Merck Sharp & Dome, Novo Nordisk, Promethera, Siemens.

AD No disclosures.

## References

1. Ayonrinde OT. Historical narrative from fatty liver in the nineteenth century to contemporary NAFLD - reconciling the present with the past. JHEP Rep. 2021;3(3):100261.
2. Ludwig J, Viggiano TR, McGill DB, Oh BJ. Nonalcoholic steatohepatitis: Mayo Clinic experiences with a hitherto unnamed disease. Mayo Clin Proc. 1980;55(7):434–8.
3. Haas JT, Francque S, Staels B. Pathophysiology and mechanisms of nonalcoholic fatty liver disease. Annu Rev Physiol. 2016;78:181–205.
4. Rinella ME, Lazarus JV, Ratziu V, Francque SM, Sanyal AJ, Kanwal F, et al. A multisociety Delphi consensus statement on new fatty liver disease nomenclature. J Hepatol. 2023;79(6):1542–56.

5. Lee BP, Dodge JL, Terrault NA. National prevalence estimates for steatotic liver disease and subclassifications using consensus nomenclature. Hepatology. 2024;79(3):666–73.
6. Eslam M, Sanyal AJ, George J, International Consensus P. MAFLD: a consensus-driven proposed nomenclature for metabolic associated fatty liver disease. Gastroenterology. 2020;158(7):1999–2014 e1.
7. Itoh S, Yougel T, Kawagoe K. Comparison between nonalcoholic steatohepatitis and alcoholic hepatitis. Am J Gastroenterol. 1987;82(7):650–4.
8. Khalifa A, Rockey DC. The utility of liver biopsy in 2020. Curr Opin Gastroenterol. 2020;36(3):184–91.
9. Khalifa A, Rockey DC. The value of liver biopsy and histology in liver disease diagnosis and patient care-a pragmatic prospective clinical practice study. J Clin Gastroenterol. 2023;58:912.
10. Seth S, Forrest EH, Morris JM, Heydtmann M, Konanahalli P, Kohnen G, Oien KA. Audit of medical (non-targeted) liver biopsy specimen quality, pathology reporting and effect on patient management. J Clin Pathol. 2022;75(7):498–502.
11. Brunt EM, Kleiner DE, Carpenter DH, Rinella M, Harrison SA, Loomba R, et al. NAFLD: reporting histologic findings in clinical practice. Hepatology. 2021;73(5):2028–38.
12. Rockey DC, Caldwell SH, Goodman ZD, Nelson RC, Smith AD. Liver biopsy. Hepatology. 2009;49(3):1017–44.
13. Palmer T, Georgiades I, Treanor D, Wright A, Shah M, Khosla R, Wyatt JI. Improved tissue sections for medical liver biopsies: a comparison of 16 vs 18 g biopsy needles using digital pathology. J Clin Pathol. 2014;67(5):415–9.
14. Vuppalanchi R, Unalp A, Van Natta ML, Cummings OW, Sandrasegaran KE, Hameed T, et al. Effects of liver biopsy sample length and number of readings on sampling variability in nonalcoholic fatty liver disease. Clin Gastroenterol Hepatol. 2009;7(4):481–6.
15. Scheuer PJ. Liver biopsy size matters in chronic hepatitis: bigger is better. Hepatology. 2003;38(6):1356–8.
16. Vibhakorn S, Cholongitas E, Kalambokis G, Manousou P, Quaglia A, Marelli L, et al. A comparison of four- versus three-pass transjugular biopsy using a 19-G Tru-cut needle and a randomized study using a cassette to prevent biopsy fragmentation. Cardiovasc Intervent Radiol. 2009;32(3):508–13.
17. Sumida Y, Nakajima A, Itoh Y. Limitations of liver biopsy and non-invasive diagnostic tests for the diagnosis of nonalcoholic fatty liver disease/nonalcoholic steatohepatitis. World J Gastroenterol. 2014;20(2):475–85.
18. Rousselet MC, Michalak S, Dupré F, Croué A, Bedossa P, Saint-André JP, Calès P. Sources of variability in histological scoring of chronic viral hepatitis. Hepatology. 2005;41(2):257–64.
19. Younossi ZM, Gramlich T, Liu YC, Matteoni C, Petrelli M, Goldblum J, et al. Nonalcoholic fatty liver disease: assessment of variability in pathologic interpretations. Mod Pathol. 1998;11(6):560–5.
20. Brunt EM, Clouston AD, Goodman Z, Guy C, Kleiner DE, Lackner C, et al. Complexity of ballooned hepatocyte feature recognition: defining a training atlas for artificial intelligence-based imaging in NAFLD. J Hepatol. 2022;76(5):1030–41.
21. Sanyal AJ, Loomba R, Anstee QM, Ratziu V, Kowdley KV, Rinella ME, et al. Utility of pathologist panels for achieving consensus in NASH histologic scoring in clinical trials: data from a phase 3 study. Hepatol Commun. 2024;8(1):e0325.
22. Goodman ZD. Role of liver biopsy in clinical trials and clinical Management of Nonalcoholic Fatty Liver Disease. Clin Liver Dis. 2023;27(2):353–62.
23. Buzzetti E, Pinzani M, Tsochatzis EA. The multiple-hit pathogenesis of non-alcoholic fatty liver disease (NAFLD). Metabolism. 2016;65(8):1038–48.
24. Kleiner DE, Brunt EM, Van Natta M, Behling C, Contos MJ, Cummings OW, et al. Design and validation of a histological scoring system for nonalcoholic fatty liver disease. Hepatology. 2005;41(6):1313–21.
25. Caldwell SH, Lee VD, Kleiner DE, Al-Osaimi AM, Argo CK, Northup PG, Berg CL. NASH and cryptogenic cirrhosis: a histological analysis. Ann Hepatol. 2009;8(4):346–52.
26. Brunt EM, Ramrakhiani S, Cordes BG, Neuschwander-Tetri BA, Janney CG, Bacon BR, Di Bisceglie AM. Concurrence of histologic features of steatohepatitis with other forms of chronic liver disease. Mod Pathol. 2003;16(1):49–56.
27. Burt AD, Mutton A, Day CP. Diagnosis and interpretation of steatosis and steatohepatitis. Semin Diagn Pathol. 1998;15(4):246–58.
28. Tandra S, Yeh MM, Brunt EM, Vuppalanchi R, Cummings OW, Ünalp-Arida A, et al. Presence and significance of microvesicular steatosis in nonalcoholic fatty liver disease. J Hepatol. 2011;55(3):654–9.
29. Germano CW, Mega PF, Mattosinho T, Dias LLC, Gestic MA, Utrini MP, et al. Microvesicular steatosis in individuals with obesity: a histological marker of non-alcoholic fatty liver disease severity. Obes Surg. 2023;33(3):813–20.
30. Tong XF, Zhao XY, Sun YM, Shi YW, Li M, Wu XN, et al. Azonal steatosis correlates with disease severity and poor outcome of nonalcoholic fatty liver disease. J Dig Dis. 2023;24(1):28–38.
31. Chalasani N, Wilson L, Kleiner DE, Cummings OW, Brunt EM, Unalp A, Network NCR. Relationship of steatosis grade and zonal location to histological features of steatohepatitis in adult patients with non-alcoholic fatty liver disease. J Hepatol. 2008;48(5):829–34.
32. Schwimmer JB, Behling C, Newbury R, Deutsch R, Nievergelt C, Schork NJ, Lavine JE. Histopathology of pediatric nonalcoholic fatty liver disease. Hepatology. 2005;42(3):641–9.
33. Brunt EM, Janney CG, Di Bisceglie AM, Neuschwander-Tetri BA, Bacon BR. Nonalcoholic steatohepatitis: a proposal for grading and stag-

ing the histological lesions. Am J Gastroenterol. 1999;94(9):2467–74.
34. Bedossa P, Poitou C, Veyrie N, Bouillot JL, Basdevant A, Paradis V, et al. Histopathological algorithm and scoring system for evaluation of liver lesions in morbidly obese patients. Hepatology. 2012;56(5):1751–9.
35. Torres DM, Williams CD, Harrison SA. Features, diagnosis, and treatment of nonalcoholic fatty liver disease. Clin Gastroenterol Hepatol. 2012;10(8):837–58.
36. Lee YA, Friedman SL. Inflammatory and fibrotic mechanisms in NAFLD-implications for new treatment strategies. J Intern Med. 2022;291(1):11–31.
37. Gadd VL, Skoien R, Powell EE, Fagan KJ, Winterford C, Horsfall L, et al. The portal inflammatory infiltrate and ductular reaction in human nonalcoholic fatty liver disease. Hepatology. 2014;59(4):1393–405.
38. Yeh MM, Brunt EM. Pathological features of fatty liver disease. Gastroenterology. 2014;147(4):754–64.
39. Kleiner DE, Makhlouf HR. Histology of nonalcoholic fatty liver disease and nonalcoholic steatohepatitis in adults and children. Clin Liver Dis. 2016;20(2):293–312.
40. Tannapfel A, Denk H, Dienes HP, Langner C, Schirmacher P, Trauner M, Flott-Rahmel B. Histopathological diagnosis of non-alcoholic and alcoholic fatty liver disease. Grade 2 consensus-based guidelines. Pathologe. 2010;31(3):225–37.
41. Lackner C. Hepatocellular ballooning in nonalcoholic steatohepatitis: the pathologist's perspective. Expert Rev Gastroenterol Hepatol. 2011;5(2):223–31.
42. Caldwell S, Lackner C. Perspectives on NASH histology: cellular ballooning. Ann Hepatol. 2017;16(2):182–4.
43. Matteoni CA, Younossi ZM, Gramlich T, Boparai N, Liu YC, McCullough AJ. Nonalcoholic fatty liver disease: a spectrum of clinical and pathological severity. Gastroenterology. 1999;116(6):1413–9.
44. Caldwell SH, Redick JA, Chang CY, Davis CA, Argo CK, Al Osaimi KA. Enlarged hepatocytes in NAFLD examined with osmium fixation: does microsteatosis underlie cellular ballooning in NASH? Am J Gastroenterol. 2006;101(7):1677–8.
45. Li YY, Zheng TL, Xiao SY, Wang P, Yang WJ, Jiang LL, et al. Hepatocytic ballooning in non-alcoholic steatohepatitis: dilemmas and future directions. Liver Int. 2023;43(6):1170–82.
46. Burt AD, Lackner C, Tiniakos DG. Diagnosis and assessment of NAFLD: definitions and histopathological classification. Semin Liver Dis. 2015;35(3):207–20.
47. Lackner C, Gogg-Kamerer M, Zatloukal K, Stumptner C, Brunt EM, Denk H. Ballooned hepatocytes in steatohepatitis: the value of keratin immunohistochemistry for diagnosis. J Hepatol. 2008;48(5):821–8.
48. Estep M, Mehta R, Bratthauer G, Alaparthi L, Monge F, Ali S, et al. Hepatic sonic hedgehog protein expression measured by computer assisted morphometry significantly correlates with features of non-alcoholic steatohepatitis. BMC Gastroenterol. 2019;19(1):27.
49. Zatloukal K, French SW, Stumptner C, Strnad P, Harada M, Toivola DM, et al. From Mallory to Mallory-Denk bodies: what, how and why? Exp Cell Res. 2007;313(10):2033–49.
50. Gill RM, Allende D, Belt PH, Behling CA, Cummings OW, Guy CD, et al. The nonalcoholic steatohepatitis extended hepatocyte ballooning score: histologic classification and clinical significance. Hepatol Commun. 2023;7(2):e0033.
51. Shami GJ, Cheng D, Verhaegh P, Koek G, Wisse E, Braet F. Three-dimensional ultrastructure of giant mitochondria in human non-alcoholic fatty liver disease. Sci Rep. 2021;11(1):3319.
52. Lee K, Jung ES, Yu E, Kang YK, Cho MY, Kim JM, et al. A scoring system for the diagnosis of non-alcoholic steatohepatitis from liver biopsy. J Pathol Transl Med. 2020;54(3):228–36.
53. Klion FM, Schaffner F. The ultrastructure of acidophilic "councilman-like" bodies in the liver. Am J Pathol. 1966;48(5):755–67.
54. Yeh MM, Belt P, Brunt EM, Kowdley KV, Wilson LA, Ferrell L. Acidophil bodies in nonalcoholic steatohepatitis. Hum Pathol. 2016;52:28–37.
55. Dhingra S, Mahadik JD, Tarabishy Y, May SB, Vierling JM. Prevalence and clinical significance of portal inflammation, portal plasma cells, interface hepatitis and biliary injury in liver biopsies from patients with non-alcoholic steatohepatitis. Pathology. 2022;54(6):686–93.
56. He YH, Pan JX, Xu LM, Gu T, Chen YW. Ductular reaction in non-alcoholic fatty liver disease: when Macbeth is perverted. World J Hepatol. 2023;15(6):725–40.
57. Eder SK, Feldman A, Strebinger G, Kemnitz J, Zandanell S, Niederseer D, et al. Mesenchymal iron deposition is associated with adverse long-term outcome in non-alcoholic fatty liver disease. Liver Int. 2020;40(8):1872–82.
58. Nelson JE, Wilson L, Brunt EM, Yeh MM, Kleiner DE, Unalp-Arida A, Kowdley KV. Relationship between the pattern of hepatic iron deposition and histological severity in nonalcoholic fatty liver disease. Hepatology. 2011;53(2):448–57.
59. Peleman C, Francque S, Berghe TV. Emerging role of ferroptosis in metabolic dysfunction-associated steatotic liver disease: revisiting hepatic lipid peroxidation. EBioMedicine. 2024;102:105088.
60. Velliou RI, Legaki AI, Nikolakopoulou P, Vlachogiannis NI, Chatzigeorgiou A. Liver endothelial cells in NAFLD and transition to NASH and HCC. Cell Mol Life Sci. 2023;80(11):314.
61. Coulon S, Heindryckx F, Geerts A, Van Steenkiste C, Colle I, Van Vlierberghe H. Angiogenesis in

chronic liver disease and its complications. Liver Int. 2011;31(2):146–62.
62. Hano H, Takasaki S, Kobayashi H, Koyama T, Lu T, Nagatsuma K. In the non-cirrhotic stage of non-alcoholic steatohepatitis, angioarchitecture of portal veins and lobular architecture are maintained. Virchows Arch. 2013;462(5):533–40.
63. McPherson S, Hardy T, Henderson E, Burt AD, Day CP, Anstee QM. Evidence of NAFLD progression from steatosis to fibrosing-steatohepatitis using paired biopsies: implications for prognosis and clinical management. J Hepatol. 2015;62(5):1148–55.
64. Kleiner DE, Brunt EM, Wilson LA, Behling C, Guy C, Contos M, et al. Association of Histologic Disease Activity with Progression of nonalcoholic fatty liver disease. JAMA Netw Open. 2019;2(10):e1912565.
65. Pelusi S, Cespiati A, Rametta R, Pennisi G, Mannisto V, Rosso C, et al. Prevalence and risk factors of significant fibrosis in patients with nonalcoholic fatty liver without steatohepatitis. Clin Gastroenterol Hepatol. 2019;17(11):2310–9.e6.
66. Singh S, Allen AM, Wang Z, Prokop LJ, Murad MH, Loomba R. Fibrosis progression in nonalcoholic fatty liver vs nonalcoholic steatohepatitis: a systematic review and meta-analysis of paired-biopsy studies. Clin Gastroenterol Hepatol. 2015;13(4):643–54.e1–9.
67. Skelly MM, James PD, Ryder SD. Findings on liver biopsy to investigate abnormal liver function tests in the absence of diagnostic serology. J Hepatol. 2001;35(2):195–9.
68. Noureddin M, Chan JL, Barradas K, Dimick-Santos L, Schabel E, Omokaro SO, et al. Attribution of nonalcoholic steatohepatitis as an etiology of cirrhosis for clinical trials eligibility: recommendations from the multi-stakeholder liver forum. Gastroenterology. 2020;159(2):422–7.e1.
69. Schuppan D, Surabattula R, Wang XY. Determinants of fibrosis progression and regression in NASH. J Hepatol. 2018;68(2):238–50.
70. Sanyal AJ, Anstee QM, Trauner M, Lawitz EJ, Abdelmalek MF, Ding D, et al. Cirrhosis regression is associated with improved clinical outcomes in patients with nonalcoholic steatohepatitis. Hepatology. 2022;75(5):1235–46.
71. Tacke F, Puengel T, Loomba R, Friedman SL. An integrated view of anti-inflammatory and antifibrotic targets for the treatment of NASH. J Hepatol. 2023;79(2):552–66.
72. Lassailly G, Caiazzo R, Ntandja-Wandji LC, Gnemmi V, Baud G, Verkindt H, et al. Bariatric surgery provides long-term resolution of nonalcoholic steatohepatitis and regression of fibrosis. Gastroenterology. 2020;159(4):1290–301.e5.
73. Wanless IR, Nakashima E, Sherman M. Regression of human cirrhosis. Morphologic features and the genesis of incomplete septal cirrhosis. Arch Pathol Lab Med. 2000;124(11):1599–607.
74. Guindi M. Liver fibrosis: the good, the bad, and the patchy-an update. Hum Pathol. 2023;141:201–11.
75. Theise ND, Jia J, Sun Y, Wee A, You H. Progression and regression of fibrosis in viral hepatitis in the treatment era: the Beijing classification. Mod Pathol. 2018;31(8):1191–200.
76. Lackner C. Prospects for a better diagnosis and prognosis of NAFLD: a pathologist's view. Hepatoma Res. 2021;7:27.
77. Pais R, Charlotte F, Fedchuk L, Bedossa P, Lebray P, Poynard T, Ratziu V. A systematic review of follow-up biopsies reveals disease progression in patients with non-alcoholic fatty liver. J Hepatol. 2013;59(3):550–6.
78. Pai RK. NAFLD histology: a critical review and comparison of scoring systems. Curr Hepatol Rep. 2019;18(4):473–81.
79. Bedossa P. Utility and appropriateness of the fatty liver inhibition of progression (FLIP) algorithm and steatosis, activity, and fibrosis (SAF) score in the evaluation of biopsies of nonalcoholic fatty liver disease. Hepatology. 2014;60(2):565–75.
80. Ong J, Younossi ZM, Reddy V, Price LL, Gramlich T, Mayes J, Boparai N. Cryptogenic cirrhosis and posttransplantation nonalcoholic fatty liver disease. Liver Transpl. 2001;7(9):797–801.
81. Francque SM, Bedossa P, Ratziu V, Anstee QM, Bugianesi E, Sanyal AJ, et al. A randomized, controlled trial of the Pan-PPAR agonist Lanifibranor in NASH. N Engl J Med. 2021;385(17):1547–58.
82. Wanless IR, Sweeney G, Dhillon AP, Guido M, Piga A, Galanello R, et al. Lack of progressive hepatic fibrosis during long-term therapy with deferiprone in subjects with transfusion-dependent beta-thalassemia. Blood. 2002;100(5):1566–9.
83. Bedossa P, Arola J, Davies S, Gouw AS, Maria G, Lackner K, et al. The EPoS staging system is a reproducible 7-tierfibrosis score for NAFLD adapted both to glass slides and digitized images (e-slides). J Hepatol. 2018;68:1.
84. Anderson EL, Howe LD, Jones HE, Higgins JP, Lawlor DA, Fraser A. The prevalence of non-alcoholic fatty liver disease in children and adolescents: a systematic review and meta-analysis. PLoS One. 2015;10(10):e0140908.
85. Wang C, Pai AK, Putra J. Paediatric non-alcoholic fatty liver disease: an approach to pathological evaluation. J Clin Pathol. 2022;75(7):443–51.
86. Alkhouri N, De Vito R, Alisi A, Yerian L, Lopez R, Feldstein AE, Nobili V. Development and validation of a new histological score for pediatric non-alcoholic fatty liver disease. J Hepatol. 2012;57(6):1312–8.
87. Brunt EM, Kleiner DE, Wilson LA, Belt P, Neuschwander-Tetri BA. Nonalcoholic fatty liver disease (NAFLD) activity score and the histopathologic diagnosis in NAFLD: distinct clinicopathologic meanings. Hepatology. 2011;53(3):810–20.
88. Francque SM. Towards precision medicine in non-alcoholic fatty liver disease. Rev Endocr Metab Disord. 2023;24(5):885–99.

89. Ratziu V, Francque S, Sanyal A. Breakthroughs in therapies for NASH and remaining challenges. J Hepatol. 2022;76(6):1263–78.
90. Dulai PS, Singh S, Patel J, Soni M, Prokop LJ, Younossi Z, et al. Increased risk of mortality by fibrosis stage in nonalcoholic fatty liver disease: systematic review and meta-analysis. Hepatology. 2017;65(5):1557–65.
91. Francque SM, van der Graaff D, Kwanten WJ. Non-alcoholic fatty liver disease and cardiovascular risk: pathophysiological mechanisms and implications. J Hepatol. 2016;65(2):425–43.
92. Targher G, Byrne CD, Lonardo A, Zoppini G, Barbui C. Non-alcoholic fatty liver disease and risk of incident cardiovascular disease: a meta-analysis. J Hepatol. 2016;65(3):589–600.
93. Rinella ME, Tacke F, Sanyal AJ, Anstee QM. Report on the AASLD/EASL joint workshop on clinical trial endpoints in NAFLD. J Hepatol. 2019;71(4):823–33.
94. Loomba R, Ratziu V, Harrison SA. Expert panel review to compare FDA and EMA guidance on drug development and endpoints in nonalcoholic steatohepatitis. Gastroenterology. 2022;162(3):680–8.
95. Brunt EM. Nonalcoholic steatohepatitis: definition and pathology. Semin Liver Dis. 2001;21(1):3–16.
96. Marchesini G, Christopher DP, Dufour J-F, Canbay A, Nobili V, Ratziu V, et al. EASL-EASD-EASO clinical practice guidelines for the management of non-alcoholic fatty liver disease. J Hepatol. 2016;64(6):1388–402.
97. Siddiqui MS, Harrison SA, Abdelmalek MF, Anstee QM, Bedossa P, Castera L, et al. Case definitions for inclusion and analysis of endpoints in clinical trials for nonalcoholic steatohepatitis through the lens of regulatory science. Hepatology. 2018;67(5):2001–12.
98. Brunt EM, Kleiner DE, Wilson LA, Unalp A, Behling CE, Lavine JE, Neuschwander-Tetri BA. Portal chronic inflammation in nonalcoholic fatty liver disease (NAFLD): a histologic marker of advanced NAFLD-Clinicopathologic correlations from the nonalcoholic steatohepatitis clinical research network. Hepatology. 2009;49(3):809–20.
99. Sanyal AJ, Van Natta ML, Clark J, Neuschwander-Tetri BA, Diehl A, Dasarathy S, et al. Prospective study of outcomes in adults with nonalcoholic fatty liver disease. N Engl J Med. 2021;385(17):1559–69.
100. Younossi ZM, Ratziu V, Loomba R, Rinella M, Anstee QM, Goodman Z, et al. Obeticholic acid for the treatment of non-alcoholic steatohepatitis: interim analysis from a multicentre, randomised, placebo-controlled phase 3 trial. Lancet. 2019;394(10215):2184–96.
101. Harrison SA, Bedossa P, Guy CD, Schattenberg JM, Loomba R, Taub R, et al. A phase 3, randomized, controlled trial of Resmetirom in NASH with liver fibrosis. N Engl J Med. 2024;390(6):497–509.
102. Newsome PN, Sejling AS, Sanyal AJ. Semaglutide or placebo for nonalcoholic steatohepatitis. Reply N Engl J Med. 2021;385(2):e6.
103. Brunt EM, Kleiner DE, Wilson LA, Sanyal AJ, Neuschwander-Tetri BA. Improvements in histologic features and diagnosis associated with improvement in fibrosis in nonalcoholic steatohepatitis: results from the nonalcoholic steatohepatitis clinical research Network treatment trials. Hepatology. 2019;70(2):522–31.
104. Ratziu V, Harrison S, Francque S, Bedossa P, Anstee Q, Serfaty L, et al. A post-hoc analysis ofthe Golden505 trial demonstrates histological and Cardiometabolic efficacy of Elafibranor-120 mg in patients with moderate or severe Nash that are eligible for pharmacotherapy. J Hepatol. 2016;62(2):1.
105. Ratziu V, Sanyal A, Harrison SA, Wong VW, Francque S, Goodman Z, et al. Cenicriviroc treatment for adults with nonalcoholic steatohepatitis and fibrosis: final analysis of the phase 2b CENTAUR study. Hepatology. 2020;72(3):892–905.
106. Anstee QM, Lucas KJ, Francque S, Abdelmalek MF, Sanyal AJ, Ratziu V, et al. Tropifexor plus cenicriviroc combination versus monotherapy in nonalcoholic steatohepatitis: results from the phase 2b TANDEM study. Hepatology. 2023;78(4):1223–39.
107. Harrison SA, Abdelmalek MF, Caldwell S, Shiffman ML, Diehl AM, Ghalib R, et al. Simtuzumab is ineffective for patients with bridging fibrosis or compensated cirrhosis caused by nonalcoholic steatohepatitis. Gastroenterology. 2018;155(4):1140–53.
108. Harrison SA, Wong VW, Okanoue T, Bzowej N, Vuppalanchi R, Younes Z, et al. Selonsertib for patients with bridging fibrosis or compensated cirrhosis due to NASH: results from randomized phase III STELLAR trials. J Hepatol. 2020;73(1):26–39.
109. Sanyal AJ, Loomba R, Anstee Q, Ratziu V, Kowdley KV, Rinella ME, et al. Topline results from a new analysis of the REGENERATE trial of obeticholic acid for the treatment of nonalcoholic steatohepatitis. Hepatology. 2022;76
110. Harrison SA, Francque SM, Zevallos OC, Cejvanovic V, Cortez-Pinto H, Krarup N, et al. Artificial intelligence-powered digital pathology model supports that fibrosis is reduced by semaglutide in patients with NASH. J Hepatol. 2022;74
111. Ratziu V, Charlotte F, Heurtier A, Gombert S, Giral P, Bruckert E, et al. Sampling variability of liver biopsy in nonalcoholic fatty liver disease. Gastroenterology. 2005;128(7):1898–906.
112. Selvaraj EA, Mózes FE, Jayaswal ANA, Zafarmand MH, Vali Y, Lee JA, et al. Diagnostic accuracy of elastography and magnetic resonance imaging in patients with NAFLD: a systematic review and meta-analysis. J Hepatol. 2021;75(4):770–85.
113. Canivet CM, Zheng MH, Qadri S, Vonghia L, Chuah KH, Costentin C, et al. Validation of the blood test MACK-3 for the noninvasive diagnosis of fibrotic nonalcoholic steatohepatitis: an international study with 1924 patients. Clin Gastroenterol Hepatol. 2023;21(12):3097–106.e10.
114. Harrison SA, Ratziu V, Boursier J, Francque S, Bedossa P, Majd Z, et al. A blood-based biomarker

panel (NIS4) for non-invasive diagnosis of nonalcoholic steatohepatitis and liver fibrosis: a prospective derivation and global validation study. Lancet Gastroenterol Hepatol. 2020;5(11):970–85.
115. Loomba R, Sanyal AJ, Nakajima A, Neuschwander-Tetri BA, Goodman ZD, Harrison SA, et al. Pegbelfermin in patients with nonalcoholic steatohepatitis and stage 3 fibrosis (FALCON 1): a randomized phase 2b study. Clin Gastroenterol Hepatol. 2024;22(1):102–12.e9.
116. Rinella ME, Dufour JF, Anstee QM, Goodman Z, Younossi Z, Harrison SA, et al. Non-invasive evaluation of response to obeticholic acid in patients with NASH: results from the REGENERATE study. J Hepatol. 2022;76(3):536–48.
117. Roerecke M, Vafaei A, Hasan OSM, Chrystoja BR, Cruz M, Lee R, et al. Alcohol consumption and risk of liver cirrhosis: a systematic review and meta-analysis. Am J Gastroenterol. 2019;114(10):1574–86.
118. Arab JP, Arrese M, Singal AK. Diagnosis of alcohol-associated hepatitis: when is liver biopsy required? Clin Liver Dis. 2021;25(3):571–84.
119. Lackner C, Tiniakos D. Fibrosis and alcohol-related liver disease. J Hepatol. 2019;70(2):294–304.
120. Roth NC, Qin J. Histopathology of alcohol-related liver diseases. Clin Liver Dis. 2019;23(1):11–23.
121. Nakano M, Fukusato T. Histological study on comparison between NASH and ALD. Hepatol Res. 2005;33(2):110–5.
122. Lackner C, Stauber RE, Davies S, Denk H, Dienes HP, Gnemmi V, et al. Development and prognostic relevance of a histologic grading and staging system for alcohol-related liver disease. J Hepatol. 2021;75(4):810–9.
123. Altamirano J, Miquel R, Katoonizadeh A, Abraldes JG, Duarte-Rojo A, Louvet A, et al. A histologic scoring system for prognosis of patients with alcoholic hepatitis. Gastroenterology. 2014;146(5):1231–9.e1–6.
124. Sandahl TD, Laursen TL, Munk DE, Vilstrup H, Weiss KH, Ott P. The prevalence of Wilson's disease: an update. Hepatology. 2020;71(2):722–32.
125. Guindi M. Wilson disease. Semin Diagn Pathol. 2019;36(6):415–22.
126. Gerosa C, Fanni D, Congiu T, Piras M, Cau F, Moi M, Faa G. Liver pathology in Wilson's disease: from copper overload to cirrhosis. J Inorg Biochem. 2019;193:106–11.
127. Ordóñez A, Snapp EL, Tan L, Miranda E, Marciniak SJ, Lomas DA. Endoplasmic reticulum polymers impair luminal protein mobility and sensitize to cellular stress in alpha1-antitrypsin deficiency. Hepatology. 2013;57(5):2049–60.
128. Mitten EK, Rutherford A. How Hepatologists use liver biopsy in the evaluation of liver disease? Surg Pathol Clin. 2023;16(3):443–56.
129. Fu DA, Campbell-Thompson M. Immunohistochemistry staining for human Alpha-1 antitrypsin. Methods Mol Biol. 2017;1639:139–43.
130. Synoracki S, Kathemann S, Schmid KW, Jastrow H, Baba HA. Lysosomal acid lipase deficiency (LAL-D) : Diagnostic and therapeutic options in an underdiagnosed disease. Pathologe. 2018;39(3):249–54.
131. Pericleous M, Kelly C, Wang T, Livingstone C, Ala A. Wolman's disease and cholesteryl ester storage disorder: the phenotypic spectrum of lysosomal acid lipase deficiency. Lancet Gastroenterol Hepatol. 2017;2(9):670–9.
132. Hůlková H, Elleder M. Distinctive histopathological features that support a diagnosis of cholesterol ester storage disease in liver biopsy specimens. Histopathology. 2012;60(7):1107–13.
133. Mihajlovic M, Vinken M. Mitochondria as the target of hepatotoxicity and drug-induced liver injury: molecular mechanisms and detection methods. Int J Mol Sci. 2022;23(6):3315.
134. Zhang H, Rios RS, Boursier J, Anty R, Chan WK, George J, et al. Hepatocyte apoptosis fragment product cytokeratin-18 M30 level and non-alcoholic steatohepatitis risk diagnosis: an international registry study. Chin Med J. 2023;136(3):341–50.
135. Kleiner DE, Chalasani NP, Lee WM, Fontana RJ, Bonkovsky HL, Watkins PB, et al. Hepatic histological findings in suspected drug-induced liver injury: systematic evaluation and clinical associations. Hepatology. 2014;59(2):661–70.
136. Allende DS, Kleiner DE. Fatty liver disease that is neither metabolic nor alcoholic. Hum Pathol. 2023;141:212–21.
137. Teramoto T, Shinohara T, Takiyama A. Computer-aided classification of hepatocellular ballooning in liver biopsies from patients with NASH using persistent homology. Comput Methods Prog Biomed. 2020;195:105614.
138. Allaume P, Rabilloud N, Turlin B, Bardou-Jacquet E, Loréal O, Calderaro J, et al. Artificial intelligence-based opportunities in liver pathology-a systematic review. Diagnostics (Basel). 2023;13(10):1799.
139. Takahashi Y, Dungubat E, Kusano H, Fukusato T. Artificial intelligence and deep learning: new tools for histopathological diagnosis of nonalcoholic fatty liver disease/nonalcoholic steatohepatitis. Comput Struct Biotechnol J. 2023;21:2495–501.
140. Ratziu V, Hompesch M, Petitjean M, Serdjebi C, Iyer JS, Parwani AV, et al. Artificial intelligence-assisted digital pathology for non-alcoholic steatohepatitis: current status and future directions. J Hepatol. 2024;80(2):335–51.
141. Lee J, Westphal M, Vali Y, Boursier J, Petta S, Ostroff R, et al. Machine learning algorithm improves the detection of NASH (NAS-based) and at-risk NASH: a development and validation study. Hepatology. 2023;78(1):258–71.
142. Loomba R, Noureddin M, Kowdley KV, Kohli A, Sheikh A, Neff G, et al. Combination therapies including cilofexor and firsocostat for bridging fibrosis and cirrhosis attributable to NASH. Hepatology (Baltimore, MD). 2021;73(2):625–43.

143. Xu S, Wang Y, Tai DCS, Wang S, Cheng CL, Peng Q, et al. qFibrosis: a fully-quantitative innovative method incorporating histological features to facilitate accurate fibrosis scoring in animal model and chronic hepatitis B patients. J Hepatol. 2014;61(2):260–9.
144. Wang Y, Wong GL, He FP, Sun J, Chan AW, Yang J, et al. Quantifying and monitoring fibrosis in non-alcoholic fatty liver disease using dual-photon microscopy. Gut. 2020;69(6):1116–26.
145. Naoumov NV, Brees D, Loeffler J, Chng E, Ren Y, Lopez P, et al. Digital pathology with artificial intelligence analyses provides greater insights into treatment-induced fibrosis regression in NASH. J Hepatol. 2022;77(5):1399–409.

# MASLD as a Multisystemic Disease

# 7

Chantal Jacqueline Córdova-Gallardo,
Andres Manuel Vargas-Beltran,
Mariana M. Ramírez Mejía,
and Nahum Méndez-Sánchez

## 7.1 Introduction

Metabolic dysfunction-associated steatotic liver disease (MASLD) has become the main cause of chronic liver disease with an increasing prevalence worldwide, affecting 25% of the general population and more than 50% of patients with metabolic syndrome [1, 2]. Due to the increasing prevalence of obesity with more of 30% of the general population affected (>600 million people) and the growing number of children with obesity, it is thought that the prevalence of MASLD will increase exponentially [3]. The risk of overall and liver-related mortality is increased in these patients closely related to fibrosis stage [4]. The concern in addition to liver disease lies in the fact that this disease does not only affect the liver, but there is growing evidence that it represents a multisystem disease with a wide spectrum of extrahepatic manifestations, affecting the heart, kidney, endocrine glands, brain, and increasing the risk of gastrointestinal cancer. The most prevalent and studied extra-hepatic manifestation is cardiovascular disease, representing the main cause of death in these patients [5] (Fig. 7.1). The risk of serious infections in general is higher in patients with MASLD compared to individuals without the disease, which is another important factor to keep in mind in these patients [6].

C. J. Córdova-Gallardo · A. M. Vargas-Beltran
Hepatology, General Surgery Department, General Hospital Dr. Manuel Gea González,
Mexico City, Mexico

M. M. Ramírez Mejía · N. Méndez-Sánchez (✉)
Faculty of Medicine, National Autonomous University of Mexico, Mexico City, Mexico

Liver Research Unit, Medica Sur Clinic and Foundation, Mexico City, Mexico
e-mail: nmendez@medicasur.org.mx



N. Méndez-Sánchez, X. Qi (eds.), *Metabolic Dysfunction-Associated Steatotic Liver Disease*,
https://doi.org/10.1007/978-981-97-9519-2_7

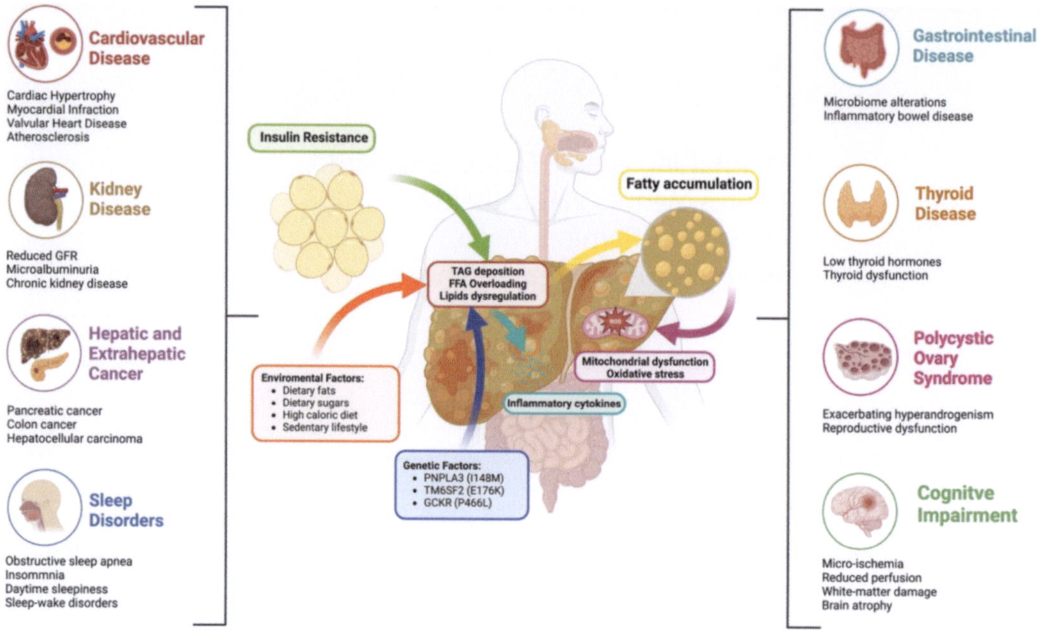


**Fig. 7.1** Mechanisms implicated in MASLD patients and their associations with extrahepatic diseases. Genetic factors, a high-sugar, and high-fat diet are some of the mechanisms that lead to a disruption of hepatic metabolism. Insulin resistance is one major factor that contributes to the onset of MASLD. These conditions cause lipid dysregulation in the liver, which contributes to fatty accumulation and oxidative stress. Consequently, inflammatory cytokines are released, promoting inflammation and the onset of MASLD. However, this condition can act as a multisystemic disease, with a wide spectrum of extrahepatic manifestations, including the heart, kidneys, brain, thyroid gland, intestines and increasing the risk of gastrointestinal cancer

## 7.2 Cardiovascular Implications and Risk Factors

MASLD is associated with cardiovascular disease (CVD). These complications are the predominant cause of mortality in these patients. It is a multifactorial etiology that includes different mechanisms for cardiovascular implications, such as dyslipidemia, IR, hypertension, inflammation, dysfunction of gut-liver axis and fat deposition [7].

1. Dyslipidemia: MASLD patients experience alterations in lipid levels. Triglyceride elevation is related to formation of coronary plaques. Additionally, higher cholesterol and triglycerides levels have been described as a risk of developing aortic valve stenosis [8].
2. Insulin resistance: Evidence show that hepatic damage activates different mechanisms that increase oxidative stress, endothelial dysfunction, and dyslipidemia. Consequently, it facilitates the formation of atherosclerosis for cardiovascular disease. Liver fibrosis is correlated with insulin resistance [9].
3. Hypertension: It is a strong risk factor for developing cardiovascular complications, including peripheral vascular disease, valvular heart disease and stroke. It has been demonstrated that exists a relationship between the severity of MASLD and risk of cardiovascular complications [10].
4. Inflammation: Fat deposition induces liver inflammation and cell death, which leads to macrophages activation. Kupffer cells are increased to regulate inflammatory responses. Consequently, there is a release of proinflammatory cytokines, including IL-1, IL-6, and IL-20. They cause a disruption of vascular tone to induce formation of plaques [11].
5. Obesity: Adipokines are biological proteins released by fat storage deposits. They impair metabolism pathways and are implicated in

cardiovascular disease pathogenesis. Leptin levels correlated with vascular disease, such as myocardial infarction or heart failure. It has been said that epicardial fat is increased in obesity and is strongly associated with the progression of coronary calcification [12].

6. Microbiome dysfunction: Intestinal barrier disruption occurs in MASLD patients and correlates with the degree of hepatic steatosis. As a result, permeability increases circulating bacterial products, leading to hepatocyte activation of proinflammatory marker. These changes are reported to be associated with risk of fatal and nonfatal cardiovascular events [13].

MASLD increases the risk of developing coronary artery calcification over time and exists a relationship with cardiomyopathy. This condition results in epicardial fat accumulation leading to irregular metabolism, and results in left ventricular diastolic dysfunction. This condition leads to fibrosis formation, which can worsen congestion and cardiac function [14].

There is evidence that MASLD severity correlates with increased risk of myocardial infarction, coronary atherosclerosis, and valvular heart disease. A cohort study from South Korea has recently demonstrated that patients with MASLD had a 1.5 times higher risk of developing nonfatal and fatal complications than those without MASLD. Noncalcified plaques are associated with these patients and indicate a higher risk of acute coronary events, leading to a sudden cardiac event [12, 15].

There are many hypotheses explaining cardiac complications. For example, release of proinflammatory factors in MASLD patients contributes to valvular heart disease. Endothelial damage is caused by an impairment of vasodilation and higher levels of biomarkers that leads to a dysfunction of endothelial barrier. As a result, it reduces antioxidant capacity and contributes to cardiovascular complications [16].

## 7.3 MASLD Impact on Kidney Function

MASLD induces a low-grade inflammation that activates oxidative stress and leads to fibrosis. It increases the release of pro-inflammatory pathways and causes endothelial dysfunction. Consequently, it decreases renal function by glomerular permeability damage and microalbuminuria, causing chronic kidney disease (CKD) [17].

Some evidence demonstrates a stronger association of MASLD with CKD patients. Mechanisms linking these two conditions include metabolic dysfunction, genetic predisposition, and environmental factors. Additionally, systemic inflammation and vascular dysfunction act as mediators in extrahepatic diseases, including CKD [18]. A meta-analysis has shown that MASLD was associated with 1.5 times higher risk for development of CKD stage >3 over a period of 9.7 years, and liver fibrosis was related to early renal dysfunction [19].

MASLD has been related to high levels of fatty acid-binding protein 4 (FABP4), a molecule secreted by adipocytes which acts as an adipokine. It has been shown that this protein is associated with tubulointerstitial and glomerular injury, decreasing glomerular filtration rate [20]. Furthermore, liver inflammation is a relevant source of profibrogenic and antifibrinolytic molecules, including fibroblast growth factor 2, tumor necrosis factor-$\alpha$, fetuin-A and transforming growth factor-$\beta$, which promote kidney dysfunction [21]. Finally, adipokines dysregulation, such as reduced adiponectin levels and elevated FABP4, has been documented in individuals with MASLD, potentially leading to renal dysfunction, atherosclerosis, and cardiovascular events, associated with metabolic inflammation [20].

## 7.4 MASLD and Cognitive Impairment

It is well known that MASLD is a multisystem disease, nevertheless the pathological mechanism of neurological affection has not yet been completely elucidated. Cognitive dysfunction is due to several mechanisms, among them a reduction in brain volume, cerebral perfusion, and white matter lesions [22].

It is thought that the endothelial dysfunction and vascular alterations present in MASLD patients cause a cognitive decline due to systemic inflammatory factors that penetrate the central nervous system (CNS) causing a neurotoxic effect and the formation of beta-amyloid plaques that provokes neuronal death and cognitive dysfunction [23]. The release of free fatty acids and IR is thought to impact memory function due to a reduction of neuronal plasticity, an altered neuronal metabolism and growth causing hippocampus damage [22].

Orexin, a neuropeptide crucial for cognitive function, is altered due to lipotoxicity, causing memory loss and learning difficulties [24]. Gut dysbiosis, by vagal stimulation, affects neuronal function causing the activation of stress mechanisms within the brain increasing the release of corticotrophin releasing hormone (CRH) in the hypothalamus with the consequent secretion of adrenocorticotropic hormone (ACTH) (in the pituitary gland) and cortisol in the adrenal glands, the secondary hypercortisolism provoke the activation of glucocorticoid receptors in the amygdala and hypocampus affecting cognitive function and memory [25].

## 7.5 MASLD and Body Composition

Body composition evaluation is an important reference for individuals' health and physical status. These two associations have been rarely studied. Nevertheless, MASLD has been linked with body composition. These changes are mainly caused by sarcopenia and fat-muscle interchange, without metabolic abnormalities. Body water, resistance and skeletal muscle mass are significantly lower in MASLD obese patients [26].

These two conditions share mechanisms that cause higher rates of mortality. In men, body mass index (BMI), fat index and waist circumference show associations with fat-free mass index. In contrast, in females, BMI and fat index appear as significant factors related to fat-free mass index. Thus, BMI and fat index serve as reliable indicators for assessing decreased muscle mass in patients with MASLD, suggesting that lower BMI may pose a risk of skeletal muscle deterioration in individuals with MASLD [27].

Evidence shows that MASLD individuals have muscle mass dysfunction. Sarcopenia is a risk factor for developing liver fibrosis and cardiovascular events. Myosteatosis, the infiltration of fat in skeletal muscle, was significantly related to increased liver stiffness in MASLD obese patients [28].

Adipose-muscle-liver axis disruption has an important role in body composition alteration. Abnormal metabolic pathways in MASLD patients result in fatty accumulation in liver and muscle, which lead to insulin resistance. Body composition indexes of nonobese subjects were significantly lower than MASLD obese subjects, with a different metabolic profile [29].

## 7.6 MASLD and Thyroid

There is a relationship between liver and thyroid function. Liver participates in metabolizing, transporting, and activating thyroid hormones. In patients with MASLD, alterations in hepatocyte function and hepatic metabolism may significantly influence these activities, which could affect thyroid function [30].

A previous study demonstrated that hypothyroidism was significantly associated with MASLD severity. In addition, reduced thyroid hormone levels are markedly linked to higher risk of cardiovascular mortality among MASLD patients [31].

The exact mechanism connecting changes in plasma thyroid hormone levels and MASLD is not fully understood. Nevertheless, it may involve a disruption of mitochondrial homeostasis, endoplasmic reticulum stress, decreased insulin sensitivity, and chronic inflammation. Low levels of free thyroxine (FT4) can trigger the release of biomarkers and inflammatory pathways, exacerbating hepatic fatty infiltration [32].

## 7.7 MASLD and Gastrointestinal Diseases

MASLD patients have an increased prevalence of gastrointestinal infections, with an adjusted odds ratio (OR) of 1.36. They are especially prone to infections, particularly *Clostridium difficile*, *Escherichia coli*, and *Salmonella*. These may be due to the observed dysbiosis, alterations in intestinal permeability and compromised immunity in MASLD patients [33].

In addition, there is a high prevalence of MASLD in patients with inflammatory bowel disease (IBD), reaching up to 55% in patients with Crohn's disease (CD) and 39.5% in patients with ulcerative colitis (UC). IBD risk factors described for developing MASLD are parenteral nutrition, disease activity and duration, medications used, type and extension of surgeries, as well as the microbiota diversity. Surgical interventions involving the ascending colon increase the risk of MASLD due to reduced insulin sensitivity and increased insulin secretion. In addition, surgeries involving ileum resection reduce FGF19 levels, leading to decreased bile acid reabsorption and altered metabolism, increased triglyceride synthesis and decreased hepatic lipid beta-oxidation. Dysbiosis aggravates the situation by promoting overexpression of proinflammatory bacterial metabolites, while reducing protective short-chain fatty acids produced by enterocytes. This dysregulation increases intestinal permeability and facilitates the passage of microbial products, such as lipopolysaccharide, through the portal vein [34].

## 7.8 MASLD and Polycystic Ovary Syndrome

The relationship between MASLD and polycystic ovary syndrome (PCOS) has attracted considerable attention due to shared metabolic dysregulations and overlapping clinical features. PCOS, a prevalent endocrine disorder among women of reproductive age, is characterized by hormonal imbalances, ovarian dysfunction and metabolic disturbances [35]. Studies have highlighted a bidirectional association between MASLD and PCOS. Individuals with PCOS are at an elevated risk of developing MASLD due to common underlying factors such as IR, hyperandrogenism and obesity. Conversely, women with MASLD show a higher prevalence of PCOS compared to the general population [36].

IR plays a central role in the pathogenesis of both conditions. In PCOS, IR contributes to hyperinsulinemia, which stimulates ovarian androgen production, exacerbating hyperandrogenism. Moreover, hyperandrogenism, a hallmark of PCOS, may further exacerbate metabolic dysfunction in MASLD by promoting hepatic lipid synthesis and impairing lipid metabolism [37]. The coexistence of MASLD and PCOS poses significant clinical implications. Women with both conditions may experience more severe metabolic disturbances, including worsened IR, dyslipidemia, and increased cardiovascular risk. Additionally, the presence of MASLD in PCOS patients may exacerbate reproductive dysfunction and complicate fertility treatments [38].

## 7.9 MASLD and Sleep Disorders

Sleep disorders such as insomnia and circadian rhythm disorders have been observed to coexist with MASLD at a higher prevalence compared to the general population. This association suggests that sleep disorders may not only coexist with MASLD but may also aggravate its progression. These sleep disorders could contribute to metabolic dysregulation, thus influencing the development and severity of MASLD [39]. Obstructive sleep apnea (OSA) is the most commonly studied sleep disorder in relation to MASLD. The association between MASLD and OSA underscores the intricate interplay between metabolic disorders and sleep disturbances. OSA, characterized by recurrent episodes of upper airway obstruction during sleep, has become an important comorbidity in people with MASLD [40, 41]. This relationship is further complicated by the presence of intermittent hypoxia, a hallmark of OSA, which can exacerbate liver injury by inducing oxidative stress, systemic inflammation and IR, all key pathological processes in the progression of MASLD to more severe stages of the disease [42]. Interventional studies have suggested that treatment of OSA may have a beneficial effect on liver outcomes in patients with MASLD. For example, the use of continuous positive airway pressure (CPAP) therapy, which relieves OSA symptoms by preventing airway closure during sleep, has been associated with a reduction in hepatic steatosis and fibrosis. This improvement is likely due to reduced hypoxic stress, which decreases the hepatic inflammatory response and improves metabolic regulation in the liver [43].

## 7.10 MASLD and Cancer

Hepatocellular carcinoma (HCC) is the most frequent type of primary liver cancer and is closely associated with chronic liver diseases such as MASLD, viral hepatitis (hepatitis B and C) and alcoholic liver disease [44]. Although HCC is often associated with liver cirrhosis resulting from these conditions, recent research has highlighted the increasing incidence of HCC in patients with MASLD who do not have cirrhosis, suggesting a direct link between MASLD and the development of liver cancer [45]. In addition to HCC, MASLD has also been implicated in the development of extrahepatic cancers, particularly gastrointestinal cancers such as colorectal cancer and pancreatic cancer. The precise mechanisms linking MASLD to extrahepatic cancers are still being elucidated, but it is believed that systemic inflammation, insulin resistance, dyslipidemia, and alterations in the gut microbiota associated with MASLD may contribute to increased risk of these cancers [46, 47].

## References


1. Kaya E, Yilmaz Y. Metabolic-associated fatty liver disease (MAFLD): a multi-systemic disease beyond the liver. J Clin Transl Hepatol. 2022;10(2):329–38.
2. Pipitone RM, Ciccioli C, Infantino G, La Mantia C, Parisi S, Tulone A, et al. MAFLD: a multisystem disease. Ther Adv Endocrinol Metab. 2023;14:20420188221145549.
3. Sangro P, de la Torre AM, Sangro B, D'Avola D. Metabolic dysfunction-associated fatty liver disease (MAFLD): an update of the recent advances in pharmacological treatment. J Physiol Biochem. 2023;79(4):869–79.
4. Dulai PS, Singh S, Patel J, Soni M, Prokop LJ, Younossi Z, et al. Increased risk of mortality by fibrosis stage in nonalcoholic fatty liver disease: systematic review and meta-analysis. Hepatology. 2017;65(5):1557–65.
5. Byrne CD, Targher G. NAFLD: a multisystem disease. J Hepatol. 2015;62(1 Suppl):S47–64.
6. Ebrahimi F, Simon TG, Hagström H, Söderling J, Wester A, Roelstraete B, Ludvigsson JF. Risk of severe infection in patients with biopsy-proven nonalcoholic fatty liver disease - a population-based cohort study. Clin Gastroenterol Hepatol. 2023;21(13):3346–55.e19.
7. Nakashima M, Nakamura K, Nishihara T, Ichikawa K, Nakayama R, Takaya Y, et al. Association between cardiovascular disease and liver disease, from a clinically pragmatic perspective as a cardiologist. Nutrients. 2023;15(3):748.
8. Kaltoft M, Langsted A, Nordestgaard BG. Triglycerides and remnant cholesterol associated with risk of aortic valve stenosis: Mendelian randomization in the Copenhagen general population study. Eur Heart J. 2020;41(24):2288–99.
9. Dongiovanni P, Rametta R, Meroni M, Valenti L. The role of insulin resistance in nonalcoholic steatohepatitis and liver disease development--a potential therapeutic target? Expert Rev Gastroenterol Hepatol. 2016;10(2):229–42.
10. Dongiovanni P, Paolini E, Corsini A, Sirtori CR, Ruscica M. Nonalcoholic fatty liver disease or metabolic dysfunction-associated fatty liver disease diagnoses and cardiovascular diseases: from epidemiology to drug approaches. Eur J Clin Investig. 2021;51(7):e13519.
11. He Y, Hwang S, Ahmed YA, Feng D, Li N, Ribeiro M, et al. Immunopathobiology and therapeutic tar-

gets related to cytokines in liver diseases. Cell Mol Immunol. 2021;18(1):18–37.
12. Lee H, Lee YH, Kim SU, Kim HC. Metabolic dysfunction-associated fatty liver disease and incident cardiovascular disease risk: a Nationwide cohort study. Clin Gastroenterol Hepatol. 2021;19(10):2138–47.e10.
13. De Cól JP, de Lima EP, Pompeu FM, Cressoni Araújo A, de Alvares GR, Bechara MD, et al. Underlying mechanisms behind the brain-gut-liver axis and metabolic-associated fatty liver disease (MAFLD): an update. Int J Mol Sci. 2024;25(7):3694.
14. Chun HS, Lee M, Lee JS, Lee HW, Kim BK, Park JY, et al. Metabolic dysfunction associated fatty liver disease identifies subjects with cardiovascular risk better than non-alcoholic fatty liver disease. Liver Int. 2023;43(3):608–25.
15. Lee SB, Park GM, Lee JY, Lee BU, Park JH, Kim BG, et al. Association between non-alcoholic fatty liver disease and subclinical coronary atherosclerosis: An observational cohort study. J Hepatol. 2018;68(5):1018–24.
16. Theofilis P, Vordoni A, Nakas N, Kalaitzidis RG. Endothelial dysfunction in nonalcoholic fatty liver disease: a systematic review and meta-analysis. Life (Basel). 2022;12(5):718.
17. Nardolillo M, Rescigno F, Bartiromo M, Piatto D, Guarino S, Marzuillo P, et al. Interplay between metabolic dysfunction-associated fatty liver disease and renal function: An intriguing pediatric perspective. World J Gastroenterol. 2024;30(15):2081–6.
18. Kwon SY, Park J, Park SH, Lee YB, Kim G, Hur KY, et al. MAFLD and NAFLD in the prediction of incident chronic kidney disease. Sci Rep. 2023;13(1):1796.
19. Mantovani A, Petracca G, Beatrice G, Csermely A, Lonardo A, Schattenberg JM, et al. Non-alcoholic fatty liver disease and risk of incident chronic kidney disease: an updated meta-analysis. Gut. 2022;71(1):156–62.
20. Tanaka M, Takahashi S, Higashiura Y, Sakai A, Koyama M, Saitoh S, et al. Circulating level of fatty acid-binding protein 4 is an independent predictor of metabolic dysfunction-associated fatty liver disease in middle-aged and elderly individuals. J Diabetes Investig. 2022;13(5):878–88.
21. Tanaka M, Mori K, Takahashi S, Higashiura Y, Ohnishi H, Hanawa N, Furuhashi M. Metabolic dysfunction-associated fatty liver disease predicts new onset of chronic kidney disease better than fatty liver or nonalcoholic fatty liver disease. Nephrol Dial Transplant. 2023;38(3):700–11.
22. Medina-Julio D, Ramírez-Mejía MM, Cordova-Gallardo J, Peniche-Luna E, Cantú-Brito C, Mendez-Sanchez N. From liver to brain: how MAFLD/MASLD impacts cognitive function. Med Sci Monit. 2024;30:e943417.
23. Kjærgaard K, Mikkelsen ACD, Wernberg CW, Grønkjær LL, Eriksen PL, Damholdt MF, et al. Cognitive dysfunction in non-alcoholic fatty liver disease-current knowledge, mechanisms and perspectives. J Clin Med. 2021;10(4):673.
24. Duffy CM, Hofmeister JJ, Nixon JP, Butterick TA. High fat diet increases cognitive decline and neuroinflammation in a model of orexin loss. Neurobiol Learn Mem. 2019;157:41–7.
25. Forsythe P, Bienenstock J, Kunze WA. Vagal pathways for microbiome-brain-gut axis communication. Adv Exp Med Biol. 2014;817:115–33.
26. Juárez E, López I, Bernal K, Velázquez A, Maldonado A, Ramos MH, et al. O-18 differences in body composition of MAFLD patients according to body mass index and metabolic profile. Ann Hepatol. 2024;29:101268.
27. Onishi S, Fukuda A, Matsui M, Ushiro K, Nishikawa T, Asai A, et al. Body composition analysis in patients with metabolic dysfunction-associated fatty liver disease. Nutrients. 2023;15(18):3878.
28. Nachit M, Lanthier N, Rodriguez J, Neyrinck AM, Cani PD, Bindels LB, et al. A dynamic association between myosteatosis and liver stiffness: results from a prospective interventional study in obese patients. JHEP Rep. 2021;3(4):100323.
29. Altajar S, Baffy G. Skeletal muscle dysfunction in the development and progression of nonalcoholic fatty liver disease. J Clin Transl Hepatol. 2020;8(4):414–23.
30. Chen YL, Tian S, Wu J, Li H, Li S, Xu Z, et al. Impact of thyroid function on the prevalence and mortality of metabolic dysfunction-associated fatty liver disease. J Clin Endocrinol Metab. 2023;108(7):e434–e43.
31. Mantovani A, Nascimbeni F, Lonardo A, Zoppini G, Bonora E, Mantzoros CS, Targher G. Association between primary hypothyroidism and nonalcoholic fatty liver disease: a systematic review and meta-analysis. Thyroid. 2018;28(10):1270–84.
32. Lim S, Kim JW, Targher G. Links between metabolic syndrome and metabolic dysfunction-associated fatty liver disease. Trends Endocrinol Metab. 2021;32(7):500–14.
33. Patel J, Sohal A, Bains K, Chaudhry H, Kohli I, Khanna T, et al. Association of metabolic dysfunction-associated fatty liver disease with gastrointestinal infections: insights from National Inpatient Sample Database. BMJ Open Gastroenterol. 2024;11(1):e001224.
34. Maresca R, Mignini I, Varca S, Calvez V, Termite F, Esposto G, et al. Inflammatory bowel diseases and non-alcoholic fatty liver disease: piecing a complex puzzle together. Int J Mol Sci. 2024;25(6):3278.
35. Patel S. Polycystic ovary syndrome (PCOS), an inflammatory, systemic, lifestyle endocrinopathy. J Steroid Biochem Mol Biol. 2018;182:27–36.
36. Gutierrez-Grobe Y, Ponciano-Rodríguez G, Ramos MH, Uribe M, Méndez-Sánchez N. Prevalence of non alcoholic fatty liver disease in premenopausal, posmenopausal and polycystic ovary syndrome women. The role of estrogens Ann Hepatol. 2010;9(4):402–9.
37. Salva-Pastor N, Chávez-Tapia NC, Uribe M, Nuño-Lámbarri N. Understanding the association of polycystic ovary syndrome and non-alcoholic

fatty liver disease. J Steroid Biochem Mol Biol. 2019;194:105445.
38. Macut D, Božić-Antić I, Bjekić-Macut J, Tziomalos K. MANAGEMENT OF ENDOCRINE DISEASE: polycystic ovary syndrome and nonalcoholic fatty liver disease. Eur J Endocrinol. 2017;177(3):R145–r58.
39. Bu LF, Xiong CY, Zhong JY, Xiong Y, Li DM, Hong FF, Yang SL. Non-alcoholic fatty liver disease and sleep disorders. World J Hepatol. 2024;16(3):304–15.
40. Xu S, Wan Y, Xu M, Ming J, Xing Y, An F, Ji Q. The association between obstructive sleep apnea and metabolic syndrome: a systematic review and meta-analysis. BMC Pulm Med. 2015;15:105.
41. Preshy A, Brown J. A bidirectional association between obstructive sleep apnea and metabolic-associated fatty liver disease. Endocrinol Metab Clin N Am. 2023;52(3):509–20.
42. Paschetta E, Belci P, Alisi A, Liccardo D, Cutrera R, Musso G, Nobili V. OSAS-related inflammatory mechanisms of liver injury in nonalcoholic fatty liver disease. Mediat Inflamm. 2015;2015:815721.
43. Sheng W, Ji G, Zhang L. Management of non-alcoholic fatty liver disease patients with sleep apnea syndrome. World J Gastroenterol. 2022;28(43):6099–108.
44. Villanueva A. Hepatocellular Carcinoma. N Engl J Med. 2019;380(15):1450–62.
45. Bae SDW, George J, Qiao L. From MAFLD to hepatocellular carcinoma and everything in between. Chin Med J. 2022;135(5):547–56.
46. Mantovani A, Petracca G, Beatrice G, Csermely A, Tilg H, Byrne CD, Targher G. Non-alcoholic fatty liver disease and increased risk of incident extrahepatic cancers: a meta-analysis of observational cohort studies. Gut. 2022;71(4):778–88.
47. Mitsala A, Tsalikidis C, Romanidis K, Pitiakoudis M. Non-alcoholic fatty liver disease and extrahepatic cancers: a wolf in Sheep's clothing? Curr Oncol. 2022;29(7):4478–510.

# MASLD and Hepatic/Extrahepatic Cancers: Understanding the Complex Relationship

**8**

Jan Best, Bernd Schnabl, and Ali Canbay

## 8.1 Introduction

The global prevalence of metabolic dysfunction-associated steatotic liver disease (MASLD) formerly known as nonalcoholic fatty liver disease (NAFLD) is estimated at 25% in the adult population, although this figure is likely to be underestimated due to the high number of unreported cases [2]. It is defined as steatotic liver disease in the presence of metabolic risk factors, particularly type 2 diabetes and obesity. If diagnosed in the early stages of fibrosis, it is potentially reversible with lifestyle changes and treatment of predisposing factors [19]. It is also associated with malignant morbidity; approximately 10–15% of patients with MASLD may progress to metabolic dysfunction-associated steatohepatitis (MASH), which in turn can lead to high-grade inflammatory liver fibrosis and, in the final stage, to cirrhosis and hepatocellular carcinoma (HCC) or various other extrahepatic cancers even in absence of fibrosis [1, 35]. Therefore, early detection of MASLD is imperative because of the risk of undertreatment and subsequent progression to cirrhosis or cancer. Only early identification of high-risk patients can reduce liver-related mortality from MASLD. Identification of these individuals is necessary to effectively treat patients and prevent progression to fibrosis, thereby reducing liver-related and all-cause mortality. In MASLD current evidence suggests the potential necessity of screening for extrahepatic malignancy, in particular in the gastrointestinal tract, irrespective of fibrosis. Once progression from MASLD to MASH fibrosis has occurred, appropriate surveillance strategies need to be implemented to facilitate early detection of MASH-related HCC. Only establishment of adopted cancer-specific screening algorithms can assure early diagnosis and consecutively curative treatment options.

J. Best
Department of Gastroenterology, Hepatology and Transplant Medicine, Medical Faculty, University of Duisburg-Essen, Essen, Germany
e-mail: Jan.best@uk-essen.de

B. Schnabl
Department of Medicine, VA San Diego Healthcare System, San Diego, CA, USA
e-mail: beschnabl@health.ucsd.edu

A. Canbay (✉)
Department of Medicine, Universitätsklinikum Knappschaftskrankenhaus Bochum, Ruhr University Bochum, Bochum, Germany
e-mail: Ali.canbay@rub.de

## 8.2 Hepatocellular Carcinoma and MASLD

Hepatocarcinogenesis is a multistage process that typically takes several decades. HCC usually develops independently of the underlying hepatopathy, based on liver cirrhosis [9]. However, in chronic hepatitis B virus (HBV) and MASH,


N. Méndez-Sánchez, X. Qi (eds.), *Metabolic Dysfunction-Associated Steatotic Liver Disease*,
https://doi.org/10.1007/978-981-97-9519-2_8

HCC can develop even in the absence of cirrhosis, highlighting the diverse mechanisms of hepatocarcinogenesis [10, 28, 39].

Recent epidemiological studies suggest that MASLD is the major cause of the steadily increasing incidence of HCC in Western industrialized countries [37]. An analysis of the American Liver Transplant Registry from 2002 to 2007 showed that the prevalence of HCC patients awaiting liver transplantation (LT) increased by 15.6% over the last 15 years, from 6.4% in 2002 to 22% in 2017. MASLD was found to be the fastest growing cause. The proportion of MASH as a cause of HCC increased 8.5-fold during the study period, from 2.1% in 2002 to 17.9% in 2017 [40]. As mentioned above, it should be noted that many HCCs arise from MASH in the absence of cirrhosis, a population that has not yet been subjected to international consensus screening for early detection of HCC [10].

Recent data from a US cohort study with over 500,000 participants showed a 10-year cumulative risk of HCC of 1.7 per 1000 patients in the MASLD cohort. In MASLD patients, the risk of HCC was 8.6 times higher than in healthy individuals. Patients with MASLD-associated cirrhosis had an even higher risk of developing HCC, with an annual incidence of 0.8–2.3% per year. Notably, approximately 20% of all MASH-associated HCC cases occurred in the absence of cirrhosis [14].

A German single-center study in 2015, which included 1119 patients with HCC of all etiologies, showed that there are relevant differences between patients with HCC due to MASH and those with other hepatopathies. Patients with HCC due to MASH were older at initial diagnosis than those with other predisposing hepatopathies (67.6 years vs. 65 years). In addition, the MASH-HCC cohort had a higher prevalence of obesity (31.1% vs. 14.7%) and type II diabetes mellitus (T2DM) (66.7% vs. 37.85%). Interestingly, HCC based on MASH showed a trend towards more frequent multifocality (80% vs. 69.7%) with larger overall lesions (6 cm vs. 4.8 cm) and a trend towards an increased rate of extrahepatic metastasis at initial diagnosis. It was also significant that the MASH-HCC patients had better global liver function despite a higher tumor burden at initial diagnosis. It is possible that the initial diagnosis of HCC in these patients was made at later stages of the tumor because they were monitored less intensively due to the absence of cirrhosis or less advanced cirrhosis [36].

A recent large meta-analysis estimated pooled incidence rates of HCC in MASLD (18 studies, 470,404 patients from 1950 through 2020). In patients with MASLD at a stage earlier than cirrhosis, the incidence rate of HCC was 0.03 per 100 person-years (95% confidence interval [CI], 0.01–0.07; I2 = 98%). In patients with cirrhosis, the incidence rate was 3.78 per 100 person-years (95% CI, 2.47–5.78; I2 = 93%). Here the authors conclude, that patients with MASLD-related cirrhosis have a risk of developing HCC similar to that reported for patients with cirrhosis from other etiologies [21].

## 8.3 Extrahepatic Cancers and MASLD

MASLD is a multisystem disease that leads to liver-related complications, such as liver failure, cirrhosis, and HCC, as well as extrahepatic complications, including cardiovascular diseases, chronic kidney disease, and various types of cancer. An association between MASLD and extrahepatic cancers affecting the gastrointestinal organs, genitourinary system, thyroid gland, lungs, and hematological [3]. Indeed, malignancy is the second most common cause of mortality in MASLD Objective evidence demonstrates that the incidence of malignant extrahepatic tumors is significantly higher in MASLD patients compared to the normal population. In contrast to HCC this development is already apparent in MASLD without the presence of predisposing liver fibrosis (Fig. 8.1).

According to a meta-analysis published in 2022 (including 64 studies), the incidence rate of HCC in the MASLD population was 1.25 per 1000 person-years (95% CI 1.01–1.49; I2 = 94.8%), while incidence of HCC was more than ten times higher at 14.46 per 1000 person-years (95% CI 10.89–18.04; I2 = 91.3%) in the

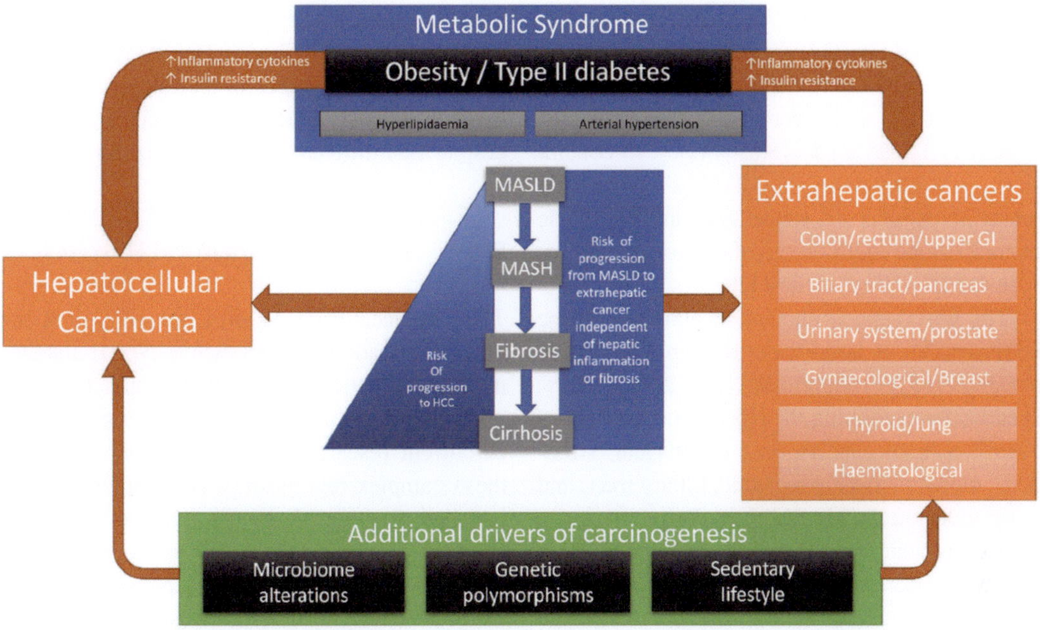


**Fig. 8.1** MASLD is the hepatic manifestation of metabolic syndrome, comprising of obesity, type II diabetes mellitus, hyperlipidemia, and arterial hypertension. The progression of MASLD to the inflammatory form, MASH, can occur through the development of liver fibrosis and cirrhosis, ultimately leading to HCC (hepatocellular carcinoma). Type II diabetes and obesity are both independent risk factors for the development of HCC and extrahepatic carcinomas. The risk of hepatocarcinogenesis increases with the severity of liver disease, while any form of MASLD is also an independent risk factor for the development of extrahepatic tumors. It is important to note that these risk factors are well-established and should be taken into consideration when assessing the overall risk of cancer in patients with these conditions

presence of MASLD-associated fibrosis or cirrhosis. In contrast, the pooled rate of MASLD-associated extrahepatic tumors was 10.58 per 1000 person-years (95% CI 8.14–13.02; I2 = 97.1%) regardless of fibrosis status. Notably, the most frequently occurring extrahepatic cancers were uterine cancer (4.27 per 1000 person-years), breast cancer (4.02 per 1000 person-years), prostate cancer (1.44 per 1000 person-years), colorectal cancer (1.43 per 1000 person-years), and lung cancer (1.35 per 1000 person-years). In summary, extrahepatic cancers have been shown to be over eight times more common than HCC in MASLD [33].

Another meta-analysis of ten cohort studies with 182,202 middle-aged individuals (24.8% with MASLD) and 8485 incident cases of extrahepatic malignancy over a median follow-up of 5.8 years (until December 2020) unequivocally established a significant association between MASLD and an increased risk of developing gastrointestinal cancers, with a risk increase of nearly 1.5–2 times. All risks were independent of confounders such as age, sex, smoking, obesity, type II diabetes mellitus. Insufficient data prevented a determination of any correlation between the severity of liver disease and an increase in extrahepatic cancer incidence rates [18].

In a Swedish nationwide, matched cohort study 10,568 individuals with biopsy-confirmed MASLD were included and matched to general population comparators ($n$ = 49,925) by age, sex, calendar year and county. Compared with controls, MASLD patients revealed significantly increased overall mortality (16.9 vs. 28.6 per 1000 person-years; aHR =1.93, 95% CI = 1.86–2.00). The MASLD-associated mortality was primarily related to extrahepatic cancer (4.5 per 1000 patient-years, aHR = 2.16, 95% CI = 2.03–2.30), followed by cirrhosis (2.7 per 1000 person-years, aHR =18.15, 95% CI =14.78–22.30), cardiovascular disease (1.4 per 1000 person-years, aHR = 1.35, 95% CI = 1.26–1.44), and hepatocellular carcinoma (HCC) (1.2 per 1000 person-years, aHR = 11.12, 95% CI = 8.65–14.30). In conclusion, excess mortality in MASLD was mainly related to extrahepatic cancer and cirrhosis, while in contrast, the contributions of cardiovascular disease and HCC were modest [29].

The observations mentioned above could be confirmed in a large-scale Korean nationwide study (5,265,590 individuals, age 20–39 years) specifically examining the risk of young-onset of gastrointestinal cancers (i.e., esophageal, stomach, colorectal, liver, pancreatic, biliary tract, and gallbladder) in the MASLD population. In result, 14,565 patients were newly diagnosed with GI-tract cancer. MASLD was associated with an increased risk of overall digestive tract (adjusted hazard ratio [aHR], 1.16; 95% CI, 1.10–1.22), stomach (aHR, 1.14; 95% CI, 1.06–1.24), colorectal (aHR, 1.14; 95% CI, 1.06–1.22), liver (aHR, 1.13; 95% CI, 1.12–1.52), pancreatic (aHR, 1.23; 95% CI, 1.09–1.40), biliary tract (aHR, 1.29; 95% CI, 1.00–1.66), and gallbladder (aHR, 1.53; 95% CI, 1.01–2.31) cancer. These associations were not confounded by age, sex, smoking status, alcohol consumption or obesity [22].

In conclusion, these findings strongly support the importance of preventing MASLD and detecting cancer early in adults with MASLD, irrespective of the presence of fibrosis or cirrhosis. The majority of studies had in common, that age, sex, education level, smoking, alcohol consumption are not confounding the clear correlation between extrahepatic cancers and MASLD.

## 8.4 Shared Pathways and Mechanisms

The association between gastrointestinal tract tumors and the metabolic syndrome, specifically diabetes mellitus type II and obesity, is a well-established fact. The severity of metabolic syndrome-related MASLD-associated liver disease strongly correlates with the risk of hepatocarcinogenesis. Additionally, MASLD increases the risk of carcinogenesis in the development of other gastrointestinal tumors, even in the absence of underlying progression to fibrosis. However, both tumor entities show similarities in the role of inflammation and obesity as the most significant drivers, despite their different carcinogenic pathways.

### 8.4.1 Sequence from MASLD to HCC

The sequence from MASLD to HCC and the influence of additive risks such as type II diabetes mellitus, genetic polymorphisms, and the stool microbiome are increasingly becoming the focus of current research [27]. Our understanding of these complex relationships is constantly evolving, and it is considered certain, that inflammation plays a pivotal role as a trigger in MASLD-related hepatocarcinogenesis, even without underlying liver cirrhosis. The progression from simple steatotic liver to MASH and, in the worst-case scenario, HCC is caused by the interplay of genetic variations, mitochondrial dysfunction, altered immune response, and microbiome imbalance, in addition to altered lipid and glucose metabolism in the context of metabolic syndrome.

Human hepatocarcinogenesis is always a multifactorial process. However, by understanding the various environmental influences (such as alcohol and smoking) and host factors (such as age, gender, familial predisposition, obesity, diabetes, and fibrosis) that interact with genetic, immunological, and viral factors, we can gain a better understanding of the development of HCC. It is important to note that DNA sequence changes in the form of mutations can lead to a resistance of proliferating hepatocytes to programmed cell death, or apoptosis, which allows mutated cells to proliferate unhindered.

### 8.4.2 Genetic Factors in Hepatocarcinogenesis

Genetic factors play a crucial role in the development of MASLD and its progression to MASH-fibrosis. Specifically, certain gene polymorphisms have been found to have a direct correlation with the prevalence of MASLD and the risk of progression to fibrosis. The Patatin-like phospholipase domain-containing 3 (PNPLA3)-gene polymorphism, for instance, has been shown to cause increased hepatic lipid accumulation and alteration of retinol storage in the liver. Research has shown that there is a three-fold increased risk of HCC, independent of potential confounding factors such as body mass index (BMI), diabetes, and advanced fibrosis [13]. This highlights the importance of considering these factors when assessing the risk of HCC. The correlation between the extent of steatosis and the progression of fibrosis in MASH has been established, regardless of obesity, diabetes, and PNPLA3 genotype. Increased genetic instability in MASH patients compared to MASLD also favors the development of HCC. Epigenetic changes cause aberrant DNA methylation and the expression of various microRNAs, such as miR-21, miR-29, miR-23, miR-155, miR-221, miR-222, miR-106, miR-93, and miR-519, which are all drivers of carcinogenesis. Here there is a direct and indirect influence on the most important tumor-associated signaling cascades (transforming growth factor beta (TGF-$\beta$), wingless and INT-1 (Wnt) / $\beta$-catenin, mitogen-activated protein kinase (MAPK) and phosphatidylinositol 3-kinase (PI3K)/AKT/mammalian target of rapamycin (mTOR) [16].

### 8.4.3 Immunological Signaling Pathways in HCC Development

Mitochondrial dysfunction and cellular stress play a significant role in the immunological mechanisms underlying the pathogenesis of HCC. The progression of MASLD is associated with various mechanisms, including insulin resistance and dysbiosis, which result in the formation of reactive oxygen species (ROS) and lipid peroxidation products. These, in turn, trigger the release of several pro-inflammatory cytokines, such as TNF-α, IL-1, and IL-6.

TNF-α activates procarcinogenic processes through the JNK/IκKb signaling pathway. IL-6 expression leads to the activation of STAT-3, an oncogenic transcription factor that plays a crucial role in the development of HCC in MASH patients, as demonstrated in various studies. Kupffer cells, which are liver-specific macrophages, release cytokines upon activation, leading to the activation of NK cells. This additional inflammatory stimulus significantly contributes to carcinogenesis. Inflammasomes, an important part of the innate immune defense, also play a crucial role in the progression of MASH [26].

Leptin activation has been shown to trigger several profibrotic and pro-oncogenic signaling cascades, including the Janus kinase (JAK)/STAT, mitogen-activated protein kinase (MAPK), telomerase reverse transcriptase (TERT), and PI3K pathways. Additionally, low adiponectin levels in the presence of peripheral insulin resistance can activate TNF-α and IL-6, reducing its anti-inflammatory effect (39).

Insulin resistance plays a crucial role in the development of metabolic syndrome and MASH. The induction of insulin-like growth factor-1 (IGF-1) also significantly contributes to this process by activating the PI3K and MAPK signaling pathways. The PI3K signaling pathway activation in hepatocarcinogenesis affects the cell cycle via cyclin D1, apoptosis via mouse double minute homolog 2 (MDM2)/p53, and cell growth via m-Tor. The MAPK signaling pathway also impacts tumor growth through the proto-oncogenes c-fos and c-jun. Furthermore, the Wnt/ß-catenin signaling pathway is activated.

Insulin resistance causes lipotoxicity of excess free fatty acids in the liver by activating lipolysis from visceral adipose tissue. This leads to the accumulation of reactive oxygen species (ROS), endoplasmic reticulum (ER) stress, and the induction of apoptosis. Glutathione peroxidase activation also results in the accumulation of free iron, which has a carcinogenic effect. Autophagy, as the cell's own recycling mechanism, plays a crucial role in the progression of MASH to HCC. Autophagy is a vital component in tumor control.

### 8.4.4 Influence of Gut Microbiome on HCC Risk

The gut microbiome plays a crucial role orchestrating the production of various metabolites, such as bile acids, and the regulation of metabolic pathways. It has been observed that dysbiosis, which refers to the alteration of the gut microbiome, is linked to MASLD, MASH, progression to cirrhosis, and associated complications.

Over the past decade, studies have demonstrated relevant alterations in the intestinal microbiome in relation to obesity. It has been observed that a leptin deficiency in obese mice is linked to an increased abundance of Firmicutes and a reduced expression of Bacteroidetes. This relationship has also been observed in further studies involving obese patients and has been associated with an improved energy yield from food and the formation of short-chain fatty acids (SCFA). It has been observed that the synthesis of deoxycholic acid (DCA), a secondary bile acid, is linked to an increased abundance of Firmicutes in Western diets. DCA is synthesized in the gut by Bacteroidetes and Clostridia from primary bile acids cholic acid (CA) and chenodeoxycholic acid (CDCA) [31].

Several rodent models have demonstrated that hepatic tumorigenesis can be reduced by intestinal sterilization, and bile acids such as DCA are considered significant metabolites. Hence, it can be said that the microbiome and its function in bile acid metabolism have a significant impact on the liver-gut axis, specifically on the bile acid receptor (FXR), which is a vital metabolic signaling pathway in hepatic carcinogenesis in MASH.

### 8.4.5 Extrahepatic Cancers in MASLD

In analogy to HCC, an increased rate of extrahepatic gastrointestinal malignancies is also seen in obesity-associated MASLD, and it is assumed that common mechanisms can contribute to carcinogenesis.

A common feature of both types of malignancy is obesity-related chronic inflammation, including NF-κB activation, as pivotal drivers of cancer [17]. Activation of NF-κB in immune cells is initiated by specific factors, including TNF-α, IL-1, and various pathogen-associated or damage-associated molecular patterns. This results in the production of pro-inflammatory cytokines, chemokines, and growth factors, such as TNF-α, IL-1, IL-6, and vascular endothelial growth factor (VEGF).

As mentioned above, adipokine signaling is a known factor in hepatocarcinogenesis, and it is possible that other pathways may also increase the risk of extrahepatic cancers through this mechanism. Adiponectin and leptin are prototypic adipokines with opposing effects. Adiponectin has substantial anti-inflammatory and insulin-sensitizing effects, while leptin favors a proinflammatory milieu [15]. The significant reduction in mortality after weight reduction by bariatric surgery impressively demonstrates the role of obesity-related adipokine alterations in the carcinogenesis of various gastrointestinal tumor entities [5]. Of note, gastric and colorectal cancers are typical examples of inflammation-dependent cancers, both associated with lowered plasma adiponectin concentrations [7].

The pivotal role of adiponectin in CRC carcinogenesis is highlighted by preclinical studies. By activating adenosine monophosphate-activated protein kinase (AMPK) and mTOR, this adipokine can effectively inhibit CRC cell growth [11]. MASLD may not be the only cause of adipokine disturbances that promote carcinogenesis. Again, in close analogy to HCC tumorigenesis, other mechanisms, such as increased production of ROS, IGF-1, or insulin resistance, may also contribute to this process. These mechanisms are activated through other inflammatory pathways, such as MAPK p38 signaling pathway.

## 8.5 Surveillance and Early Detection of MASLD-Related Cancers

In recent decades, there has been a steady increase in MASLD/MASH-associated tumor diseases predominantly of the gastrointestinal tract. While internationally agreed guidelines define the surveillance strategy for MASLD-associated HCC, there are no conclusive surveillance strategies for MASLD-associated extrahepatic gastrointestinal tumors despite a clear carcinogenic association.

### 8.5.1 Screening for HCC in MASLD

In Western industrialized countries, the incidence of HCC is increasing in proportion to the rising prevalence of MASLD. Late initial diagnosis contributes to the high mortality rate. A more effective monitoring strategy is needed to improve early detection and treatment outcomes. However, cure is possible in very early tumor stages through partial liver resection, ablation or liver transplantation. Current monitoring strategies, often based on liver sonography, are not very sensitive, especially in MASLD. Scoring systems based on biomarkers and risk factors can effectively stratify patients into risk groups and predict HCC before a tumor lesion in the liver is detectable by imaging techniques. This will enable more personalized monitoring intervals based on individual risk in the future. This will help to avoid overdiagnosis, which is psychosocially distressing for patients, and ensure the earliest possible detection of tumors. Patients undergoing liver transplantation due to a diagnosis of HCC can also benefit from such a risk stratification model, as the assessment of the risk of tumor recurrence after transplantation can be used to identify those patients who will significantly benefit from such an intervention. Established biomarkers and molecular genetic changes associated with the progression of fatty liver to HCC can optimize existing surveillance strategies in the future. An international surveillance strategy is needed for patients with MASH-associated HCC, given the increasing incidence of this disease worldwide. Surveillance is justified due to the high risk of HCC, despite the lack of a clear consensus among international guidelines for patients with non-cirrhotic MASH.

The American Association for the Study of Liver Diseases (AASLD) HCC guideline does not recommend surveillance for MASLD/MASH alone; only MASH cirrhotics should be offered sonography with or without alpha- fetoprotein (AFP) determination. Patients with MASLD but without cirrhosis, especially those with advanced fibrosis, will benefit from risk stratification tools to identify those at highest risk. Surveillance should be considered for selected patients with advanced fibrosis, particularly if there is clinical suspicion of potentially understaged fibrosis by noninvasive markers or biopsy [30].

A German retrospective single-center study showed that 41.7% of MASH-HCCs were in non-cirrhotic livers [10]. In addition, sensitivity of ultrasound-based monitoring in MASH patients is limited by both obesity and hepatic steatosis. In these patients, it is often not possible to adequately assess all liver segments. An Italian study showed that a BMI >25 was associated with a significantly reduced HCC detection rate [8]. Whether sonography alone can actually achieve a significant reduction in HCC-associated mortality in MASH patients has not been conclusively established [34].

Several early detection strategies have been tested to provide HCC patients with curative treatment options through earlier diagnosis. It is important to note that recent HCC guidelines tend to favor ultrasound alone over biomarker-based diagnostics, due to the cost-benefit ratio being a significant factor in the high-risk population.

A meta-analysis conducted in the USA investigated the sensitivity of sonography in detecting hepatocellular carcinoma (HCC) in a group of 13,367 patients at risk of HCC due to any etiology, with or without simultaneous AFP determination. The study found that ultrasound alone had a sensitivity of only 45%, which could be significantly increased to 63% by adding AFP. However, further research is required to establish whether sonography alone can reduce HCC-associated mortality. Prospective studies are urgently needed to clarify this issue [34].

The GALAD score was developed to improve the unsatisfactory performance of sonography-based HCC surveillance. This score includes age, gender, and the biomarkers AFP, AFP isoform L3 (AFP-L3), and des-7-gamma-carboxy-prothrombin (DCP). A recent multicenter study conducted in Japan and Germany demonstrated that the GALAD score can detect HCC with high sensitivity and good specificity in MASLD/MASH patient collectives, both in the presence and absence of cirrhosis. Early-stage HCC can be reliably detected [4]. However, due to the lack of prospective phase III data on the performance of the GALAD score in detecting HCC in MASH patients, its use in HCC surveillance is not currently recommended in the guidelines.

Further investigation is required to elucidate the role of technologies that may complement current biomarker-based surveillance strategies. Identifying a subset of patients at the highest risk is critical to concentrate the effort and resources of regular HCC screening [12]. Chromosomal aberrations, epigenetic abnormalities, and changes in gene expression play a pivotal role in hepatocarcinogenesis. Omics profiling, including transcriptomics, proteomics, and metabolomics, has identified several candidate biomarkers for HCC risk, which can improve HCC screening by enabling individual risk-stratified patient management. Transcriptomic dysregulations in chronic liver diseases indicate the functional molecular status that supports carcinogenesis. Circulating nucleic acids, proteins, and metabolites serve as measures of molecular HCC risk. Genetic and epigenetic abnormalities, gene expression profiles, and proteomics provide a wealth of data on HCC risk. Bioinformatics and network medicine play a crucial role in organizing and analyzing accumulated data [24]. These analyses enable the identification of a specific niche of application for each individual biomarker with confidence.

### 8.5.2 Screening for CRC in MASLD

Of all extrahepatic tumors, colorectal cancer has the most commonly described association with MASLD. However, it remains unclear whether this supports clear risk-stratified adaptations of previous CRC screening recommendations in the MASLD population.

An Asian meta-analysis of relevant observational studies (eight cross-sectional and three longitudinal) to quantify the magnitude of the association between MASLD and risk of colorectal adenoma and cancer (January 2000 to November 2017) suggests that MASLD is independently associated with a moderately increased prevalence and incidence of colorectal adenoma and cancer.

Another population-based study from Taiwan showed that patients with MASLD may have a 1.259-fold increased risk of CRC compared with those without MASLD (95% confidence interval [CI]: 1.047–1.486, $P = 0.003$) [38].

However, current data are insufficient to justify adjusting current screening intervals for CRC in MASLD patients. Due to the concomitant risk of HCC and CRC in the MASLD population, potential combined surveillance for both tumor entities may be significant in the future.

## 8.6 Clinical Implications and Patient Care

Both HCC and extrahepatic tumor diseases exhibit particular treatment limitations due to MASLD per se and associated metabolic comorbidities, both in curative and palliative therapy.

### 8.6.1 HCC Treatment in MASLD Patients

MASLD, as the underlying etiology, has special features that are relevant in both planned partial hepatectomy and in liver transplantation (LT).

The planning of a partial liver resection or listing for LT for HCC is already characterized by special features in MASH compared to other etiologies. Metabolic syndrome (especially T2DM and obesity), coronary artery disease and chronic renal insufficiency are known to be predictors of poorer postoperative and long-term outcomes.

Patients with MASH on the LT waiting list face several challenges: an overall higher age at listing, comorbidities and a lower MELD score compared to other etiologies. In the context of obesity and transplantation, the results of different meta-analyses are very different: some studies report worse post-LT survival in patients with a high BMI, while other studies report similar long-term outcomes as in normal-weight patients. It is clear that postoperative complication rates are higher in obese patients. Whether bariatric surgery combined with LT improves overall survival needs to be investigated in larger randomized trials. However, T2DM should be highlighted as a predictor of poor long-term graft and patient survival. In the future, the integrated weighting of MASH-associated comorbidities in the selection of MASH-HCC patients for potential LT listing will be a major challenge [20].

Systemic therapy is the preferred treatment for treating irresectable lesions in BCLC stage C HCC, although locoregional therapies may be possible in selected cases. Combination therapies that include immune checkpoint inhibitors (such as Atezolizumab + Bevacizumab or Durvalumab + Tremelimumab) are the recommended first-line treatment for HCC. It is important to note that there are initial indications that immune checkpoint inhibitors may be less effective in treating HCC related to MASLD than in HCC caused by other factors. A meta-analysis of three randomized phase III clinical trials has been conducted to test immune checkpoint inhibitors (ICI) in over 1600 patients with advanced HCC. The analysis has revealed that ICI therapy does not improve overall survival (OS) in patients with HCC of nonviral etiology. Furthermore, in two additional cohorts, patients with MASH-related HCC who received ICI treatment exhibited poorer OS compared to patients with other etiologies. These data strongly suggest that MASH-associated HCC may be less responsive to ICI treatment. Aberrant T-cell activation related to MASH is the likely cause of tissue damage and immune surveillance suppression [25]. Insufficient data prevents international clinical practice guidelines from drawing specific conclusions or recommending modifications to the current management of patients with HCC based on the underlying cause.

### 8.6.2 Cytotoxic Chemotherapy for Extrahepatic Neoplasia in MASLD

The steatotic liver is not only a therapeutic hurdle in the treatment of HCC; the use of cytotoxic chemotherapy can also have significant limitations in the treatment of a large number of extrahepatic gastrointestinal tumors.

A relevant number of patients develop mostly reversible chemotherapy-induced acute steatohepatitis (CASH) in the short-term following the application of cytoreductive chemotherapy. This entity is most frequently described in patients with colorectal liver metastases, most of whom received prior irinotecan or oxaliplatin-containing treatment regimens. However, methotrexate, 5-fluorouracil, tamoxifen and l-asparaginase can also induce this form of steatohepatitis. The CASH-inducing mechanism has not yet been fully clarified, but the triggering focus appears to be mitochondrial dysfunction with subsequent cascade from stellate-cell activation to inflammation. The predisposing risk factors appear to overlap significantly with those of MASH, namely all features of the metabolic syndrome, excessive alcohol consumption and previous liver damage of any genesis [23]. Interestingly, in analogy to MASH, similar predisposing gene polymorphisms, such as the PNPLA3 p.I148 M risk allele, appear to be present [6].

If there is pre-therapeutic evidence of altered liver function, such as elevated liver enzymes, steatosis on ultrasound, or even evidence of fibrosis (e.g., assessed by FIB-4 test, VCTE), and this cannot be readily explained by liver involvement by the tumor, then close monitoring of enzymes and liver function tests should be performed and biopsy may be considered in unclear cases. Some authors recommend quantification of histological changes observed in the liver by using a uniform scoring system, such as modified hepatitis activity scores [32].

## 8.7 Conclusion

In conclusion, pre-therapeutic damage to the liver parenchyma caused by steatosis must always be considered as an additive mortality factor when making treatment decisions, both in the treatment of primary liver cancer and extrahepatic tumors. Future prospective studies must help to stratify patients with MASLD/MASH into risk groups so that dose and treatment regimens can be adapted as necessary.

## References


1. Angulo P. Nonalcoholic fatty liver disease. N Engl J Med. 2002;346:1221–31.
2. Araujo AR, Rosso N, Bedogni G, Tiribelli C, Bellentani S. Global epidemiology of non-alcoholic fatty liver disease/non-alcoholic steatohepatitis: what we need in the future. Liver Int. 2018;38(Suppl 1):47–51.
3. Armstrong MJ, Adams LA, Canbay A, Syn WK. Extrahepatic complications of nonalcoholic fatty liver disease. Hepatology. 2014;59:1174–97.
4. Best J, Bechmann LP, Sowa JP, Sydor S, Dechene A, Pflanz K, Bedreli S, Schotten C, Geier A, Berg T, Fischer J, Vogel A, Bantel H, Weinmann A, Schattenberg JM, Huber Y, Wege H, Von Felden J, Schulze K, Bettinger D, Thimme R, Sinner F, Schutte K, Weiss KH, Toyoda H, Yasuda S, Kumada T, Berhane S, Wichert M, Heider D, Gerken G, Johnson P, Canbay A. GALAD score detects early hepatocellular carcinoma in an international cohort of patients with nonalcoholic steatohepatitis. Clin Gastroenterol Hepatol. 2020;18(3):728–735.e4.
5. Carlsson LMS, Sjoholm K, Jacobson P, Andersson-Assarsson JC, Svensson PA, Taube M, Carlsson B, Peltonen M. Life expectancy after bariatric surgery in the Swedish obese subjects study. N Engl J Med. 2020;383:1535–43.
6. Casper M, Zimmermann S, Weber SN, Arslanow A, Lammert F, Krawczyk M. Risk of chemotherapy-associated liver injury (CALI) in PNPLA3 p.148M allele carriers: preliminary results of a transient elastography-based study. Dig Liver Dis. 2020;52:102–6.
7. Coussens LM, Werb Z. Inflammation and cancer. Nature. 2002;420:860–7.
8. Del Poggio P, Olmi S, Ciccarese F, Di Marco M, Rapaccini GL, Benvegnu L, Borzio F, Farinati F, Zoli M, Giannini EG, Caturelli E, Chiaramonte M, Trevisani F, Italian Liver Cancer (ITA.LI.CA) Group. Factors that affect efficacy of ultrasound surveillance for early stage hepatocellular carcinoma in patients with cirrhosis. Clin Gastroenterol Hepatol. 2014;12(11):1927–33.e2.
9. El-Serag HB, Rudolph KL. Hepatocellular carcinoma: epidemiology and molecular carcinogenesis. Gastroenterology. 2007;132:2557–76.
10. Ertle J, Dechene A, Sowa JP, Penndorf V, Herzer K, Kaiser G, Schlaak JF, Gerken G, Syn WK, Canbay A. Non-alcoholic fatty liver disease progresses to hepatocellular carcinoma in the absence of apparent cirrhosis. Int J Cancer. 2011;128:2436–43.
11. Fujisawa T, Endo H, Tomimoto A, Sugiyama M, Takahashi H, Saito S, Inamori M, Nakajima N, Watanabe M, Kubota N, Yamauchi T, Kadowaki T, Wada K, Nakagama H, Nakajima A. Adiponectin suppresses colorectal carcinogenesis under the high-fat diet condition. Gut. 2008;57:1531–8.
12. Fujiwara N, Qian T, Koneru B, Hoshida Y. Omics-derived hepatocellular carcinoma risk biomarkers for precision care of chronic liver diseases. Hepatol Res. 2020;50:817–30.
13. Hassan MM, Kaseb A, Etzel CJ, El-Serag H, Spitz MR, Chang P, Hale KS, Liu M, Rashid A, Shama M, Abbruzzese JL, Loyer EM, Kaur H, Hassabo HM, Vauthey JN, Wray CJ, Hassan BS, Patt YZ, Hawk E, Soliman KM, Li D. Genetic variation in the PNPLA3 gene and hepatocellular carcinoma in USA: risk and prognosis prediction. Mol Carcinog. 2013;52(Suppl 1):E139–47.
14. Kanwal F, Kramer JR, Mapakshi S, Natarajan Y, Chayanupatkul M, Richardson PA, Li L, Desiderio R, Thrift AP, Asch SM, Chu J, El-Serag HB. Risk of hepatocellular cancer in patients with non-alcoholic fatty liver disease. Gastroenterology. 2018;155(6):1828–1837.e2.
15. Kucukoglu O, Sowa JP, Mazzolini GD, Syn WK, Canbay A. Hepatokines and adipokines in NASH-related hepatocellular carcinoma. J Hepatol. 2021;74:442–57.
16. Kutlu O, Kaleli HN, Ozer E. Molecular pathogenesis of nonalcoholic steatohepatitis- (NASH-) related hepatocellular carcinoma. Can J Gastroenterol Hepatol. 2018;2018:8543763.
17. Mantovani A, Allavena P, Sica A, Balkwill F. Cancer-related inflammation. Nature. 2008;454:436–44.
18. Mantovani A, Petracca G, Beatrice G, Csermely A, Tilg H, Byrne CD, Targher G. Non-alcoholic fatty liver disease and increased risk of incident extrahepatic cancers: a meta-analysis of observational cohort studies. Gut. 2022;71:778–88.
19. Margini C, Dufour JF. The story of HCC in NAFLD: from epidemiology, across pathogenesis, to prevention and treatment. Liver Int. 2016;36:317–24.
20. Mikolasevic I, Filipec-Kanizaj T, Mijic M, Jakopcic I, Milic S, Hrstic I, Sobocan N, Stimac D, Burra P. Nonalcoholic fatty liver disease and liver transplantation - where do we stand? World J Gastroenterol. 2018;24:1491–506.
21. Orci LA, Sanduzzi-Zamparelli M, Caballol B, Sapena V, Colucci N, Torres F, Bruix J, Reig M, Toso C. Incidence of hepatocellular carcinoma in patients with nonalcoholic fatty liver disease: a systematic review, meta-analysis, and meta-regression. Clin Gastroenterol Hepatol. 2022;20(2):283–292.e10.
22. Park JH, Hong JY, Shen JJ, Han K, Park JO, Park YS, Lim HY. Increased risk of young-onset digestive tract cancers among young adults age 20-39 years with nonalcoholic fatty liver disease: a nationwide cohort study. J Clin Oncol. 2023;41:3363–73.
23. Paternostro R, Sieghart W, Trauner M, Pinter M. Cancer and hepatic steatosis. ESMO Open. 2021;6:100185.
24. Pei Y, Zhang T, Renault V, Zhang X. An overview of hepatocellular carcinoma study by omics-based methods. Acta Biochim Biophys Sin Shanghai. 2009;41:1–15.

25. Pfister D, Nunez NG, Pinyol R, Govaere O, Pinter M, Szydlowska M, Gupta R, Qiu M, Deczkowska A, Weiner A, Muller F, Sinha A, Friebel E, Engleitner T, Lenggenhager D, Moncsek A, Heide D, Stirm K, Kosla J, Kotsiliti E, Leone V, Dudek M, Yousuf S, Inverso D, Singh I, Teijeiro A, Castet F, Montironi C, Haber PK, Tiniakos D, Bedossa P, Cockell S, Younes R, Vacca M, Marra F, Schattenberg JM, Allison M, Bugianesi E, Ratziu V, Pressiani T, D'alessio A, Personeni N, Rimassa L, Daly AK, Scheiner B, Pomej K, Kirstein MM, Vogel A, Peck-Radosavljevic M, Hucke F, Finkelmeier F, Waidmann O, Trojan J, Schulze K, Wege H, Koch S, Weinmann A, Bueter M, Rossler F, Siebenhuner A, De Dosso S, Mallm JP, Umansky V, Jugold M, Luedde T, Schietinger A, Schirmacher P, Emu B, Augustin HG, Billeter A, Muller-Stich B, Kikuchi H, Duda DG, Kutting F, Waldschmidt DT, Ebert MP, Rahbari N, Mei HE, Schulz AR, Ringelhan M, Malek N, Spahn S, Bitzer M, Ruiz De Galarreta M, Lujambio A, Dufour JF, Marron TU, Kaseb A, Kudo M, Huang YH, Djouder N, Wolter K, Zender L, Marche PN, Decaens T, Pinato DJ, Rad R, Mertens JC, Weber A, Unger K, et al. NASH limits anti-tumour surveillance in immunotherapy-treated HCC. Nature. 2021;592:450–6.
26. Pierantonelli I, Svegliati-Baroni G. Nonalcoholic fatty liver disease: basic pathogenetic mechanisms in the progression from NAFLD to NASH. Transplantation. 2019;103:e1–e13.
27. Reimer KC, Wree A, Roderburg C, Tacke F. New drugs for NAFLD: lessons from basic models to the clinic. Hepatol Int. 2020;14:8–23.
28. Seyda Seydel G, Kucukoglu O, Altinbasv A, Demir OO, Yilmaz S, Akkiz H, Otan E, Sowa JP, Canbay A. Economic growth leads to increase of obesity and associated hepatocellular carcinoma in developing countries. Ann Hepatol. 2016;15:662–72.
29. Simon TG, Roelstraete B, Khalili H, Hagstrom H, Ludvigsson JF. Mortality in biopsy-confirmed nonalcoholic fatty liver disease: results from a nationwide cohort. Gut. 2021;70:1375–82.
30. Singal AG, Llovet JM, Yarchoan M, Mehta N, Heimbach JK, Dawson LA, Jou JH, Kulik LM, Agopian VG, Marrero JA, Mendiratta-Lala M, Brown DB, Rilling WS, Goyal L, Wei AC, Taddei TH. AASLD practice guidance on prevention, diagnosis, and treatment of hepatocellular carcinoma. Hepatology. 2023;78:1922–65.
31. Sydor S, Best J, Messerschmidt I, Manka P, Vilchez-Vargas R, Brodesser S, Lucas C, Wegehaupt A, Wenning C, Assmuth S, Hohenester S, Link A, Faber KN, Moshage H, Cubero FJ, Friedman SL, Gerken G, Trauner M, Canbay A, Bechmann LP. Altered microbiota diversity and bile acid signaling in cirrhotic and noncirrhotic NASH-HCC. Clin Transl Gastroenterol. 2020;11:e00131.
32. Tannapfel A, Reinacher-Schick A. Chemotherapy associated hepatotoxicity in the treatment of advanced colorectal cancer (CRC). Z Gastroenterol. 2008;46:435–40.
33. Thomas JA, Kendall BJ, Dalais C, Macdonald GA, Thrift AP. Hepatocellular and extrahepatic cancers in non-alcoholic fatty liver disease: a systematic review and meta-analysis. Eur J Cancer. 2022;173:250–62.
34. Tzartzeva K, Obi J, Rich NE, Parikh ND, Marrero JA, Yopp A, Waljee AK, Singal AG. Surveillance imaging and alpha fetoprotein for early detection of hepatocellular carcinoma in patients with cirrhosis: a meta-analysis. Gastroenterology. 2018;154(6):1706–1718.e1.
35. Vernon G, Baranova A, Younossi ZM. Systematic review: the epidemiology and natural history of non-alcoholic fatty liver disease and non-alcoholic steatohepatitis in adults. Aliment Pharmacol Ther. 2011;34:274–85.
36. Weinmann A, Alt Y, Koch S, Nelles C, Duber C, Lang H, Otto G, Zimmermann T, Marquardt JU, Galle PR, Worns MA, Schattenberg JM. Treatment and survival of non-alcoholic steatohepatitis associated hepatocellular carcinoma. BMC Cancer. 2015;15:210.
37. Wong RJ, Cheung R, Ahmed A. Nonalcoholic steatohepatitis is the most rapidly growing indication for liver transplantation in patients with hepatocellular carcinoma in the U.S. Hepatology. 2014;59:2188–95.
38. Wu PH, Chung CH, Wang YH, Hu JM, Chien WC, Cheng YC. Association between nonalcoholic fatty liver disease and colorectal cancer: a population-based study. Medicine (Baltimore). 2023;102:e33867.
39. Xiang X, You XM, Zhong JH, Li LQ. Hepatocellular carcinoma in the absence of cirrhosis in patients with chronic hepatitis B virus infection. J Hepatol. 2017;67:885–6.
40. Younossi Z, Stepanova M, Ong JP, Jacobson IM, Bugianesi E, Duseja A, Eguchi Y, Wong VW, Negro F, Yilmaz Y, Romero-Gomez M, George J, Ahmed A, Wong R, Younossi I, Ziayee M, Afendy A, Global Nonalcoholic Steatohepatitis Council. Nonalcoholic steatohepatitis is the fastest growing cause of hepatocellular carcinoma in liver transplant candidates. Clin Gastroenterol Hepatol. 2019;17(4):748–755.e3.

# 9 Current Standards in Therapeutic Management

Jesse Pustjens and Willem P. Brouwer

## 9.1 Introduction

As we have seen, MASLD is a complex disease influenced by many genetic and environmental factors. Likewise, the clinical manifestation of MASLD can range from a subclinical disease to a progressive disease with hepatic and extra-hepatic conditions, such as liver cirrhosis and cardiovascular disease. With respect to this complexity, it becomes clear that there is no "one-size-fits-all" therapeutic approach (Fig. 9.1). To date, drug that effectively improve steatosis and fibrosis are limited, and it is reasonable to believe that there will no one drug will be able to completely cure the complex and multifaceted disease that is MASLD [1]. Rather, a successful therapeutic approach should be multidisciplinary and tailored to a patient's specific lifestyle and disease burden. Ultimately, the goal of treatment should be to decrease MASH-related mortality, reduce progression to cirrhosis or HCC and improvement of general cardiometabolic health [2]. For the majority of those with MASLD, lifestyle modification will form the primary method to reach these goals, but pharmacological or surgical options can be considered under certain conditions.

J. Pustjens · W. P. Brouwer (✉)
Department of Gastroenterology and Hepatology, Erasmus University Medical Center Rotterdam, Rotterdam, The Netherlands
e-mail: j.pustjens@erasmusmc.nl; w.p.brouwer@erasmusmc.nl



N. Méndez-Sánchez, X. Qi (eds.), *Metabolic Dysfunction-Associated Steatotic Liver Disease*,
https://doi.org/10.1007/978-981-97-9519-2_9

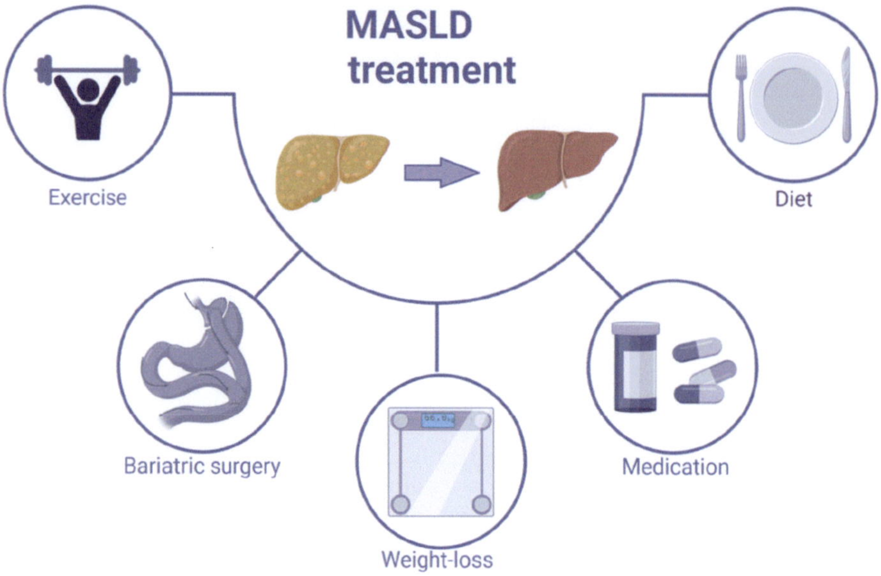


**Fig. 9.1** Current proposed treatments for MASLD. Although specific therapeutical options are limited, general strategies have been proposed to manage it include: physical exercise, bariatric surgery, weight loss, medication, and diet

## 9.2 Lifestyle Modifications: Diet, Exercise, and Weight Loss

Due to the intricate relation between MASLD, adiposity and insulin resistance, weight loss should be a key goal in any lifestyle modification program for overweight individuals (BMI ≥25 kg/M$^2$). Clinical practice guidelines recommend 7–10% total weight loss in order to improve hepatic steatosis, MASH and fibrosis [2, 3]. However, even modest weight loss (>5%) has been shown to reduce hepatic steatosis and insulin resistance [4]. Caloric deficits of 500–1000 kcal/day are suggested to reach a weight loss of around 500–1000 g/week [3]. Sustained weight reduction is however challenging for many, and warrants for long-term guidance with a multidisciplinary approach with respect to patient-specific barriers, and may include consultation of nutritionists, dietitians, health psychologists and consideration of family engagement and socioeconomic status [5].

In MASLD patients with a healthy BMI, where weight loss might be less of a priority, improved diet composition should still be promoted as this has been shown to lead to improved liver health [6]. Some data even suggests that nonobese MASLD patients benefit from modest weight loss as this can achieve steatosis remission [7]. Furthermore, these "lean" MASLD appear to be more likely to maintain their weight reduction compared to their obese counterparts.

In MASLD patients, the degree of weight reduction correlates strongly with disease regression, regardless of the method used [4]. However, different dietary approaches exist that are associate with MASLD, independent of total energy intake. Four researched dietary approaches are highlighted here, but many others exist.

### 9.2.1 Western Diet (WD)

The WD, prevalent in many developed countries, is marked by its predominant consumption of animal products such as red meat, processed meats, lards, and dairy items, as well as junk foods, sodas, and sugary snacks. Conversely, it tends to be poor in foods like whole grains, fruits, vegetables, and fish. This dietary pattern often results in an overconsumption of calories and an unbalanced nutrient profile, characterized by excessive intake of saturated fats, refined sugars, and salts. Numerous studies have demonstrated its association with adverse health outcomes, including a heightened risk of obesity, insulin resistance, and MASLD [8]. Consequently, individuals with MASLD should avoid or significantly modify this dietary pattern.

### 9.2.2 Mediterranean Diet (MD)

Characterized by high intake of fruits, vegetables, legumes, cereals, fish, and with extra virgin olive oil as is primary source of fat, the MD is widely recognized as a healthy dietary pattern. Studies have demonstrated its effectiveness in promoting weight loss, improving metabolic parameters, and reducing the risk of cardiovascular disease [1]. In the context of MASLD, the MD has been shown to be associated with regression of hepatic steatosis and fibrosis, and even HCC [8]. The health benefits of the MD are largely attributed to its high content of polyphenols, bioactive compounds abundant in plant-based foods central to the MD. Polyphenols have been suggested to be protective against several malignancies, cardiovascular diseases, diabetes, as well as MASLD [1]. However, there remains an unmet need for high-quality randomized controlled trials to further substantiate these findings.

### 9.2.3 Dietary Approaches to Stopping Hypertension (DASH)

The DASH diet has been used to treat and prevent hypertension since the 1990s. It stands out by a low saturated fat and salts content, while being high in proteins and fiber. This dietary approach emphasizes the consumption of fruits, vegetables, fish, whole grains, nuts, seeds, legumes, low-fat dairy products and minimizes the intake of fats, red meat and refined sugars. In general, DASH emphasizes the consumption of minimally processed and fresh foods. Its protective effects in cardiovascular disease has been well established, and evidence is now emerging to support the use of DASH as a preventive tool for MASLD [8].

### 9.2.4 Intermittent Calorie Restriction

Rather than a diet based on nutrient guidelines, periodic caloric restriction is a dietary approach based around restricting the feeding period. Various patterns exist, in which fasting periods are followed by intervals with ad-libitum food consumption. Besides leading to a reduced calorie intake, periodic fasting seems to provoke several physiological changes that are associated with several health benefits [6]. Concerning MASLD, periodic fasting has demonstrated its effects in reduction of hepatic steatosis, improvement of fibrosis-scores and liver enzymes, although more clinical trials are needed to corroborate these findings [8].

Alongside a balanced diet, physical exercise plays a crucial role in treating MASLD. Remarkably, even without weight loss, exercise can produce a 20–30% relative reduction in hepatic steatosis [9]. This effect is attributed to several factors, including enhanced peripheral insulin sensitivity, reduced visceral fat, and increased clearance of very low-density lipoprotein (VLDL) [4]. Current clinical practice guidelines recommend ≥150 min of moderate-intensity physical exercise per week [2]. Various forms of exercise (aerobic exercise, resistance exercise, or high intensity intermittent exercise) seem to yield similar results for reducing hepatic steatosis [9]. Therefore, the choice of exercise should be tailored to individual patient preferences and capabilities. The beneficial effects of physical exercise should not be underestimated as they are far-reaching, especially in the cardiometabolic domain. Nevertheless, the impact of physical exercise on hepatic steatosis remains modest when compared to weight reduction, which has the potential to reduce steatosis by >80% [10].

## 9.3 Pharmacological Interventions: Beyond Metformin and Statins

Currently, pharmacological options aimed specifically at MASH are emerging. Additionally, several agents that are approved for other indications, have shown their potential in reducing hepatic steatosis and even fibrosis.

### 9.3.1 Resmetirom

The urgent need for approved drugs that target MASLD or MASH specifically, makes for exciting times. Recently, Resmetirom emerged as the first approved drug to treat MASH with liver fibrosis [11]. Resmetirom is an oral, liver-directed thyroid hormone receptor selective agonist that targets mitochondrial function and β-oxidation of fatty acids. It has demonstrated its efficacy in MASH resolution and improvement of liver fibrosis. It also improved dyslipidemia, but otherwise had an overall neutral effects on body weight, insulin resistance, glycemia, heart rate, and blood pressure. The safety profile is acceptable, with only nausea, vomiting, and diarrhea occurring more often with Resmetirom compared to the placebo. Although this represents a major step in MASH treatment, the placebo-subtracted effect of Resmetirom is overall modest (approximately 2 of 10 patients treated will have MASH resolution and approximately 1 of 10 patients treated will have fibrosis improvement). Therefore, treatment should be combined with other aforementioned therapeutic options.

### 9.3.2 GLP-1 Receptor Agonists (GLP1-RA)

GLP-1 is a hormone released after food intake that promotes insulin secretion and suppresses glucagon secretion. It also reduces gastric emptying and enhances feelings of satiety. Besides its indication as a glucose lowering drug in diabetic patients, it is also able to induce significant weight loss (on average 3–5 kg) [12]. Due to the overlapping pathophysiology of diabetes and MASLD, GLP1-RAs are subject of clinical studies, but it has not yet been approved in the treatment of MASH. In studies on MASH patients, GLP1-RAs reduced fibrosis progression compared to a placebo, with a dose-dependent response [13]. Overall, most studies on GLP1-RAs in MASLD or MASH favor their effectiveness and safety, but prospective data are needed to conform treatment dose and duration [12]. Additionally, careful consideration of its side effects are needed, which are predominantly gastrointestinal such as diarrhea, vomiting, and obstipation, but also pancreatitis.

### 9.3.3 Vitamin E

Vitamin E has potent antioxidative effects and has demonstrated some beneficial effects in MASLD treatments under certain circumstances [3]. The therapeutic mechanisms of vitamin E are believed to be diverse, including improved lipid and glucose metabolism and reduction of oxidative stress [14]. In a clinical trial involving nondiabetic MASH patients, treatment with 800 IU of vitamin E per day for 96 weeks resulted in significant improvements in serum liver enzymes and certain histological features compared to placebo [15]. Data regarding its effects in diabetic patients is however still lacking, as well as its effect on fibrosis reduction. However, a retrospective study on MASH patients with advanced fibrosis suggested that vitamin E use was associated with decreased risks of hepatic decompensation and increased transplant free survival. Despite these promising results, caution is warranted in prescribing long-term vitamin E therapy, particularly due to yet-to-be elucidated associations with hemorrhagic stroke and prostate cancer [16, 17].

### 9.3.4 Sodium-Glucose Cotransporter-2 Inhibitors (SGLT-2i)

SGLT-2i have emerged as an effective oral glucose lowering drug in the treatment of diabetes mellitus type 2. This class of drug exert their effects by inhibiting glucose reabsorption in the kidneys, thereby promoting urinary glucose excretion. Besides lowering blood glucose levels, this induces a 2–3% weight loss, attributed to a negative energy balance and increased lipid metabolism [13, 18]. As a result of these effects, SGLT-2i have become subject of research in the field of MASLD. Animal MASH models demonstrated potential beneficial effects of SGLT-2i on liver steatosis, inflammation and fibrosis, findings now gaining support from clinical studies [18]. Treatment with SGLT-2i inhibitors have been shown to decrease serum transaminase, GGT levels as well as hepatic steatosis in MASLD patients [19]. Additionally, SGLT-2i have demonstrated cardiovascular and renal protective effects, which could be particularly advantageous in patients with MASLD who often have concomitant metabolic and cardiovascular comorbidities. However, the hepatoprotective effects of SLGT-2i still have to be confirmed in a large RCT setting and with histological outcomes, before they will be approved in the treatment of MASLD. Furthermore, their safety profile needs to be investigated in this patient group, as they are known to be associated with hypoglycemia, ketoacidosis, and urinary tract infections [20].

## 9.4 Role of Bariatric Surgery in MASLD Management

For those MASLD patients with insufficient response to lifestyle modifications and pharmacological treatment, bariatric surgery can be an alternative for achieving weight reduction and managing metabolic complications [2]. Current guidelines dictate that individuals with a BMI $\geq$40 kg/m$^2$ can be considered for bariatric surgery, irrespective of metabolic comorbidities. Additionally, in those with a BMI $\geq$35 kg/m$^2$, in combination with (pre-) diabetes mellitus type 2, uncontrolled hypertension, osteoarthritis of hip or knee or urinary incontinence, surgery may also be considered. Currently, MASH is gaining recognition as comorbidity that also stands to benefit from bariatric surgery [3]. The vast majority those that are eligible for bariatric surgery under current guidelines have MASLD (86.6%), and many suffer from its more severe form of MASH (36.7%) [21].

The cardiometabolic benefits of bariatric surgery are mainly associated with the amount of realized weight loss that comes forth from restriction of the gastric volume and malabsorption of nutrients [1]. It can induce sustained weight loss up 30%, and improve insulin resistance, hypertension, dyslipidemia and obstructive sleep apnea [22]. Importantly, the therapeutic effects of bariatric surgery on MASLD and MASH resolution are profound and conformed with histological outcomes, including fibrosis. Studies have shown that following bariatric surgery, there is a resolution of steatosis in 56%, hepatocyte ballooning in 49%, inflammation in 45% and fibrosis in 25% of postoperative liver biopsies [23]. This indicates that bariatric surgery could be recommended as a treatment of MASLD in patients with obesity. However, if substantial weight loss is not achieved following bariatric surgery, MASH is likely to persist [24].

Commonly used bariatric procedures include laparoscopic sleeve gastrectomy, laparoscopic Roux-en-Y gastric bypass and laparoscopic adjustable gastric banding. Data comparing outcomes of these different procedures are limited, but it is well accepted that Roux-en-Y gastric bypass offers greater advantages over laparoscopic sleeve gastrectomy in terms of diabetes remission, weight loss, and hypertension control [23]. However, some evidence indicate that laparoscopic sleeve gastrectomy may have a greater impact on steatosis and fibrosis incidence [25].

Needless to say, potential benefits of surgical intervention must be weighed against the risk of perioperative a postoperative complications. Proper patient selection is key in this regard. Fortunately, MASH does not appear to influence the complication rate of bariatric surgery [26]. However, in cirrhotic patients, caution is warranted as they have a 2.67 times higher risk of perioperative complications. Meta-analyses have indicated that in cases of compensated cirrhosis, bariatric surgery is considered both effective and safe, contrasting with decompensated cirrhosis where mortality rates are notably higher (0.9% vs. 18.2%) [27].

## 9.5 Collaborative Care Models and Patient Empowerment

MASLD is a complex and multisystem disease and successful treatment can be a challenging feat for health care providers. With limited effective pharmaceutical treatments, lifestyle modifications remain the cornerstone in most treatment strategies. While advise on weight loss, physical exercise and dietary approaches are easily given, they are famously difficult to adhere to. To maximize therapeutic success, many stakeholders should play a role MASLD treatment. Although data on this subject is limited, a multidisciplinary approach to MASLD has been shown to be clinically effective and potentially cost-effective [28]. Treatment should be patient centered and consulting specialties should be chosen with respect to patient-specific needs but may include diabetologists, cardiologists, nephrologists, psychiatrists, physiatrists, dentists, nutritionists, and pharmacists [29].

## References


1. Mantovani A, Dalbeni A. Treatments for NAFLD: state of art. Int J Mol Sci. 2021;22(5):2350.
2. European Association for the Study of the L, European Association for the Study of D, European Association for the Study of O. EASL-EASD-EASO clinical practice guidelines for the management of non-alcoholic fatty liver disease. J Hepatol. 2016;64(6):1388–402.
3. Rinella ME, Neuschwander-Tetri BA, Siddiqui MS, Abdelmalek MF, Caldwell S, Barb D, et al. AASLD practice guidance on the clinical assessment and management of nonalcoholic fatty liver disease. Hepatology. 2023;77(5):1797–835.
4. Romero-Gomez M, Zelber-Sagi S, Trenell M. Treatment of NAFLD with diet, physical activity and exercise. J Hepatol. 2017;67(4):829–46.
5. Lowe MR, Miller-Kovach K, Phelan S. Weight-loss maintenance in overweight individuals one to five years following successful completion of a commercial weight loss program. Int J Obes Relat Metab Disord. 2001;25(3):325–31.
6. Semmler G, Datz C, Reiberger T, Trauner M. Diet and exercise in NAFLD/NASH: beyond the obvious. Liver Int. 2021;41(10):2249–68.
7. Wong VW, Wong GL, Chan RS, Shu SS, Cheung BH, Li LS, et al. Beneficial effects of lifestyle intervention in non-obese patients with non-alcoholic fatty liver disease. J Hepatol. 2018;69(6):1349–56.
8. Torres-Pena JD, Arenas-de Larriva AP, Alcala-Diaz JF, Lopez-Miranda J, Delgado-Lista J. Different dietary approaches, non-alcoholic fatty liver disease and cardiovascular disease: a literature review. Nutrients. 2023;15(6):1483.
9. Hashida R, Kawaguchi T, Bekki M, Omoto M, Matsuse H, Nago T, et al. Aerobic vs. resistance exercise in non-alcoholic fatty liver disease: a systematic review. J Hepatol. 2017;66(1):142–52.
10. Thoma C, Day CP, Trenell MI. Lifestyle interventions for the treatment of non-alcoholic fatty liver disease in adults: a systematic review. J Hepatol. 2012;56(1):255–66.
11. Harrison SA, Bedossa P, Guy CD, Schattenberg JM, Loomba R, Taub R, et al. A phase 3, randomized, controlled trial of Resmetirom in NASH with liver fibrosis. N Engl J Med. 2024;390(6):497–509.
12. Rong L, Zou J, Ran W, Qi X, Chen Y, Cui H, et al. Advancements in the treatment of non-alcoholic fatty liver disease (NAFLD). Front Endocrinol (Lausanne). 2022;13:1087260.
13. Newsome PN, Buchholtz K, Cusi K, Linder M, Okanoue T, Ratziu V, et al. A placebo-controlled trial of subcutaneous Semaglutide in nonalcoholic steatohepatitis. N Engl J Med. 2021;384(12):1113–24.
14. He W, Xu Y, Ren X, Xiang D, Lei K, Zhang C, et al. Vitamin E ameliorates lipid metabolism in mice with nonalcoholic fatty liver disease via Nrf2/CES1 signaling pathway. Dig Dis Sci. 2019;64(11):3182–91.
15. Sanyal AJ, Chalasani N, Kowdley KV, McCullough A, Diehl AM, Bass NM, et al. Pioglitazone, vitamin E, or placebo for nonalcoholic steatohepatitis. N Engl J Med. 2010;362(18):1675–85.
16. Gaziano JM, Sesso HD, Christen WG, Bubes V, Smith JP, MacFadyen J, et al. Multivitamins in the prevention of cancer in men: the Physicians' Health Study II randomized controlled trial. JAMA. 2012;308(18):1871–80.
17. Neuhouser ML, Barnett MJ, Kristal AR, Ambrosone CB, King IB, Thornquist M, et al. Dietary supplement use and prostate cancer risk in the carotene and retinol efficacy trial. Cancer Epidemiol Biomarkers Prev. 2009;18(8):2202–6.
18. Katsiki N, Perakakis N, Mantzoros C. Effects of sodium-glucose co-transporter-2 (SGLT2) inhibitors on non-alcoholic fatty liver disease/non-alcoholic steatohepatitis: ex quo et quo vadimus? Metabolism. 2019;98:iii.
19. Mantovani A, Petracca G, Csermely A, Beatrice G, Targher G. Sodium-glucose Cotransporter-2 inhibitors for treatment of nonalcoholic fatty liver disease: a meta-analysis of randomized controlled trials. Meta. 2020;11(1):22.
20. Mascolo A, Di Napoli R, Balzano N, Cappetta D, Urbanek K, De Angelis A, et al. Safety profile of sodium glucose co-transporter 2 (SGLT2) inhibitors: a brief summary. Front Cardiovasc Med. 2022;9:1010693.
21. Mazzini GS, Augustin T, Noria S, Romero-Marrero C, Li N, Hameed B, et al. ASMBS position statement

on the impact of metabolic and bariatric surgery on nonalcoholic steatohepatitis. Surg Obes Relat Dis. 2022;18(3):314–25.
22. Nguyen NT, Varela JE. Bariatric surgery for obesity and metabolic disorders: state of the art. Nat Rev Gastroenterol Hepatol. 2017;14(3):160–9.
23. Zhou H, Luo P, Li P, Wang G, Yi X, Fu Z, et al. Bariatric surgery improves nonalcoholic fatty liver disease: systematic review and meta-analysis. Obes Surg. 2022;32(6):1872–83.
24. Lassailly G, Caiazzo R, Ntandja-Wandji LC, Gnemmi V, Baud G, Verkindt H, et al. Bariatric surgery provides long-term resolution of nonalcoholic steatohepatitis and regression of fibrosis. Gastroenterology. 2020;159(4):1290–301 e5.
25. de Barros F, Fonseca ABM. Bariatric surgery during the evolution of fatty liver-a randomized clinical trial comparing gastric bypass and sleeve gastrectomy based on transient elastography. Clin Obes. 2020;10(6):e12393.
26. Weingarten TN, Swain JM, Kendrick ML, Charlton MR, Schroeder BJ, Lee RE, et al. Nonalcoholic steatohepatitis (NASH) does not increase complications after laparoscopic bariatric surgery. Obes Surg. 2011;21(11):1714–20.
27. Bai J, Jia Z, Chen Y, Li Y, Zheng S, Duan Z. Bariatric surgery is effective and safe for obese patients with compensated cirrhosis: a systematic review and meta-analysis. World J Surg. 2022;46(5):1122–33.
28. Moolla A, Motohashi K, Marjot T, Shard A, Ainsworth M, Gray A, et al. A multidisciplinary approach to the management of NAFLD is associated with improvement in markers of liver and cardio-metabolic health. Frontline Gastroenterol. 2019;10(4):337–46.
29. Yoneda M, Kobayashi T, Iwaki M, Nogami A, Saito S, Nakajima A. Nonalcoholic fatty liver disease as a systemic disease and the need for multidisciplinary care. Gut Liver. 2023;17(6):843–52.

# 10 Revolutionary Breakthroughs

Nahum Méndez-Sánchez
and Mariana M. Ramírez-Mejía

## 10.1 Introduction

Metabolic dysfunction-associated steatotic liver disease (MASLD) encompasses a spectrum of liver diseases ranging from simple steatosis to metabolic steatohepatitis (MASH), which involves inflammation and possible progression to fibrosis, cirrhosis and even hepatocellular carcinoma (HCC) [1]. Traditional approaches to the treatment of MASLD have focused on lifestyle modifications, such as diet and exercise, aimed at reducing obesity and insulin resistance (IR) [2]. Although these interventions remain key strategies, they are often insufficient, especially in patients with advanced stages of the disease or resistant to lifestyle changes [3]. As the MASLD and MASH epidemic grows, the search for new drug targets and treatment strategies is becoming increasingly imperative [4]. The identification of novel drug targets in MASLD and MASH represents a promising avenue for therapeutic innovation. These targets span a wide range of biological pathways involved in disease pathogenesis, offering diverse opportunities for intervention (Fig. 10.1) [5].

N. Méndez-Sánchez (✉) · M. M. Ramírez-Mejía
Faculty of Medicine, National Autonomous University of Mexico, Mexico City, Mexico

Liver Research Unit, Medica Sur Clinic and Foundation, Mexico City, Mexico
e-mail: nmendez@medicasur.org.mx



N. Méndez-Sánchez, X. Qi (eds.), *Metabolic Dysfunction-Associated Steatotic Liver Disease*,
https://doi.org/10.1007/978-981-97-9519-2_10

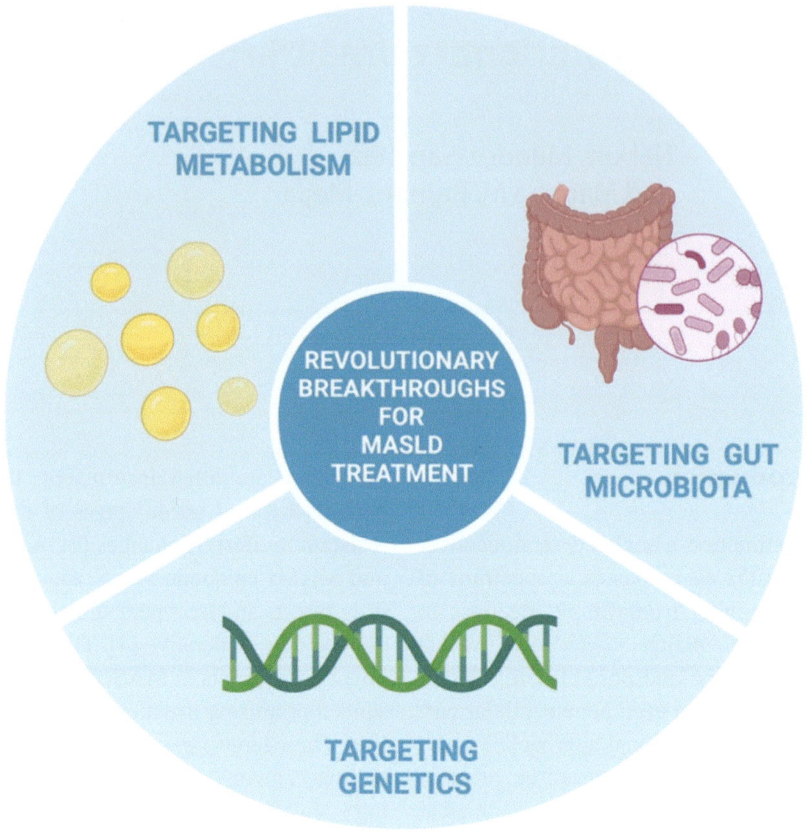


**Fig. 10.1** This figure illustrates the key therapeutic strategies and breakthroughs in the treatment of metabolic dysfunction-associated steatotic liver disease (MASLD). The figure highlights three major therapeutic approaches: targeting hepatic lipid metabolism, modulating gut microbiota, and gene therapies

## 10.2 Targeting Hepatic Lipid Metabolism

Dysregulation of lipid metabolism constitutes a central pillar in the pathogenesis of MASLD. Targeting hepatic lipid metabolism represents a crucial avenue for the development of new therapies in the treatment of MASLD [6]. New therapies, targeting specific enzymes, receptors and pathways involved in hepatic lipid metabolism, aim to restore lipid homeostasis, mitigate liver injury and halt liver disease progression [7].

### 10.2.1 Targeting Enzymes

#### 10.2.1.1 ACC Inhibitors

One promising approach is the inhibition of lipogenesis pathways, specifically targeting key enzymes such as acetyl-CoA carboxylase (ACC) and stearoyl-CoA desaturase-1 (SCD-1). ACC is involved in the ATP-dependent transformation of acetyl-coenzyme A (CoA) to malonyl-CoA, which is a crucial and limiting step in de novo lipogenesis (DNL) [8]. It has been observed that pharmacological inhibition of ACC reduced hepatic malonyl-CoA levels and enhanced hepatic ketogenesis, inhibiting DNL and fatty acid accumulation in the liver. The consequent reduction in polyunsaturated fatty acids (PUFAs) in the liver, due to diminished malonyl-CoA, results in PUFAs deficiency. This shortage triggers the activation of SREBP-1c, which subsequently elevates GPAT1 levels and increases very low density lipoprotein (VLDL) secretion. This sequence of events contributes to the occurrence of hypertriglyceridemia, recognized as the main adverse effect related to the use of ACC inhibitors (iACC) [9–11]. Recent advancements in the field have led to the development of innovative approaches aimed at mitigating the adverse effects associated with iACC [12]. The coadministration of iACC with diacylglycerol acyltransferase 2 (DGAT2) inhibitors presents a promising strategy. This combination has been shown to significantly reduce hepatic fat accumulation and liver injury, without the undesirable elevation of serum triglycerides that occurs when iACCs are administered alone [11].

#### 10.2.1.2 DGAT2 Inhibitors

DGAT2 is a crucial enzyme for the final step of triglyceride synthesis, in which it catalyzes the addition of a fatty acid to diacylglycerol (DAG) to form triglycerides. Since triglyceride accumulation is a hallmark of MASLD, inhibiting DGAT2 activity has been proposed as a strategy to reduce hepatic lipid accumulation, which could reverse or prevent MASLD progression [13, 14]. Inhibition of DGAT2 not only directly prevents the final step of triglyceride synthesis in hepatocytes, but also triggers adaptive responses in the liver that further mitigate lipid accumulation. These responses include downregulation of genes encoding lipogenic enzymes and induction of pathways involved in fatty acid oxidation [15, 16]. Clinical exploration of DGAT2 inhibitors has yielded promising initial results. Small molecule inhibitors, such as ervogastat, have been the subject of clinical trials, showing notable reductions in hepatic fat content in short-term studies [16, 17]. In addition, antisense oligonucleotides (ASOs) targeting DGAT2, such as IONIS-DGAT2rx, represent an innovative gene silencing approach to reduce hepatic fat content, offering an alternative to small molecule inhibitors [18].

#### 10.2.1.3 FASN Inhibitors

Fatty acid synthase (FAS), another enzyme involved in DNL, is also considered a potential therapeutic target [19]. FAS is responsible for the last stage of DNL, transforming acetyl-CoA and malonyl-CoA into palmitate [20]. Recent research has highlighted that platensimycin (PTM) is a potent inhibitor of FAS, offering a novel approach to address the complexities of MASLD [21]. PTM, especially when formulated in liposome-based nanoformulations, not only markedly attenuated weight gain and reduced total triglyceride and plasma glucose levels, but also significantly decreased liver steatosis [19].

#### 10.2.1.4 SCD-1 Inhibitors

In the other side, SCD-1 catalyzes the conversion of saturated fatty acids to monounsaturated fatty acids (MUFAs), which are critical components of triglycerides, phospholipids and cholesterol esters [22]. Modulation of SCD-1 activity has been shown to influence the fluidity of cellular lipid membranes, affecting not only lipid storage and mobilization, but also the insulin sensitivity of liver cells [23, 24]. It has been observed that pharmacological inhibition of SCD-1 reduced liver steatosis, liver lipid droplet accumulation and insulin resistance in high-fat diet (HFD)-fed mice [5]. Clinical trials evaluating the efficacy of Aramchol, a novel synthetic molecule targeting SCD-1, in patients with MASLD have yielded mixed results. Although Aramchol has been found to be safe and tolerable, its efficacy in reducing biochemical markers of liver disease compared to placebo has not been conclusively demonstrated. This highlights the complexity of MASLD as a multifactorial disease and the difficulties of treatment targeting a single enzyme or pathway [25].

### 10.2.2 Targeting Nuclear Receptors

Nuclear receptors (NRs) are a superfamily of transcription factors that play an essential role in various physiological processes such as cell growth, differentiation, apoptosis, metabolism, and gene expression [26]. These receptors are predominantly triggered by a wide variety of small, lipid-soluble molecules, encompassing a range of both internal and external lipids such as steroids, retinoids, and phospholipids [27]. NRs play a key role in the development and progression of liver disease, as they influence crucial functions such as hepatic lipid and glucose metabolism, bile acid regulation, drug detoxification, inflammation, liver regeneration, fibrosis, and tumor formation [28], making them key therapeutic targets for MASLD.

#### 10.2.2.1 Farsenoid X Receptor

In healthy individuals, farsenoid X receptor (FXR) plays a key role in maintaining bile acid levels within a narrow physiological range. FXR activation inhibits bile acid synthesis in the liver and increases bile acid excretion from the liver to the intestine, thereby reducing the liver's exposure to bile acids [29]. Nevertheless, in the context of MASLD, FXR functionality is compromised. This impairment is multifaceted, as it involves not only a reduction in FXR expression, but also alterations in its activation by bile acids. This dysfunction leads to an accumulation of toxic bile acids in the liver, which aggravates liver injury. This accumulation is a critical factor contributing to the progression of simple steatosis to the more severe form of the disease [30]. FXR agonists, have been investigated for their therapeutic potential in the treatment of MASLD due to their multifunctional roles in regulating liver health. By activating FXR, these agonists not only modulate bile acid synthesis and secretion, but also have significant effects in reducing inflammation and mitigating fibrosis [31, 32]. Although, global FXR activation causes adverse effects such as cholesterol homeostasis imbalance and pruritus [30].

#### 10.2.2.2 Peroxisome Proliferator-Activated Receptors

Peroxisome proliferator-activated receptors (PPARs) are key regulators of lipid metabolism and energy homeostasis [33]. PPARα activation enhances fatty acid oxidation, which can help reduce liver fat [34]. PPARγ, on the other hand, improves insulin sensitivity and decreases inflammation [35]. PPARß/δ activation has shown potential in increasing HDL cholesterol, reducing triglycerides, and improving insulin sensitivity [36]. Clinical trials of PPAR-targeted drugs have shown promising results, with some agents demonstrating significant improvements in liver histology, biochemical markers of liver function, and metabolic parameters associated with MASLD [37].

#### 10.2.2.3 Liver X Receptor

Liver X receptors (LXRs) are involved in cholesterol homeostasis and inflammation. They are involved in the regulation of lipid and glucose metabolism in the liver [38]. The therapeutic potential of LXRs in the treatment of MASLD lies in their ability to modulate various metabolic pathways. LXRs can influence lipid metabolism by regulating the expression of genes involved in cholesterol efflux, fatty acid synthesis, and lipogenesis. This regulation helps to reduce lipid accumulation in the liver [5]. In addition, it has been demonstrated that LXR agonists can reduce hepatic inflammation caused by lipopolysaccharide (LPS) in a high-fat diet (HFD)-induced MASLD mouse model. This reduction in inflammation is due to a decrease in the proinflammatory activities of macrophages, marked by a decrease in the levels of TNF-α and inducible nitric oxide synthase (iNOS) [39]. LXRs also help regulate the liver's inflammatory response by influencing the transcription of inflammatory cytokines [26].

### 10.2.3 Challenges and Future Perspective

While targeting liver lipid metabolism holds promise for the treatment of MASLD, several challenges and future considerations must be addressed to translate these therapeutic strategies into clinical practice. One of these is the need to improve the specificity and selectivity of pharmacological agents directed against lipid metabolism enzymes and nuclear receptors. Many of the compounds currently under investigation may have undesirable effects or lack specificity for the intended target, which may result in adverse effects or limited therapeutic efficacy [7]. In addition, the development of combination therapies targeting multiple pathways involved in hepatic lipid metabolism may offer synergistic effects and greater efficacy compared to monotherapy. The combination of agents targeting different enzymes, receptors or signaling pathways involved in the pathogenesis of MASLD could address the multifactorial nature of the disease and provide more comprehensive therapeutic benefits [40].

## 10.3 Gut Microbiota Modulation for MASLD Treatment

Modulation of the gut microbiota offers a promising approach to treat MASLD. The gut-liver axis, which represents the pathway through which endotoxins, microbial metabolites and dietary components from the gut reach the liver, is a critical focus for innovative therapeutic strategies to address this prevalent liver disease [41]. Several strategies for modulating the gut microbiota include the use of probiotics, prebiotics, synbiotics and dietary modifications and fecal microbiota transplantation (FMT).

### 10.3.1 Probiotics and Prebiotics

In healthy individuals, the gut microbiota is mainly composed of Firmicutes and Bacteroidetes phyla, with Actinobacteria and Proteobacteria also present in smaller quantities. Nevertheless, in MASLD cases, dysbiosis is evident through reduced microbial diversity, which is defined by an increased relative abundance of species of the Proteobacteria and Bacteroidetes phyla, along with increases in the Enterobacteriaceae family and the Escherichia genus [42]. Addressing these imbalances through the use of probiotics and prebiotics offers a potential therapeutic avenue for MASLD.

#### 10.3.1.1 Probiotics

According with the International Scientific Association for Probiotics and Prebiotics, probiotics are live microorganisms that, when administered in adequate amounts, confer a health benefit on the host [43]. These benefits encompass enhanced barrier function, stimulation of the intestinal immune system, and protection against pathogens. Currently, the main probiotic bacterial genera studied are *Lactobacillus, Bifidobacterium*, and *Streptococcus*, which can be found in different foods and supplements [44]. Specific strains of probiotics have demonstrated their potential to reduce liver enzymes, improve lipid profiles and decrease insulin resistance, such as *Lactobacillus acidophilus*, *Bifidobacterium lactis*, *Lactobacillus rhamnosus*, and *Streptococcus thermophilus* [45]. For example, *Lactobacillus acidophilus* has been associated with decreased levels of liver enzymes, improved steatosis and reduced insulinemia and liver glycogen [46, 47]. *Bifidobacterium lactis* has been particularly noted for its role in improving immune function and reducing inflammatory responses [48, 49]. *Lactobacillus rhamnosus* offers promising results in reducing hepatic fat accumulation and improving insulin sensitivity [50, 51]. In addition, *Streptococcus thermophilus* has been shown to help improve intestinal barrier function and reduce the translocation of harmful bacteria and toxins to the liver, further alleviating inflammatory and metabolic stress on liver tissues [45, 47].

#### 10.3.1.2 Prebiotics

Prebiotics are defined as selectively fermented ingredient that results in specific changes in the composition and/or activity of the gastrointestinal microbiota, thus conferring benefit(s) upon host health [43, 52]. Prebiotics play a key role in modulating the intestinal environment to foster a beneficial microbial community. Through the process of selective fermentation, prebiotics promote the growth of beneficial intestinal bacteria such as *Bifidobacteria* and *Lactobacilli* [53]. This change in microbial balance may also result in increased production of beneficial metabolites, including short-chain fatty acids (SCFA) such as butyrate, known for their protective effects on the liver [54]. The most studied prebiotics for MASLD are fructooligosaccharides (FOS) and inulin. It has been observed that FOS can reshape the gut microbiota by increasing levels of beneficial bacteria such as *Klebsiella variicola*, *Lactobacillus gasseri*, and *Clostridium perfringens*. Furthermore, FOS administration has been associated with the downregulation of genes linked to lipid metabolism and inflammation, including ACC1, PPARγ, CD36, MTTP, APOC3, IL-6, and IL-1β [55]. Regarding inulin, studies have shown its potential in preventing MASLD by influencing the gut microbiota and inhibiting the inflammatory pathway involving Lipopolysaccharide-Toll-like receptor 4-Mψ-Nuclear factor-κB-nod-like receptor protein 3 through the gut-liver axis [56].

### 10.3.2 Fecal Microbiota Transplantation

Fecal microbiota transplantation (FMT) has gained attention as a potential therapeutic approach to treat MASLD. This procedure involves transferring fecal matter from a healthy donor to the gastrointestinal tract of a recipient, with the aim of restoring a balanced and beneficial composition of the gut microbiota. By introducing a diverse and healthy microbiota through FMT, it may help restore gut microbial balance, improve intestinal barrier function, and mitigate systemic inflammation, thereby alleviating MASLD progression [57]. Clinical trials have demonstrated that FMT can effectively reduce liver fat accumulation and improve liver function in patients with MASLD, particularly in those who are lean rather than obese [58].

### 10.3.3 Challenges and Future Perspective

Although FMT shows promise as a therapeutic approach for MASLD, several challenges and future considerations must be addressed to fully exploit its potential. A major challenge is the standardization of donor screening and selection criteria. Ensuring that fecal donors are healthy and free of infectious diseases or conditions that may adversely affect the recipient is essential to the safety and efficacy of FMT. The development of standardized protocols for donor screening, including rigorous pathogen testing and assessment of microbial composition, will be crucial in establishing guidelines for FMT procedures [59]. The long-term safety and efficacy of FMT should also be carefully evaluated. Although clinical trials have demonstrated promising short-term results, the potential for adverse effects and the durability of therapeutic effects over time remain uncertain. Longitudinal studies evaluating the microbiota composition, metabolic parameters, and liver health of FMT recipients are necessary to monitor the long-term consequences of FMT and identify any potential risks or complications [60].

## 10.4 Gene Therapies and the Potential for Personalized Medicine

The intersection of gene therapies and personalized medicine in the context of MASLD represents a transformative approach to medical treatment. As MASLD affects a significant portion of the world's population and often progresses to more severe liver disease, personalized gene therapies promise more targeted and effective interventions. This approach tailors treatments based on individual genetic background, which could significantly improve outcomes over standard therapies [61].

The emergence of gene therapies offers unprecedented opportunities to address the underlying molecular mechanisms that cause MASLD. These therapies aim to correct genetic defects, modulate gene expression, or enhance protective pathways involved in liver health [62]. One promising avenue of gene therapy involves the delivery of therapeutic nucleic acids, such as small interfering RNA (siRNA) or antisense oligonucleotides (ASOs), to silence or modulate specific genes associated with MASLD. Targeting the I148M variant of PNPLA3 by ASOs at the RNA level shows promise for long-term suppression of risk-associated variants in carriers, and liver-targeted administration together with triantennal N-acetyl galactosamine has shown efficacy in reducing hepatic lipogenesis and steatosis in murine models [63, 64].

### 10.4.1 Challenges and Future Perspective

Although gene therapy holds great promise for the treatment of MASLD, several challenges must be addressed to realize its full potential. One of these is the development of safe and effective delivery methods for therapeutic nucleic acids. Efficient delivery systems are crucial to ensure that therapeutic agents reach their target cells in the liver without causing unwanted effects or triggering immune responses [65]. Another challenge is to ensure that therapeutic agents reach the liver with precision. Achieving specific targeting is essential to maximize therapeutic efficacy while minimizing unwanted effects on other organs. Strategies such as liver-targeted delivery using ligands that bind to receptors specifically expressed on hepatocytes or liver-targeted gene editing techniques are being explored to improve precision targeting [66]. Furthermore, addressing potential immune responses to gene therapy remains a major hurdle. The immune system may recognize therapeutic nucleic acids as foreign invaders, resulting in immune activation and elimination of the therapeutic agents. Strategies to circumvent immune detection, such as modifying the chemical structure of nucleic acids or incorporating immunosuppressive agents into delivery systems, are being investigated to improve immune tolerance of gene therapy [67].

## 10.5 Conclusions

The integration of various therapeutic strategies, including targeting hepatic lipid metabolism, modulating gut microbiota, and exploring gene therapies, represents a multifaceted approach to tackling the complex pathology of MASLD. These approaches offer promising avenues for the development of novel treatments that could potentially halt or reverse the progression of the disease. Furthermore, as our understanding of the molecular mechanisms underlying MASLD continues to deepen, the identification of new drug targets and therapeutic strategies is imperative. The exploration of innovative approaches, such as harnessing the potential of nanomedicine for targeted drug delivery or leveraging artificial intelligence for personalized treatment optimization, holds promise for advancing the field.

## References

1. Sangro P, de la Torre AM, Sangro B, D'Avola D. Metabolic dysfunction-associated fatty liver disease (MAFLD): an update of the recent advances in pharmacological treatment. J Physiol Biochem. 2023;79(4):869–79.
2. Stefano JT, Duarte SMB, Ribeiro Leite Altikes RG, Oliveira CP. Non-pharmacological management options for MAFLD: a practical guide. Ther. Adv Endocrinol Metab. 2023;14:20420188231160394.
3. Hallsworth K, Adams LA. Lifestyle modification in NAFLD/NASH: facts and figures. JHEP Rep. 2019;1(6):468–79.
4. Habibullah M, Jemmieh K, Ouda A, Haider MZ, Malki MI, Elzouki AN. Metabolic-associated fatty liver disease: a selective review of pathogenesis, diagnostic approaches, and therapeutic strategies. Front Med (Lausanne). 2024;11:1291501.
5. Wang GY, Zhang XY, Wang CJ, Guan YF. Emerging novel targets for nonalcoholic fatty liver disease treatment: evidence from recent basic studies. World J Gastroenterol. 2023;29(1):75–95.
6. Mendez-Sanchez N, Cruz-Ramon VC, Ramirez-Perez OL, Hwang JP, Barranco-Fragoso B, Cordova-

Gallardo J. New aspects of lipotoxicity in nonalcoholic steatohepatitis. Int J Mol Sci. 2018;19(7):2034.
7. Vitulo M, Gnodi E, Rosini G, Meneveri R, Giovannoni R, Barisani D. Current Therapeutical approaches targeting lipid metabolism in NAFLD. Int J Mol Sci. 2023;24(16):12748.
8. Neokosmidis G, Cholongitas E, Tziomalos K. Acetyl-CoA carboxylase inhibitors in non-alcoholic steatohepatitis: is there a benefit? World J Gastroenterol. 2021;27(39):6522–6.
9. Goedeke L, Bates J, Vatner DF, Perry RJ, Wang T, Ramirez R, et al. Acetyl-CoA carboxylase inhibition reverses NAFLD and hepatic insulin resistance but promotes hypertriglyceridemia in rodents. Hepatology. 2018;68(6):2197–211.
10. Kim CW, Addy C, Kusunoki J, Anderson NN, Deja S, Fu X, et al. Acetyl CoA carboxylase inhibition reduces hepatic steatosis but elevates plasma triglycerides in mice and humans: a bedside to bench investigation. Cell Metab. 2017;26(2):394–406.e6.
11. Calle RA, Amin NB, Carvajal-Gonzalez S, Ross TT, Bergman A, Aggarwal S, et al. ACC inhibitor alone or co-administered with a DGAT2 inhibitor in patients with non-alcoholic fatty liver disease: two parallel, placebo-controlled, randomized phase 2a trials. Nat Med. 2021;27(10):1836–48.
12. Bian H, Liu Y-M, Chen Z-N. New avenues for NASH therapy by targeting ACC. Cell Metab. 2022;34(2):191–3.
13. Yamaguchi K, Yang L, McCall S, Huang J, Yu XX, Pandey SK, et al. Inhibiting triglyceride synthesis improves hepatic steatosis but exacerbates liver damage and fibrosis in obese mice with nonalcoholic steatohepatitis. Hepatology. 2007;45(6):1366–74.
14. Syed-Abdul MM. Lipid metabolism in metabolic-associated steatotic liver disease (MASLD). Meta. 2023;14(1):12.
15. Yu XX, Murray SF, Pandey SK, Booten SL, Bao D, Song XZ, et al. Antisense oligonucleotide reduction of DGAT2 expression improves hepatic steatosis and hyperlipidemia in obese mice. Hepatology. 2005;42(2):362–71.
16. Amin NB, Carvajal-Gonzalez S, Purkal J, Zhu T, Crowley C, Perez S, et al. Targeting diacylglycerol acyltransferase 2 for the treatment of nonalcoholic steatohepatitis. Sci Transl Med. 2019;11(520):eaav9701.
17. Futatsugi K, Cabral S, Kung DW, Huard K, Lee E, Boehm M, et al. Discovery of Ervogastat (PF-06865571): a potent and selective inhibitor of diacylglycerol acyltransferase 2 for the treatment of non-alcoholic steatohepatitis. J Med Chem. 2022;65(22):15000–13.
18. Loomba R, Morgan E, Watts L, Xia S, Hannan LA, Geary RS, et al. Novel antisense inhibition of diacylglycerol O-acyltransferase 2 for treatment of non-alcoholic fatty liver disease: a multicentre, double-blind, randomised, placebo-controlled phase 2 trial. Lancet Gastroenterol Hepatol. 2020;5(9):829–38.
19. Su M, Cao D, Wang Z, Duan Y, Huang Y. Fatty acid synthase inhibitor platensimycin intervenes the development of nonalcoholic fatty liver disease in a mouse model. Biomedicines. 2021;10(1):5.
20. Dorn C, Riener MO, Kirovski G, Saugspier M, Steib K, Weiss TS, et al. Expression of fatty acid synthase in nonalcoholic fatty liver disease. Int J Clin Exp Pathol. 2010;3(5):505–14.
21. Singh SB, Kang L, Nawrocki AR, Zhou D, Wu M, Previs S, et al. The fatty acid synthase inhibitor Platensimycin improves insulin resistance without inducing liver steatosis in mice and monkeys. PLoS One. 2016;11(10):e0164133.
22. Paton CM, Ntambi JM. Biochemical and physiological function of stearoyl-CoA desaturase. Am J Physiol Endocrinol Metab. 2009;297(1):E28–37.
23. Dobrzyn P, Jazurek M, Dobrzyn A. Stearoyl-CoA desaturase and insulin signaling--what is the molecular switch? Biochim Biophys Acta. 2010;1797(6–7):1189–94.
24. Ntambi JM. Regulation of stearoyl-CoA desaturase by polyunsaturated fatty acids and cholesterol. J Lipid Res. 1999;40(9):1549–58.
25. Malik A, Nadeem M, Amjad W, Malik MI, Javaid S, Farooq U, et al. Effects of Aramchol in patients with nonalcoholic fatty liver disease (NAFLD). A systematic review and meta-analysis. Prz Gastroenterol. 2023;18(1):67–75.
26. Yang X, Gonzalez FJ, Huang M, Bi H. Nuclear receptors and non-alcoholic fatty liver disease: an update. Liver Research. 2020;4(2):88–93.
27. Huang P, Chandra V, Rastinejad F. Structural overview of the nuclear receptor superfamily: insights into physiology and therapeutics. Annu Rev Physiol. 2010;72:247–72.
28. Yang Z, Danzeng A, Liu Q, Zeng C, Xu L, Mo J, et al. The role of nuclear receptors in the pathogenesis and treatment of non-alcoholic fatty liver disease. Int J Biol Sci. 2024;20(1):113–26.
29. Xi Y, Li H. Role of farnesoid X receptor in hepatic steatosis in nonalcoholic fatty liver disease. Biomed Pharmacother. 2020;121:109609.
30. Henry Z, Meadows V, Guo GL. FXR and NASH: an avenue for tissue-specific regulation. Hepatol Commun. 2023;7(5):e0127.
31. Clifford BL, Sedgeman LR, Williams KJ, Morand P, Cheng A, Jarrett KE, et al. FXR activation protects against NAFLD via bile-acid-dependent reductions in lipid absorption. Cell Metab. 2021;33(8):1671–84.e4.
32. Abenavoli L, Falalyeyeva T, Boccuto L, Tsyryuk O, Kobyliak N. Obeticholic acid: a new era in the treatment of nonalcoholic fatty liver disease. Pharmaceuticals (Basel). 2018;11(4):104.
33. Chinetti G, Fruchart JC, Staels B. Peroxisome proliferator-activated receptors (PPARs): nuclear receptors at the crossroads between lipid metabolism and inflammation. Inflamm Res. 2000;49(10):497–505.
34. Burri L, Thoresen GH, Berge RK. The role of PPARα activation in liver and muscle. PPAR Res. 2010;2010:1.

35. Sharma AM, Staels B. Review: Peroxisome proliferator-activated receptor gamma and adipose tissue--understanding obesity-related changes in regulation of lipid and glucose metabolism. J Clin Endocrinol Metab. 2007;92(2):386–95.
36. Palomer X, Barroso E, Pizarro-Delgado J, Peña L, Botteri G, Zarei M, et al. PPARβ/δ: a key therapeutic target in metabolic disorders. Int J Mol Sci. 2018;19(3):913.
37. Kamata S, Honda A, Ishii I. Current clinical trial status and future prospects of PPAR-targeted drugs for treating nonalcoholic fatty liver disease. Biomol Ther. 2023;13(8):1264.
38. Bilotta MT, Petillo S, Santoni A, Cippitelli M. Liver X receptors: regulators of cholesterol metabolism, inflammation, autoimmunity, and cancer. Front Immunol. 2020;11:584303.
39. Liu Y, Han X, Bian Z, Peng Y, You Z, Wang Q, et al. Activation of liver X receptors attenuates endotoxin-induced liver injury in mice with nonalcoholic fatty liver disease. Dig Dis Sci. 2012;57(2):390–8.
40. Esler WP, Cohen DE. Pharmacologic inhibition of lipogenesis for the treatment of NAFLD. J Hepatol. 2024;80(2):362–77.
41. Bakhshimoghaddam F, Alizadeh M. Modulation of the gut microbiota represents a new management for non-alcoholic fatty liver disease. Hepatobiliary Surg Nutr. 2020;9(2):223–6.
42. Shen F, Zheng RD, Sun XQ, Ding WJ, Wang XY, Fan JG. Gut microbiota dysbiosis in patients with non-alcoholic fatty liver disease. Hepatobiliary Pancreat Dis Int. 2017;16(4):375–81.
43. Hill C, Guarner F, Reid G, Gibson GR, Merenstein DJ, Pot B, et al. Expert consensus document. The International Scientific Association for Probiotics and Prebiotics consensus statement on the scope and appropriate use of the term probiotic. Nat Rev Gastroenterol Hepatol. 2014;11(8):506–14.
44. Castillo V, Figueroa F, González-Pizarro K, Jopia P, Ibacache-Quiroga C. Probiotics and prebiotics as a strategy for non-alcoholic fatty liver disease, a narrative review. Foods. 2021;10(8):1719.
45. Carpi RZ, Barbalho SM, Sloan KP, Laurindo LF, Gonzaga HF, Grippa PC, et al. The effects of probiotics, prebiotics and synbiotics in Non-Alcoholic Fat Liver Disease (NAFLD) and Non-Alcoholic Steatohepatitis (NASH): a systematic review. Int J Mol Sci. 2022;23(15):8805.
46. Jeong JJ, Park HJ, Cha MG, Park E, Won SM, Ganesan R, et al. The lactobacillus as a probiotic: focusing on liver diseases. Microorganisms. 2022;10(2):288.
47. Abenavoli L, Scarpellini E, Rouabhia S, Balsano C, Luzza F. Probiotics in non-alcoholic fatty liver disease: which and when. Ann Hepatol. 2013;12(3):357–63.
48. Yan Y, Liu C, Zhao S, Wang X, Wang J, Zhang H, et al. Probiotic Bifidobacterium lactis V9 attenuates hepatic steatosis and inflammation in rats with non-alcoholic fatty liver disease. AMB Express. 2020;10(1):101.
49. Cristofori F, Dargenio VN, Dargenio C, Miniello VL, Barone M, Francavilla R. Anti-inflammatory and immunomodulatory effects of probiotics in gut inflammation: a door to the body. Front Immunol. 2021;12:578386.
50. Ritze Y, Bárdos G, Claus A, Ehrmann V, Bergheim I, Schwiertz A, Bischoff SC. Lactobacillus rhamnosus GG protects against non-alcoholic fatty liver disease in mice. PLoS One. 2014;9(1):e80169.
51. Wang G, Jiao T, Xu Y, Li D, Si Q, Hao J, et al. Bifidobacterium adolescentis and lactobacillus rhamnosus alleviate non-alcoholic fatty liver disease induced by a high-fat, high-cholesterol diet through modulation of different gut microbiota-dependent pathways. Food Funct. 2020;11(7):6115–27.
52. Davani-Davari D, Negahdaripour M, Karimzadeh I, Seifan M, Mohkam M, Masoumi SJ, et al. Prebiotics: definition, types, sources, mechanisms, and clinical applications. Food Secur. 2019;8(3):92.
53. Ji J, Jin W, Liu SJ, Jiao Z, Li X. Probiotics, prebiotics, and postbiotics in health and disease. MedComm (2020). 2023;4(6):e420.
54. Markowiak-Kopeć P, Śliżewska K. The effect of probiotics on the production of short-chain fatty acids by human intestinal microbiome. Nutrients. 2020;12(4):1107.
55. Huang X, Chen Q, Fan Y, Yang R, Gong G, Yan C, et al. Fructooligosaccharides attenuate non-alcoholic fatty liver disease by remodeling gut microbiota and association with lipid metabolism. Biomed Pharmacother. 2023;159:114300.
56. Bao T, He F, Zhang X, Zhu L, Wang Z, Lu H, et al. Inulin exerts beneficial effects on non-alcoholic fatty liver disease via modulating gut microbiome and suppressing the lipopolysaccharide-toll-like receptor 4-Mψ-nuclear factor-κB-nod-like receptor protein 3 pathway via gut-liver axis in mice. Front Pharmacol. 2020;11:558525.
57. Abenavoli L, Maurizi V, Rinninella E, Tack J, Di Berardino A, Santori P, et al. Fecal microbiota transplantation in NAFLD treatment. Medicina (Kaunas). 2022;58(11):1559.
58. Xue L, Deng Z, Luo W, He X, Chen Y. Effect of fecal microbiota transplantation on non-alcoholic fatty liver disease: a randomized clinical trial. Front Cell Infect Microbiol. 2022;12:759306.
59. Woodworth MH, Carpentieri C, Sitchenko KL, Kraft CS. Challenges in fecal donor selection and screening for fecal microbiota transplantation: a review. Gut Microbes. 2017;8(3):225–37.
60. Del Barrio M, Lavín L, Santos-Laso Á, Arias-Loste MT, Odriozola A, Rodriguez-Duque JC, et al. Faecal microbiota transplantation, paving the way to treat non-alcoholic fatty liver disease. Int J Mol Sci. 2023;24(7):6123.
61. Sookoian S, Pirola CJ. Precision medicine in nonalcoholic fatty liver disease: new therapeutic insights from genetics and systems biology. Clin Mol Hepatol. 2020;26(4):461–75.

62. Shi F, Zhao M, Zheng S, Zheng L, Wang H. Advances in genetic variation in metabolism-related fatty liver disease. Front Genet. 2023;14:1213916.
63. Cherubini A, Casirati E, Tomasi M, Valenti L. PNPLA3 as a therapeutic target for fatty liver disease: the evidence to date. Expert Opin Ther Targets. 2021;25(12):1033–43.
64. Lindén D, Ahnmark A, Pingitore P, Ciociola E, Ahlstedt I, Andréasson AC, et al. Pnpla3 silencing with antisense oligonucleotides ameliorates nonalcoholic steatohepatitis and fibrosis in Pnpla3 I148M knock-in mice. Mol Metab. 2019;22:49–61.
65. Yokoo T, Kamimura K, Abe H, Kobayashi Y, Kanefuji T, Ogawa K, et al. Liver-targeted hydrodynamic gene therapy: recent advances in the technique. World J Gastroenterol. 2016;22(40):8862–8.
66. Maestro S, Weber ND, Zabaleta N, Aldabe R, Gonzalez-Aseguinolaza G. Novel vectors and approaches for gene therapy in liver diseases. JHEP Rep. 2021;3(4):100300.
67. Bessis N, GarciaCozar FJ, Boissier MC. Immune responses to gene therapy vectors: influence on vector function and effector mechanisms. Gene Ther. 2004;11(Suppl 1):S10–7.

# 11 Integrative Approaches to MASLD Management

Zahra Dossaji, Tooba Laeeq, Lubaba Haque, Magnus Chun, and Robert G. Gish

## 11.1 Introduction

Fatty liver disease stands out as one of the most prevalent and rapidly growing liver disorders globally, estimated to affect approximately 38% of the world's population [38]. Since the inception of the term "nonalcoholic fatty liver disease" (NAFLD), there has been substantial debate regarding the nomenclature of fatty liver disease (FLD). Experts argue that the term "nonalcoholic" fails to accurately depict the disease's etiology, and the term "fatty" contributes to stigma and shaming [41].

In 2020, international experts issued a consensus statement proposing that the disease be renamed from NAFLD to metabolic dysfunction-associated fatty liver disease (MAFLD) [10]. The adoption of MAFLD in over 70 countries and super-regions has enhanced the ability of health-care providers to identify individuals with a higher number of risk factors and an increased likelihood of developing fibrosis [38]. Over the past 3 years, the term "metabolic dysfunction-associated steatotic liver disease" (MASLD) has gained popularity. Unlike MAFLD, MASLD diagnosis is contingent on a patient meeting just 1 of the 5 metabolic risk factors, as opposed to 2 of the 7 parameters required for MAFLD [38]. Individuals meeting the criteria for both MASLD and alcohol-related fatty liver disease (ALD) are categorized as having metALD [41]. Individuals with MASLD and steatohepatitis are designated as having metabolic dysfunction-associated steatohepatitis (MASH), which is the updated term for nonalcoholic steatohepatitis (NASH) [41].

A clear delineation of clinical and histological features among different FLD nomenclatures provides valuable insights for developing therapeutic strategies. The medical management of MASLD encompasses both pharmaceutical and non-pharmaceutical therapies while addressing the underlying metabolic disease. This chapter will specifically focus on integrative approaches, delving into complementary therapies, alternative treatments, holistic therapies, motivational interviews, and holistic care models incorporating multidisciplinary teams (Fig. 11.1).

Z. Dossaji (✉) · T. Laeeq · L. Haque · M. Chun
Department of Internal Medicine, Kirk Kerkorian School of Medicine at University of Nevada Las Vegas, Las Vegas, NV, USA
e-mail: zahra.dossaji@unlv.edu; Tooba.laeeq@unlv.edu; lubaba.haque@unlv.edu; magnus.chun@unlv.edu

R. G. Gish
Hepatitis B Foundation, Doylestown, PA, USA
e-mail: rgish@robertgish.com



N. Méndez-Sánchez, X. Qi (eds.), *Metabolic Dysfunction-Associated Steatotic Liver Disease*,
https://doi.org/10.1007/978-981-97-9519-2_11

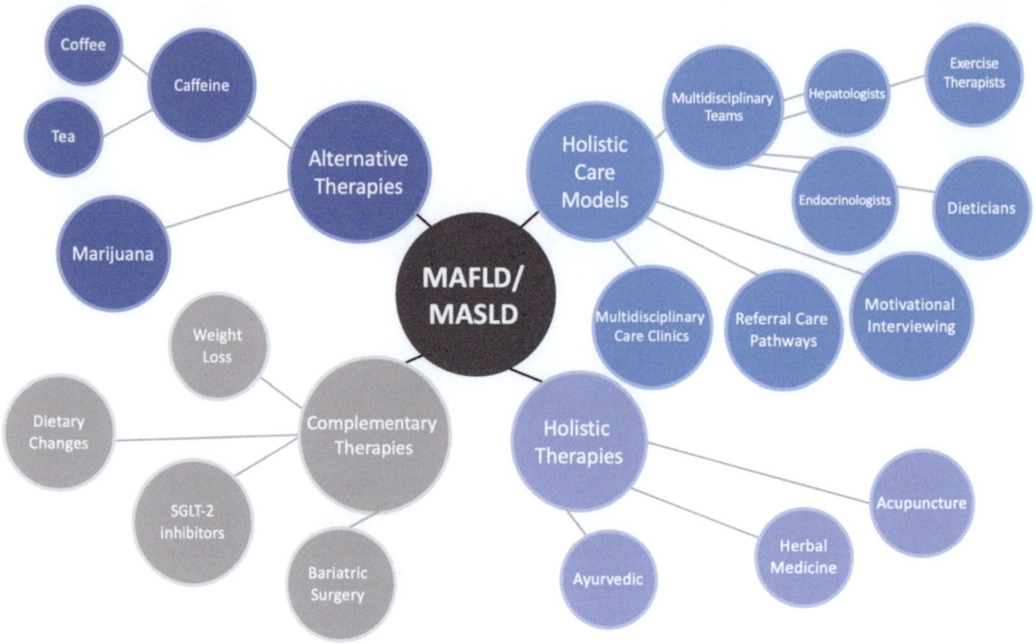


**Fig. 11.1** An overview of integrative strategies to manage MAFLD/MASLD. *MAFLD* Metabolic Associated Fatty Liver Disease, *MASLD* Metabolic dysfunction-associated steatotic liver disease

## 11.2 Complementary Therapies

There are currently no FDA-approved therapies for MASLD, despite its emerging clinical need and extrahepatic manifestations [39]. While it is well-known that MASLD is a multisystem disease, little has been established regarding its extrahepatic manifestations. The primary reason for the terminology change from NAFLD to MASLD was recent literature and the potential association between insulin resistance, diabetes mellitus, obesity, chronic kidney disease, cardiovascular disease, cancers, and fatty liver disease. This cross-talk suggests that metabolic alterations serve as a potent cause of liver disease, rather than alcohol alone [36]. Understanding this connection is crucial for improving outcomes in patients with MASLD and comorbid conditions. The management of MASLD should prioritize enhancing both quality of life and overall survival by comprehensively addressing all associated risk factors.

### 11.2.1 MASLD and Diabetes Mellitus

Fatty liver disease, reported in up to 75% of the affected population (i.e., those who are obese, overweight, and/or have diabetes), is closely linked to insulin resistance, leading to lipolysis and dyslipidemia [5]. This interaction, attributed to increased fructose consumption, significantly impacts the gut microbiome's role in obesity and dyslipidemia. Moreover, it promotes de novo lipid synthesis in the liver, contributing to FLD and increasing oxidative stress [9].

In the study of therapeutic options for steatotic liver disease and diabetes mellitus, semaglutide showed fatty liver resolution in a phase 2 clinical trial compared to placebo, though no change in fibrosis stages was observed [32]. Additionally, weight loss therapies, encompassing lifestyle modifications and dietary changes like a low-calorie carbohydrate-restrictive diet, play a crucial role in reducing insulin resistance and steatotic liver disease [42].

### 11.2.2 MASLD and Cardiovascular Disease

A chronic, systemic inflammatory state and dyslipidemia potentially contribute to cardiovascular complications in patients with MASLD, the leading cause of death in this population [34]. The relationship between MAFLD and cardiovascular disease is intricate, involving metabolic, inflammatory, and vascular pathways [23]. Common risk factors increase the chances of atherosclerotic disease in this population.

Growth differentiation factor 15 (GDF 15) emerges as a therapy for its role in obesity and cardiometabolic disease, affecting MASLD incidence through modulation of appetite-regulating hormones [48]. Bariatric surgery also shows promise, reducing cardiovascular mortality in patients with steatotic liver disease [18]. Overall, prioritizing weight loss and healthy diets for managing obesity is crucial in treating cardiovascular and metabolic syndrome [17].

### 11.2.3 MASLD and Chronic Kidney Disease

Due to the systemic inflammatory state observed in patients with MASLD and MASH, emerging data suggests that kidney involvement within this spectrum [1]. In a study of 12,571 patients, the independent association of MAFLD and NAFLD with albuminuria vs. chronic kidney disease (CKD) was analyzed. Patients with MASLD exhibited a lower estimated glomerular filtration rate (eGFR) and a higher prevalence of CKD compared to patients with NAFLD when controlled for confounding factors, suggesting a direct effect on renal function [46].

Sodium-glucose cotransporter 2 inhibitors (SGLT2i) are currently under study for their efficacy in cardiovascular disease, metabolic benefits, and CKD. SGLT2i exhibit anti-inflammatory and anti-fibrotic effects, reducing oxidative stress, among other benefits [54]. Their cardio-metabolic-renal benefits position them as an optimal treatment option for MASLD associated with CKD.

## 11.3 Alternative Treatments for MASLD

### 11.3.1 Caffeine

Coffee and tea, widely consumed beverages, are recognized for various health benefits, including cardiovascular improvement, reduced cancer risk, and lowered Parkinson's disease risk. Notably, they exhibit hepatoprotective effects, primarily attributed to chlorogenic acids (CGA), polyphenols that reduce intestinal glucose absorption and lipid accumulation and suppress liver fibrogenesis and carcinogenesis [52].

Caffeine, present in both drinks, inhibited hepatic stellate cell activation in experimental studies [43]. Additionally, bioactive compounds like flavonoids, polyphenols, theanine, and catechins influence hepatocellular health [51]. Associations between coffee and tea consumption and a reduction in hepatocellular carcinoma (HCC) have been observed [53]. Well-designed randomized controlled trials (RCTs) are crucial for further investigating the impact of these beverages on hepatocellular health and MASLD treatment.

### 11.3.2 Marijuana

Marijuana, the most used or abused (often illicit) substance in the United States, has seen increased use with its legalization in various states. Despite its association with increased calorie consumption, patients who use marijuana show a decreased risk of obesity and diabetes [16]. Cannabidiol, a primary active phytocannabinoid, acts as a partial antagonist in cannabinoid type I receptors, potentially explaining its impact on insulin sensitivity. Further research on this aspect is pending.

Considering the hypothesized beneficial effects on metabolic abnormalities, there is a theory that marijuana may assist with MASLD management. Cannabinoids, including cannabidiol and cannabigerol, help prevent the release of inflammatory cytokines and pro-inflammatory mediators, addressing insulin resistance and MASLD. These cannabinoids also possess modest anti-inflammatory properties, offering preventive measures for FLD [16].

### 11.3.3 Alcohol

Alcohol consumption can synergistically accelerate the progression of liver diseases, such as viral hepatitis, to cirrhosis. The pathophysiology involves alcohol metabolism by hepatic enzymes—alcohol dehydrogenase and aldehyde dehydrogenase. Alcohol is first converted to acetaldehyde and then to acetate, leading to NADH (nicotinamide adenine dinucleotide + hydrogen) accumulation that combines with fatty acids to form triglycerides. This accumulation results in FLD and eventual cirrhosis with ongoing hepatocellular damage [33].

Initial studies suggested moderate alcohol consumption might prevent and support liver health, but later research contradicted this, confirming alcohol's role in rapid liver disease progression. Recent studies even indicate that light and moderate alcohol consumption accelerates liver disease in individuals with preexisting MAFLD [33].

Distinguishing between MASLD and ALD is challenging, as their histological stages leading to cirrhosis appear similar. Clinical differentiation relies on a thorough history and specific biochemical tests [19] including the use of phosphatidyl ethanol (PEth) testing.

## 11.4 Holistic Therapies for MASLD

### 11.4.1 Ayurvedic

Studies have explored whether herbal and ayurvedic medicine may help alleviate hepatic oxidative stress. Exploring new avenues for MASLD treatment, Patel et al. studied the effects of withaferin A formed from *Withania somnifera* extracts. The study revealed a leptin-driven decrease in obesity, lipid profile, and liver disease, among other benefits [35]. Singhal et al. examined ayurvedic dietary regimens and physical exercise effects on liver steatosis, showing significant improvement in the group receiving ayurvedic therapy and exercise for managing MASLD [44]. Shilajit, another ayurvedic medicine that modulates cytokines, inflammation, and adipogenesis, also demonstrated a protective role in liver disease [12]. In addition, milk extracts like *Silybum marianum*, bitter melon (*Momordica charantia*), hawthorn (*Crataegus fructus*), and phytomedicines containing berberine extracts have all shown a protective role in modulating fatty liver/steatotic liver disease [40, 50].

### 11.4.2 Acupuncture

Acupuncture, a traditional Chinese medicine therapy, has been gaining recent global popularity. Experimental studies highlight acupuncture's impact on weight, glucose metabolism, lipid metabolism, sympathetic nervous system modulation, and insulin sensitivity [24]. A meta-analysis of RCTs involving 939 patients demonstrates acupuncture's superiority over traditional medicine in treating steatotic liver disease [6]. A study in mice revealed that acupuncture can downregulate apolipoproteins and lipid absorption in the small intestine, influencing steatotic liver disease incidence [13]. Additionally, evidence suggests acupuncture's role in attenuating liver inflammation and histopathological changes in steatotic liver disease via cytokine modulation [26]. However, despite promising evidence, further research is essential to establish acupuncture as a treatment modality for MASLD.

### 11.4.3 Herbal Medicine

Danzhi tiaozhi decoction (DZTZD), an ancient Chinese herbal medication known to be used for MASLD, contains 254 active compounds targeting pathways related to diabetes, lipid metabolism, and atherosclerosis. Jiang et al. demonstrated its efficacy in reducing weight, lipid accumulation, atherosclerosis, and inflammation in animal models. Additionally, DZTZD affected the JNK/AKT pathway, known to trigger insulin resistance and oxidative stress, reducing MASLD incidence [15].

Si-ni-san (SNS), another herbal formula with cooling properties, has also been used as a herbal therapy for MASLD treatment. A study on mice with a high-fat diet showed SNS downregulating fatty acid synthase expression, preventing lipid accumulation in hepatocytes and contributing to MASLD prevention [21].

Wang et al. investigated the effects of a combination of polygonati rhizoma (PR) and angelicae sinensis radix (ASR), known as jiuzhuan huangjing, in MASLD. The study found that this combination had positive effects on cellular steatosis by promoting fatty acid oxidation, enhancing mitochondrial function, and reducing oxidative stress [49].

Shenling baizhu powder (SLP), a Chinese herbal medicine with an unknown mechanism, has also been studied as a potential MASLD treatment. Song et al. revealed that rats on a high-fat diet and treated with SLP for 3 weeks showed a decrease in liver fat accumulation achieved by inhibiting genes responsible for lipid synthesis and lipid peroxidation in mitochondria [45].

Future investigations of the potential benefits of traditional medicine practices, herbal remedies, and botanical supplements in managing MASLD should explore their mechanisms of action and compatibility with conventional medical treatments.

## 11.5 Holistic Care Models and the Importance of Multidisciplinary Teams

### 11.5.1 Multidisciplinary Teams and Clinics

The intricate nature of MASLD, coupled with its association with other metabolic diseases and a heightened risk of cardiac and diabetic complications, underscores the necessity of implementing multidisciplinary care [20]. Multidisciplinary teams (MDTs) are crucial in addressing MASLD, as evident in previous studies [2, 11, 55]. An integrated MDT approach is vital, starting in outpatient settings with multidisciplinary clinics (MDCs). MDCs enhance care coordination by bringing together healthcare professionals from various disciplines to discuss patient healthcare plans collectively [11]. This approach has been successful in conditions like asthma, chronic obstructive pulmonary disease (COPD), schizophrenia [25, 29, 47], liver transplant, and liver cancer, and it has shown improved patient outcomes for MASLD. Early diagnosis through MDCs allows for prompt management plans and quick referrals to hepatologists, resulting in improved hemoglobin A1C (HbA1c), significant weight loss, reduced total cholesterol, and normalized liver enzymes [11]. Armstrong et al. [2] enrolled 64 diabetic patients in their MDC, diagnosing 30% with MASLD. Furthermore, the MDC approach appears cost-effective in enhancing liver-related and cardiometabolic health in patients with MASLD [8, 11, 27, 30].

While MDCs offer personalized patient management, better communication, and improved time/cost efficiency, challenges include geographical limitations requiring patient travel and oversaturation of tertiary centers in populated cities [55]. Despite this, studies show lowered sequential referral rates to secondary care with the MDC approach [8]. MDT providers in the MDC include gastroenterologists/hepatologists, diabetologists, bariatric/weight loss specialists, psychologists, cardiologists, and advanced practice providers like dieticians and clinical nurse specialists [55]. Bariatricians and weight loss specialists are crucial for providing valuable feedback and discussing potential bariatric surgery options [20, 37]. Patients enrolled in MDC should target a 10% total body weight loss, with diabetologists ensuring appropriate blood glucose control and proactive screening for MASLD, considering its association with increased all-cause mortality in diabetic patients [3, 11].

### 11.5.2 Referral Care Pathways

Despite the encouragement for a multidisciplinary approach, there is a paucity of published guidelines. Several clinical care models propose a range of services for managing diabetes, dyslipidemia, cardiovascular risk, lifestyle modifications, and medications for comorbid conditions in patients with MASLD [22]. These clinics, led by MDTs including hepatologists, endocrinologists, diabetes specialist nurses, dietitians, and allied health professionals, aim for holistic patient management [22]. Co-locating services streamlines patient care, reducing the need for multiple specialist visits and creating system efficiencies. Examples of these clinics, such as the one at the Royal Free Hospital in Camden and Islington (in the United Kingdom), demonstrated significant improvements in alanine transaminase (ALT), aspartate transaminase (AST), blood pressure, cholesterol, and weight loss for patients with MASLD [28]. Another MDC in London containing a hepatologist, diabetologist, dietician, and exercise therapist also saw similar results where median ALT fell from 61 to 50 and weight fell from 90.5 kg to 87.3 kg ($P < 0.001$). They used a comprehensive screening tool called the MEATLOAF consultation, assessing for dietary and exercise counseling [7].

One exemplary multidisciplinary care model is the Innovative Center for Health and Nutrition in Gastroenterology (ICHANGE) program [20]. Drawing inspiration from successful models in cancer treatment, women's health, and cardiovascular disease management, ICHANGE presents a referral algorithm with the goal of identifying risk factors for MASLD progression, fostering the creation of cohesive, personalized management plans [20]. The ICHANGE model is led by a hepatologist collaborating with an endocrinologist, cardiologist, and dietitian, collectively managing associated comorbidities. The team further comprises gastroenterologists, endobariatricians, bariatric surgeons, and advanced practice providers, aiming to streamline referrals and provide specialized care in a unified clinical setting [20]. All patients undergo diet and lifestyle counseling, receive exercise recommendations, and are presented with personalized meal plans. The target population is identified through electronic medical records and fibrosis score calculators. The referral algorithm incorporates the Fibrosis-4 (FIB-4) score or clinical/radiologic evidence of advanced fibrosis [20]. However, it is recommended that all patients at risk of MASLD be referred to the program. For those deemed low risk based on the FIB-4 score (less than 1.3), transient elastography is scheduled. Scores higher than 6.0 kPa lead to enrollment in the ICHANGE program [20]. A nurse navigator coordinates assessments and ensures follow-up at 1- to 6-month intervals, highlighting care coordination in the model's patient-centered approach.

A drawback of the ICHANGE program is the inclusion of the indeterminate FIB-4 values, which has the potential of over referrals and saturating the capacity of these clinics [55]. Efficient referral pathways for patients with MASLD ensure appropriate access to clinical services. These pathways often use noninvasive tests (NITs), involving either surrogate scores or ratios (e.g., AST to ALT ratio, FIB-4 score), and liver stiffness measurements by ultrasound or magnetic resonance imaging (MRI). The performance of NITs is influenced by pretest probability, with high negative predictive value in low-prevalence primary care settings. Combining NITs in sequential algorithms improves advanced fibrosis detection in both primary and secondary care.

In the United Kingdom, referral pathways commission primary care to identify high-risk patients for advanced liver disease specialists using NITS. Crossan et al. explored improving MASLD referral pathways by using noninvasive fibrosis tests, aiming to reduce reliance on liver biopsies and enhance patient management efficiency. Their study revealed that implementing a 2-tier noninvasive test strategy, involving an initial FIB-4 assessment followed by a second test (Fibroscan, Enhanced Liver Fibrosis Test, or FibroTest) for those with an indeterminate result, proved to be a more cost-effective approach. This approach surpassed immediate secondary care referral or liver biopsy without prior noninvasive testing, demonstrating at least a 40% cost savings compared to using liver biopsy for all patients. Referral pathways in Northeast England required a similar 2-step process with FIB-4 or followed by transient elastography before secondary care referral. An audit of 50 consecutive patients attending the follow-up hepatology clinics showed the care bundle resulted in better implementation of several aspects of patient management [31].

Future studies could delve into patient-reported outcomes and experiences in holistic MASLD treatment. They could assess the impact of a multidisciplinary approach on patient quality of life, treatment adherence, and overall satisfaction with healthcare. With the increasing digitization of healthcare, studies should also explore integrating technology, such as mobile applications, wearables, and telehealth platforms, to support multidisciplinary treatment. More data is required to ascertain the feasibility and effectiveness of technology-assisted interventions in promoting lifestyle changes and preventing the progression of MASLD.

### 11.5.3 Motivational Interviewing

Patient education and motivational interviewing are crucial in guiding patients to strengthen their motivation and commitment to change, resulting in a customized action plan for sustained weight loss. Studies on weight loss have demonstrated that motivational interviewing can significantly enhance weight loss, leading to a 3.3 lb. increase compared to control groups [14]. Furthermore, Centis and colleagues have shown that defining stages of change and motivation can improve clinical care for individuals with MASLD by tailoring programs that effectively utilize behavioral counseling [4]. The healthcare provider can begin the discussion by informing the patient about the increased risks of conditions such as type 2 diabetes, heart disease, and liver damage associated with MASLD while emphasizing the effectiveness of moderate weight loss and regular exercise in managing it. They then ask the patient a series of questions to assess their motivation and readiness for change regarding weight loss and exercise. Subsequently, the provider summarizes the patient's reasons for change, strategies for success, and overall readiness before inquiring about their intended actions. This approach, known as motivational interviewing, fosters patient engagement, empowerment, and motivation by encouraging self-reflection and commitment to change [14].

## 11.6 Conclusion

MASLD represents the hepatic manifestation of metabolic syndrome and may present with various comorbidities. Considering the significant impact of comorbidities on MASLD severity, especially with cardiovascular mortality as the primary cause of death in patients with MASLD, a comprehensive treatment approach is essential for early detection and reduced disease progression [55]. Presently, no specific pharmaceutical therapies are established for MASLD, and while holistic treatments have been considered, none have demonstrated efficacy in RCTs. We expect the approval of resmetiron by the time of this publication and the focus of treatment will initially be on patients with F2/F3 liver fibrosis pending the labeling. Furthermore, studies have yet to evaluate their sustainability and effectiveness over time. Potential future research topics could explore the impact of mind-body interventions, such as mindfulness meditation, yoga, and relaxation techniques, on MASLD outcomes. Studying their influence on metabolic parameters associated with MASLD would be intriguing, considering their potential to reduce stress and enhance mental well-being.

A multidisciplinary treatment strategy for MASLD, involving various healthcare professionals, has proven effective in enhancing liver-related and cardiovascular risk factors. Encouraging collaboration among healthcare professionals caring for patients with MASLD can lead to earlier diagnosis and improved management, addressing not only liver disease but also the extrahepatic complications of this multisystem disorder.

**Acknowledgments** The authors would like to acknowledge Kelly Schrank, MA, ELS, of Bookworm Editing Services LLC for her editorial services in preparing the manuscript for publication.

**Disclosures Human and Animal Rights**: This article does not contain any studies with human or animal subjects performed by any of the authors.

**Conflicts of Interest** Z. Dossaji: This author has nothing to disclose. T. Laeeq: This author has nothing to disclose. L. Haque: This author has nothing to disclose. M. Chun: This author has nothing to disclose. R.G. Gish: This author has served as a consultant and/or advisor for Gilead Sciences. Dr. Gish has a speaker's contract to do promotional talks for AbbVie, AstraZeneca, BMS, Diasorin, Eisai, Genentech, Gilead Sciences Inc., Intercept, Mallinckrodt, VBI Vaccines.

## References

1. Adams LA, Anstee QM, Tilg H, et al. Non-alcoholic fatty liver disease and its relationship with cardiovascular disease and other extrahepatic diseases. Gut. 2017;66(6):1138–53. https://doi.org/10.1136/gutjnl-2017-313884.
2. Armstrong MJ, Hazlehurst JM, Parker R, et al. Severe asymptomatic non-alcoholic fatty liver disease in routine diabetes care; a multi-disciplinary team approach to diagnosis and management. QJM. 2014;107(1):33–41. https://doi.org/10.1093/qjmed/hct198.
3. Bril F, Cusi K. Management of nonalcoholic fatty liver disease in patients with type 2 diabetes: a call to action. Diabetes Care. 2017;40(3):419–30. https://doi.org/10.2337/dc16-1787.
4. Centis E, Moscatiello S, Bugianesi E, et al. Stage of change and motivation to healthier lifestyle in non-alcoholic fatty liver disease. J Hepatol. 2013;58(4):771–7. https://doi.org/10.1016/j.jhep.2012.11.031.
5. Cetin EG, Demir N, Sen I. The relationship between insulin resistance and liver damage in non-alcoholic fatty liver patients. Sisli Etfal Hastan Tip Bul. 2020;54(4):411–5. https://doi.org/10.14744/semb.2018.83604.
6. Chen P, Zhong X, Dai Y, et al. The efficacy and safety of acupuncture in nonalcoholic fatty liver disease: a systematic review and meta-analysis of randomized controlled trials. Medicine (Baltimore). 2021;100(38):e27050. https://doi.org/10.1097/md.0000000000027050.
7. Cobbold JFL, Raveendran S, Peake CM, et al. Piloting a multidisciplinary clinic for the management of non-alcoholic fatty liver disease: initial 5-year experience. Frontline Gastroenterol. 2013;4(4):263–9.
8. Crossan C, Majumdar A, Srivastava A, et al. Referral pathways for patients with NAFLD based on non-invasive fibrosis tests: diagnostic accuracy and cost analysis. Liver Int. 2019;39(11):2052–60. https://doi.org/10.1111/liv.14198.
9. Drożdż K, Nabrdalik K, Hajzler W, et al. Metabolic-associated fatty liver disease (MAFLD), diabetes, and cardiovascular disease: associations with fructose metabolism and gut microbiota. Nutrients. 2022;14(1):103. https://www.mdpi.com/2072-6643/14/1/103.
10. Eslam M, Newsome PN, Sarin SK, et al. A new definition for metabolic dysfunction-associated fatty liver disease: An international expert consensus statement. J Hepatol. 2020;73(1):202–9. https://doi.org/10.1016/j.jhep.2020.03.039.
11. Eslam M, Ahmed A, Després JP, et al. Incorporating fatty liver disease in multidisciplinary care and novel clinical trial designs for patients with metabolic diseases. Lancet Gastroenterol Hepatol. 2021;6(9):743–53. https://doi.org/10.1016/s2468-1253(21)00132-1.
12. Ghezelbash B, Shahrokhi N, Khaksari M, et al. Protective roles of shilajit in modulating resistin, adiponectin, and cytokines in rats with non-alcoholic fatty liver disease. Chin J Integr Med. 2022;28(6):531–7. https://doi.org/10.1007/s11655-022-3307-3.
13. Han J, Guo X, Meng XJ, et al. Acupuncture improved lipid metabolism by regulating intestinal absorption in mice. World J Gastroenterol. 2020;26(34):5118–29. https://doi.org/10.3748/wjg.v26.i34.5118.
14. Hunt CM, Turner MJ, Gifford EJ, Britt RB, Su GL. Identifying and treating nonalcoholic fatty liver disease. Fed Pract. 2019;36(1):20–9.
15. Jiang X, Tang N, Liu Y, et al. Integrating network analysis and pharmacokinetics to investigate the mechanisms of danzhi tiaozhi decoction in metabolic-associated fatty liver disease (MAFLD). J Ethnopharmacol. 2024;318(Pt B):117008. https://doi.org/10.1016/j.jep.2023.117008.
16. Kim D, Kim W, Kwak MS, et al. Inverse association of marijuana use with nonalcoholic fatty liver disease among adults in the United States. PLoS One. 2017;12(10):e0186702.
17. Kosinski C, Jornayvaz FR. Effects of ketogenic diets on cardiovascular risk factors: evidence from animal and human studies. Nutrients. 2017;9(5):517. https://doi.org/10.3390/nu9050517.
18. Krishnan A, Hadi Y, Alqahtani SA, et al. Cardiovascular outcomes and mortality after bariatric surgery in patients with nonalcoholic fatty liver disease and obesity. JAMA Netw Open. 2023;6(4):e237188. https://doi.org/10.1001/jamanetworkopen.2023.7188.
19. Kulkarni AV, Sarin SK. The bidirectional impacts of alcohol consumption and MAFLD for progressive fatty liver disease. Ther Adv Endocrinol Metab. 2023;14:20420188231178370. https://doi.org/10.1177/20420188231178370.

20. Kumar S, Wong R, Newberry C, et al. Multidisciplinary clinic models: a paradigm of care for management of NAFLD. Hepatology. 2021;74(6):3472–8. https://doi.org/10.1002/hep.32081.
21. Lan T, Geng XJ, Zhang SJ, et al. Si-ni-san inhibits hepatic Fasn expression and lipid accumulation in MAFLD mice through AMPK/p300/SREBP-1c axis. Phytomedicine. 2023;123:155209. https://doi.org/10.1016/j.phymed.2023.155209.
22. Lazarus JV, Anstee QM, Hagström H, et al. Defining comprehensive models of care for NAFLD. Nat Rev Gastroenterol Hepatol. 2021;18(10):717–29. https://doi.org/10.1038/s41575-021-00477-7.
23. Lee HH, Lee HA, Kim EJ, et al. Metabolic dysfunction-associated steatotic liver disease and risk of cardiovascular disease. Gut. 2023;73(3):533–40. https://doi.org/10.1136/gutjnl-2023-331003.
24. Liang F, Koya D. Acupuncture: is it effective for treatment of insulin resistance? Diabetes Obes Metab. 2010;12(7):555–69. https://doi.org/10.1111/j.1463-1326.2009.01192.x.
25. Lim A, Stewart K, Abramson MJ, et al. Multidisciplinary approach to management of maternal asthma (MAMMA©): the PROTOCOL for a randomized controlled trial. BMC Public Health. 2012;12:1094. https://doi.org/10.1186/1471-2458-12-1094.
26. Ma B, Li P, An H, et al. Electroacupuncture attenuates liver inflammation in nonalcoholic fatty liver disease rats. Inflammation. 2020;43(6):2372–8. https://doi.org/10.1007/s10753-020-01306-w.
27. Mantovani A, Goyale A, Roccarina DA, et al. A multidisciplinary approach to non-alcoholic fatty liver disease (NAFLD) improves cardiovascular risk factors: the experience of a tertiary liver center in UK. Dig Liv Dis. 2020;52(suppl 1):E46. https://doi.org/10.1016/j.dld.2019.12.042.
28. Mantovani A, Goyale A, Roccarina D, et al. A multidisciplinary approach to non-alcoholic fatty liverdisease (NAFLD) improves cardiovascular risk factors. Journal of Hepatology. 2020;73:S110. https://doi.org/10.1016/S0168-8278(20)30741-8.
29. Marzolini S, Jensen B, Melville P. Feasibility and effects of a group-based resistance and aerobic exercise program for individuals with severe schizophrenia: a multidisciplinary approach. Ment Health Phys Act. 2009;2(1):29–36. https://doi.org/10.1016/j.mhpa.2008.11.001.
30. Molla A, Motohashi K, Marjot T, et al. A multidisciplinary approach to the management of NAFLD is associated with improvement in markers of liver and cardio-metabolic health. Frontline Gastroenterol. 2019;10(4):337–46. https://doi.org/10.1136/flgastro-2018-101155.
31. Neilson LJ, Macdougall L, Lee PS, et al. Implementation of a care bundle improves the management of patients with non- alcoholic fatty liver disease. Frontline Gastroenterol. 2021;12:578–85. https://doi.org/10.1136/flgastro-2020-101480.
32. Newsome PN, Buchholtz K, Cusi K, et al. A placebo-controlled trial of subcutaneous semaglutide in nonalcoholic steatohepatitis. N Engl J Med. 2021;384(12):1113–24. https://doi.org/10.1056/NEJMoa2028395.
33. Patel R, Mueller M. Alcoholic liver disease. [Updated 2023 Jul 13]. In: StatPearls [Internet]. Treasure Island, FL: StatPearls Publishing; 2024. Available via https://www.ncbi.nlm.nih.gov/books/NBK546632/.
34. Patel D, Vedamurthy D. Lipid luminations: AHA scientific statement on nonalcoholic fatty liver disease; 2020. Available via https://www.lipid.org/lipid-spin/fall-2022/lipid-luminations-aha-scientific-statement-nonalcoholic-fatty-liver-disease. Accessed 5 Feb 2024.
35. Patel DP, Yan T, Kim D, et al. Withaferin a improves nonalcoholic steatohepatitis in mice. J Pharmacol Exp Ther. 2019;371(2):360–74. https://doi.org/10.1124/jpet.119.256792.
36. Pipitone RM, Ciccioli C, Infantino G, et al. MAFLD: a multisystem disease. Ther Adv Endocrinol Metab. 2023;14:20420188221145549. https://doi.org/10.1177/20420188221145549.
37. Porayko MK, Articolo A, Cerenzia W, et al. Differences in NAFLD/NASH management by provider specialty: opportunities for optimizing multidisciplinary care. J Multidiscip Healthc. 2022;15:1533–45. https://doi.org/10.2147/jmdh.s367607.
38. Ramírez-Mejía MM, Jiménez-Gutiérrez C, Eslam M, et al. Breaking new ground: MASLD vs. MAFLD-which holds the key for risk stratification? Hepatol Int. 2023;18:168. https://doi.org/10.1007/s12072-023-10620-y.
39. Raza S, Rajak S, Upadhyay A, et al. Current treatment paradigms and emerging therapies for NAFLD/NASH. Front Biosci (Landmark Ed). 2021;26(2):206–37. https://doi.org/10.2741/4892.
40. Ren S, Ma X, Wang R, et al. Preclinical evidence of berberine on non-alcoholic fatty liver disease: a systematic review and meta-analysis of animal studies. Front Pharmacol. 2021;12:742465. https://doi.org/10.3389/fphar.2021.742465.
41. Rinella ME, Lazarus JV, Ratziu V, et al. A multisociety Delphi consensus statement on new fatty liver disease nomenclature. J Hepatol. 2023;79(6):1542–56. https://doi.org/10.1016/j.jhep.2023.06.003.
42. Roeb E, Geier A. Nonalcoholic steatohepatitis (NASH) - current treatment recommendations and future developments. Z Gastroenterol. 2019;57(4):508–17. https://doi.org/10.1055/a-0784-8827.
43. Salomone F, Galvano F, Li Volti G. Molecular bases underlying the hepatoprotective effects of coffee. Nutrients. 2017;9(1):85.
44. Singhal P, Nesari T, Gupta GS. Efficacy of herbomineral compounds and pathya (ayurvedic dietary regime and physical exercise) in the management of yakṛt roga (non-alcoholic fatty liver disease). Anc Sci Life. 2015;34(4):216–22. https://doi.org/10.4103/0257-7941.160866.
45. Song S, Zheng J, Zhao D, et al. Quantitative proteomics analysis based on data-independent acqui-

sition reveals the effect of shenling baizhu powder (SLP) on protein expression in MAFLD rat liver tissue. Clin Proteomics. 2023;20(1):55. https://doi.org/10.1186/s12014-023-09442-9.

46. Sun DQ, Jin Y, Wang TY, et al. MAFLD and risk of CKD. Metabolism. 2021;115:154433. https://doi.org/10.1016/j.metabol.2020.154433.
47. Vanfleteren LEGW, Spruit MA, Wouters EFM, et al. Management of chronic obstructive pulmonary disease beyond the lungs. Lancet Respir Med. 2016;11:911–24. https://doi.org/10.1016/s2213-2600(16)00097-7.
48. Wang D, Day EA, Townsend LK, et al. GDF15: emerging biology and therapeutic applications for obesity and cardiometabolic disease. Nat Rev Endocrinol. 2021;17(10):592–607. https://doi.org/10.1038/s41574-021-00529-7.
49. Wang T, Li YQ, Yu LP, et al. Compatibility of polygonati rhizoma and angelicae sinensis radix enhance the alleviation of metabolic dysfunction-associated fatty liver disease by promoting fatty acid β-oxidation. Biomed Pharmacother. 2023;162:114584. https://doi.org/10.1016/j.biopha.2023.114584.
50. Wat E, Wang Y, Chan K, et al. An in vitro and in vivo study of a 4-herb formula on the management of diet-induced metabolic syndrome. Phytomedicine. 2018;42:112–25. https://doi.org/10.1016/j.phymed.2018.03.028.
51. Xu J, Wei Y, Huang Y, et al. Regulatory effects and molecular mechanisms of tea and its active compounds on nonalcoholic fatty liver disease. J Agric Food Chem. 2023; https://doi.org/10.1021/acs.jafc.2c07702.
52. Xue H, Wei M, Ji L. Chlorogenic acids: a pharmacological systematic review on their hepatoprotective effects. Phytomedicine. 2023;118:154961.
53. Yu J, Liang D, Li J, et al. Coffee, green tea intake, and the risk of hepatocellular carcinoma: a systematic review and meta-analysis of observational studies. Nutr Cancer. 2023;75(5):1295–308.
54. Zelniker TA, Braunwald E. Mechanisms of cardiorenal effects of sodium-glucose cotransporter 2 inhibitors: JACC state-of-the-art review. J Am Coll Cardiol. 2020;75(4):422–34. https://doi.org/10.1016/j.jacc.2019.11.031.
55. Zoncapè M, Liguori A, Tsochatzis E. Multidisciplinary clinic models for the management of non-alcoholic fatty liver disease. Hepatobiliary Surg Nutr. 2022;11(4):586–91. https://doi.org/10.21037/hbsn-22-58.

# 12 MASLD in Special Populations

Vikrant Sood, Snehavardhan Pandey, Mohit Kehar, Alexandre Louvet, Mariana M. Ramírez-Mejía, and Nahum Méndez-Sánchez

## 12.1 MASLD in Children

Vikrant Sood, Snehavardhan Pandey, and Mohit Kehar

### 12.1.1 Introduction

Pediatric nonalcoholic fatty liver disease (NAFLD) presents as persistent hepatic steatosis in individuals aged 18 years or younger, distinct from genetic or metabolic disorders, infections, steatogenic medications, alcohol use, or malnutrition. NAFLD ranges from simple steatosis to nonalcoholic steatohepatitis (NASH), an inflammatory and progressive form advancing to NAFLD cirrhosis, becoming a significant cause of chronic liver disease in both children and adults [1, 2]. Although only 3–5% of NAFLD patients develop significant liver disease, it is anticipated to become the primary indication for liver transplantation in adults in the future [3]. Formerly considered an adult ailment, these liver disorders are increasingly prevalent among children, necessitating a thorough understanding of their epidemiology, etiology, clinical manifestations, and management. The terminology for NAFLD has evolved, with the introduction of metabolic-associated fatty liver disease (MAFLD) to encompass the intricate connection between metabolic dysfunction, obesity, and liver pathology [4]. Recently, various societies have proposed replacing NAFLD with metabolic dysfunction-associated steatotic liver disease (MASLD), defined by the presence of at least one of five cardiometabolic risk factors, with the need to rule out alternative causes of hepatic steatosis and identify coexisting conditions [5]. This evolving nomenclature underscores the complex relationship between metabolic distur-

V. Sood
Department of Pediatric Hepatology and Liver Transplantation, Institute of Liver and Biliary Sciences, New Delhi, India

S. Pandey
Department of Pediatric Hepatology & Liver Transplantation, Sahyadri Hospital, Pune, India

M. Kehar (✉)
Division of Pediatric Gastroenterology, Hepatology and Nutrition, Children Hospital of Eastern Ontario, Ottawa, ON, Canada
e-mail: MKehar@cheo.on.ca

A. Louvet (✉)
Service des maladies de l'appareil digestif, Hôpital Huriez, Lille cedex, France
e-mail: alexandre.louvet@chru-lille.fr

M. M. Ramírez-Mejía · N. Méndez-Sánchez (✉)
Faculty of Medicine, National Autonomous University of Mexico, Mexico City, Mexico

Liver Research Unit, Medica Sur Clinic and Foundation, Mexico City, Mexico
e-mail: nmendez@medicasur.org.mx



N. Méndez-Sánchez, X. Qi (eds.), *Metabolic Dysfunction-Associated Steatotic Liver Disease*,
https://doi.org/10.1007/978-981-97-9519-2_12

bances and hepatic lipid accumulation. However, the introduction of the term MASLD has primarily targeted adult patients, potentially leading to ambiguity, especially regarding the metabolic aspect. Adult hepatologists, focusing on steatosis and insulin resistance mechanisms, may interpret the metabolic term differently than pediatric hepatologists, who prioritize considering inborn errors of metabolism in younger children with fatty liver disease. To maintain clarity and avoid potential issues arising from different interpretations, this chapter will use the terminology MASLD unless referencing existing literature.

**Epidemiology**
In recent years, pediatric MASLD epidemiology has shifted significantly due to global childhood obesity increases, linked to cultural changes and sedentary lifestyles [6, 7]. Diagnostic methods, including serum ALT levels, ultrasonography, and liver biopsy, vary in reported MASLD prevalence, estimated from 3% to 10% in general pediatric populations [8]. A systematic review found a mean MASLD prevalence of 7.6%, rising to 34.2% in child obesity clinics [9]. Globally, MASLD has become a primary driver of chronic liver disease (CLD) among adolescents and young adults [7]. NHANES data from 1999 to 2016 showed a 40% increase in MASLD prevalence among 6- to 21-year olds, with significant variations across demographics [10]. Histologically confirmed MASLD prevalence data in pediatrics are limited. In autopsy samples of children and adolescents aged 2–19 years in the USA, histologically confirmed MASLD was reported at 9.6%, rising significantly to 38% in the subset of obese children [11]. Another study by Xanthakos, involving 242 adolescents undergoing bariatric surgery with a mean age of 16.9 years and mean BMI of 51.6, found that 59% had histologically confirmed MASLD, with 24% having borderline and 10% having definite NASH [12]. MASLD prevalence in children is increasing globally, with recent meta-analyses indicating rates of 12.4% in nonobese and 63.4% in obese children in India, averaging at 35.4% [13]. Similar trends are seen in Korea, Japan, and China [14–17]. Variations by race and ethnicity are notable, with Hispanics having the highest prevalence (11.8%) and African Americans the lowest (1.5%) [11]. Genetic factors like PNPLA3 variants and differences in screening patterns contribute to these disparities [18, 19]. Significant differences exist in screening and referral practices, with African Americans less likely to be referred despite abnormal labs [20]. Gender disparities are also observed, with a 2:1 male-to-female ratio, possibly linked to hormonal influences [21, 22]. Notably, recent NHANES data showed elevated ALT prevalence in males (12.4%) compared to females (3.5%) [22], suggesting potential roles of estrogen in liver protection or androgens exacerbating NASH.

### 12.1.2 Natural History

The lack of long-term studies following unselected cohorts of children into adulthood has created a substantial gap in our understanding of the natural history of pediatric MASLD and the identification of predictors for severe disease progression. To unravel the evolving nature of these disorders and pinpoint factors influencing their progression from childhood to adulthood, comprehensive, extended research is imperative. Longitudinal studies have revealed concerning trends in pediatric MASLD [23–25]. Clinical trial data indicate that over a two-year period, approximately one-third of children with MASLD exhibit histologic progression, with factors such as increasing obesity rates, elevated aminotransferase levels, and disrupted glucose homeostasis being associated with disease progression [26]. Furthermore, a significant proportion of children present with advanced fibrosis or even cirrhosis at diagnosis, highlighting the severity of the disease in this population [25, 27, 28]. While longitudinal data is limited, it's evident that many children with MASLD present with advanced disease. In a North American multicenter study of 108 children, 20% presented with advanced fibrosis [27]. Despite these findings, the epidemiological impact of MASLD on severe liver outcomes such as cirrhosis and decompensation remain unclear due to a lack of larger-scale studies. However, the rising incidence of pediatric cirrhosis underscores the urgent need for further investigation into the specific influence of NAFLD/MASLD/MAFLD on this concerning trend [29]. Comprehensive, extended research efforts are imperative to unravel the evolving nature of these disorders, identify predictors of disease progression, and inform targeted interventions to mitigate the burden of pediatric MASLD. Table 12.1 enumerates the risk factors for pediatric MASLD.

**Table 12.1** Risk factors for the development of MASLD

| Risk factor | Description |
|---|---|
| Gender | Males |
| Ethnicity | Hispanic population |
| Familial factors | Obesity, hypertension, type 2 diabetes mellitus |
| Nutritional factors | Overweight, obese, protein energy malnutrition [75, 76] |
| Dietary factors | Consumption of foods with high glucose and fructose, long chain unsaturated fatty acids, processed foods & beverages [77] |
| Lifestyle-related factors | Sedentary lifestyle, increased screen time, lack of physical activity |
| Underlying disorders | Prolonged bedridden states, cerebral palsy, stroke, etc. |
| Genetic factors | PNPLA3, GCKR, TM6SF2 [79–81]. Table 12.2 Enumerates common genetic variants associated with NAFLD in children |
| Epigenetic factors | Maternal—Obesity, gestational diabetes, hypothyroidism<br>Perinatal & postnatal: Low birth weight, large for gestation, decreased duration of breast feeding, early introduction of sugars [81] |
| Psychological factors | Personality disorders—Depression, low self-esteem |
| Endocrine disorders | High androgenic states—Peripubertal age, PCOS |
| Drugs | Steroids, antipsychotics, antidepressants, anticonvulsants (valproate), chemotherapeutic drugs (methotrexate) |
| Other | Obstructive sleep apnea syndrome (OSAS) [82] |

**Table 12.2** Genetic variants in pediatric MASLD

| |
|---|
| PNPLA3 (Patatin-like phospholipase domain containing 3) |
| GCKR (Glucokinase regulatory protein) |
| TM6SF2 (transmembrane 6 superfamily member 2) |
| TRAPPC9 (C8orf17/ potassium channel, subfamily K, member 9) |
| NCAN (Neurocan) |
| LCP1 (lymphocyte cytosolic protein 1) |
| ACTR5 (ARP5 actin-related protein 5 homolog) |
| IL17RA (interleukin 17 receptor A) |

### 12.1.3 Pathophysiological Variations Between Adult and Pediatric MASLD

The pathophysiology of MASLD in children is complex, with factors such as diet, environment, genetics, epigenetics, and microbiota playing a role (Fig. 12.1) [30, 31]. While the detailed pathophysiology of MASLD has been extensively discussed in previous chapters, it is worth noting that the risk factors of pediatric MASLD appears to parallel that of adult MASLD. Notably, there are no distinct animal models specifically designed to study pediatric MASLD. However, there are some key differences between adult and pediatric MASLD, which will be outlined below. Pediatric NASH exhibits two distinct histologic patterns: Type 1, commonly seen in adults, features steatosis, ballooning degeneration, and perisinusoidal fibrosis; while Type 2, more prevalent in children, is characterized by steatosis, portal inflammation, and portal fibrosis. Notably, Type 1 MASH tends to emerge at an older age (mean age of 13.5), while Type 2 MASH is more likely to manifest in younger children (mean age of 11.5) [32]. The difference in histology between children and adults complicates the use of scoring systems like NASH CRN, widely used in adults for MASLD biopsies. One challenge is that the MASH used in these systems considers lobular but not portal inflammation. Additionally, ballooning, a significant feature in adult MASH associated with disease progression, is less clear in children. In adults, fibrosis typically starts

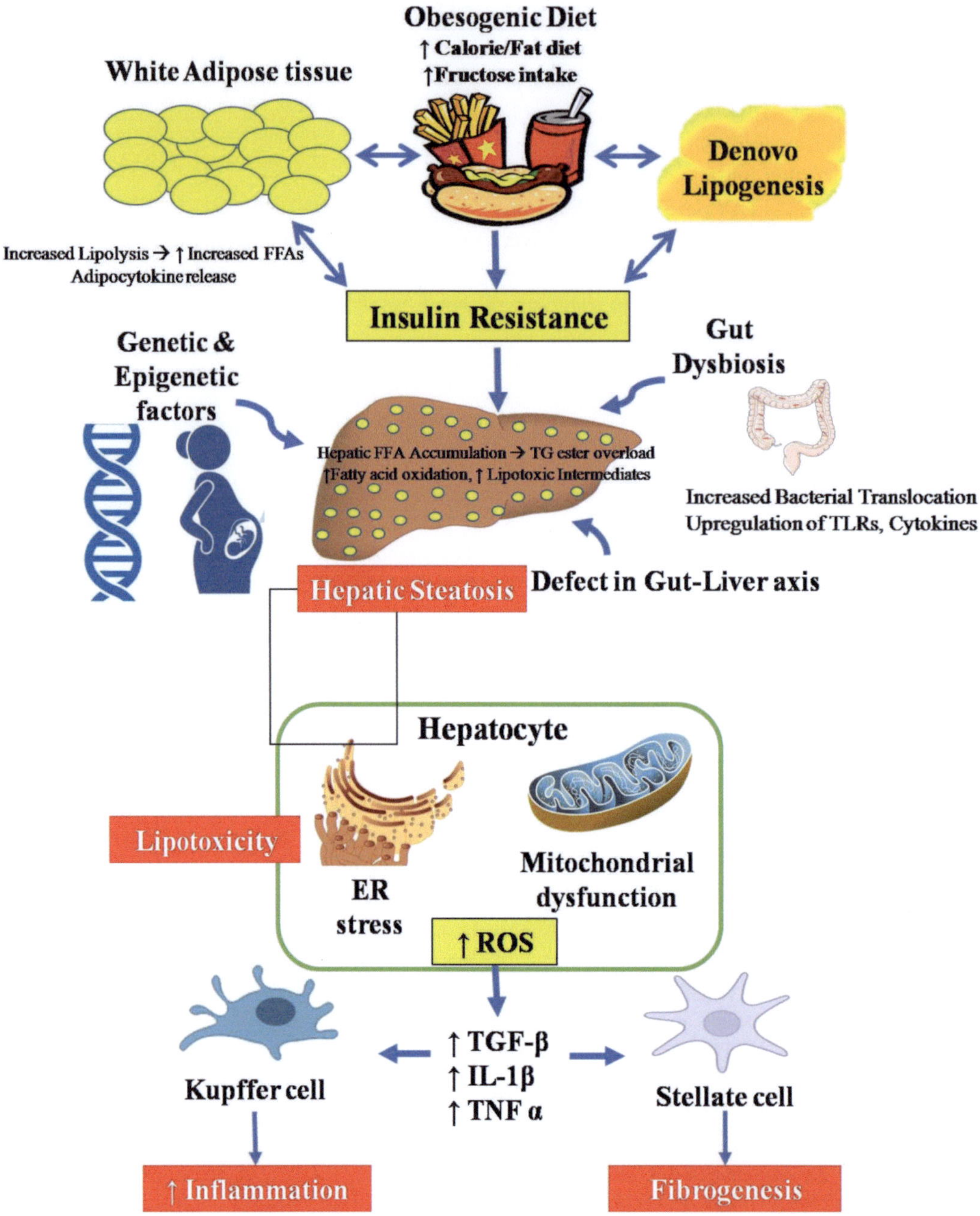


**Fig. 12.1** Pathogenesis of MASLD: The development of metabolic dysfunction-associated steatotic liver disease (MASLD) involves multiple factors. Insulin resistance is a key player promoting increased de novo lipogenesis. The composition of one's diet and its individual components has an impact on the intestinal microbiota influencing both hepatic inflammation and steatosis. Increased lipogenesis and free cholesterol contribute to cellular stress causing mitochondrial dysfunction and endoplasmic reticulum (ER) stress and release of reactive oxygen species (ROS) known as lipotoxicity. Lipopolysaccharides activate hepatic Kupffer cells, triggering the production of pro-inflammatory cytokines. Various mechanisms collectively induce inflammation, marked by the production of pro-inflammatory cytokines, activating stellate cells to produce collagen and promote fibrogenesis. *ER* endoplasmic reticulum, *FFA* free fatty acids, *IL-1β* interleukin 1β, *ROS* reactive oxygen species, *TG* triglyceride, *TGF-β* transforming growth factor-β, *TNF-α* tumor necrosis factor-α, *TLR* toll-like receptor

around hepatocytes in zone 3, forming pericellular "chicken wire" fibrosis. In contrast, children often exhibit zone 1 damage and a dominant portal-periportal fibrosis pattern, though pericellular and perisinusoidal fibrosis may also occur. The prevalence of cirrhosis at presentation in children, although typically noted to be around 1–2%, may vary across studies and has not been systematically studied, unlike in adults where it ranges from 5% to 10%. These observed distinctions suggest the potential existence of diverse disease pathophysiological processes influenced by age. Obtaining pediatric-specific data is crucial to address these knowledge gaps, providing insights into the unique progression of MASLD in the pediatric population and guiding tailored interventions and management approaches in this age group.

### 12.1.4 Signs and Symptoms in Pediatric MASLD

Pediatric MASLD often presents as asymptomatic, with diagnosis typically incidental during routine medical check-ups or investigations. Symptoms, when present, are nonspecific, including fatigue, malaise, and vague abdominal discomfort. Routine blood tests may reveal elevated liver enzymes, notably ALT, but normal levels do not exclude MASLD. This aspect remains contentious, given that some children with ultrasound-confirmed MASLD may have normal ALT levels, and cases of advanced fibrosis have been documented in children with normal liver enzymes [33]. Hepatomegaly may be present but not always palpable, requiring imaging for confirmation. Identification of metabolic risk factors such as obesity, signs of insulin resistance, and components of metabolic syndrome is crucial in diagnosis.

### 12.1.5 Differential Diagnosis

Differentiating MASLD from other liver disorders is crucial in pediatric age. Viral hepatitis and drug-induced liver injury could present as elevated transaminases in an overweight or healthy child and thought to be due to underlying MASLD [34]. Similarly, metabolic liver diseases can show fatty liver on an ultrasound or on liver biopsy. Table 12.3 shows an elaborate list of conditions that need to be considered and evaluated as per relevant clinical scenario. The differentiating points towards an organic disease are presence of younger age at presentation, significant jaundice, splenomegaly, ascites especially early in the course of disease and microvesicular steatosis on liver biopsy. Table 12.3 shows a tabulated representation of hepatic steatosis in children.

### 12.1.6 Diagnostics

The diagnostic landscape for pediatric MASLD involves a comprehensive approach integrating clinical evaluation, imaging studies, and laboratory assessments. Initial indicators include routine blood tests, notably revealing elevated liver enzymes, while ultrasound provides insights into hepatic steatosis. However, normal enzyme

**Table 12.3** Differential diagnosis of MASLD

| Disease category | Specific disorders |
|---|---|
| Underlying liver disease | |
| Disorders of amino acid metabolism. | Tyrosinemia, urea cycle defects |
| Disorders of carbohydrate metabolism. | Glycogen storage disorders, galactosemia, hereditary fructose intolerance |
| Disorders of lipid metabolism. | Lysosomal storage disorders, fatty acid oxidation disorders, cholesterol ester storage disorders |
| Others. | Wilson disease, mitochondrial disorders, citrin deficiency, bile acid synthetic disorders, congenital disorders of glycosylation |
| Drugs | Steroids, methotrexate, antidepressants, anticonvulsant |
| Infection | Hepatitis C |
| Nutrition & lifestyle | Anorexia nervosa, sudden weight loss, total parenteral nutrition |
| Others | Cystic fibrosis, turner syndrome, celiac disease |

levels do not exclude MASLD, necessitating advanced modalities such as liver biopsy and emerging noninvasive tools for a thorough understanding of the disease spectrum. The NASPGHAN practice guideline recommends MASLD screening in children aged 9–11, particularly targeting those who are obese or overweight with additional risk factors [1]. The AASLD does not recommend screening overweight and obese children due to insufficient data regarding the long-term benefits and cost-effectiveness of such measures [35]. Screening typically involves ALT testing, with sex-specific upper limits of normal. Controversy exists over routine ultrasound (US) due to cases of US confirmed MASLD with normal ALT levels. The proposed pediatric MAFLD definition requires evidence of steatosis, detectable through various methods, along with one of several specified criteria related to excess adiposity, prediabetes or type 2 diabetes, or signs of metabolic dysregulation. These factors encompass increased waist circumference, hypertension, hypertriglyceridemia, low serum HDL cholesterol levels, impaired fasting glucose, and an elevated triglyceride-to-HDL cholesterol ratio [4] (Fig. 12.2). MASLD diagnosis involves identifying steatotic liver disease (SLD) via imaging or biopsy, confirming at least one of five cardiometabolic criteria, and ruling out other causes of steatosis [5].

***Liver biopsy:*** Liver biopsy stands out as the gold standard for diagnosing MASLD, grading hepatic steatosis, diagnosis of MASH, ruling out other causes and staging disease (fibrosis) severity. However, the procedure's invasiveness, with potential complications such as pain, internal bleeding, bile leakage, and pneumothorax, limits its widespread use. Moreover, sampling errors due to the small liver area sampled and variability in pathologist interpretation pose diagnostic challenges [36]. Despite its drawbacks, liver biopsy is advised in patients at increased risk of MASH and advanced fibrosis. NASPGHAN guidelines recommend performing a liver biopsy in patients who have increased risk of MASH and/or advanced fibrosis such as those with high ALT levels (>80 U/L), splenomegaly, or an aspartate aminotransferase (AST) to ALT ratio of >1 [1]. Pediatric MASH diagnosis is challenging due to distinct histological patterns, where overlapping features of adult MASH types 1 and 2 are common in children. Various scoring systems, such as the Brunt score and NAFLD activity score (NAS), aim to standardize histological grading, although the pediatric MASLD histological score exists, it is more relevant for research than clinical practice [37].

***Assessment and detection of steatosis on imaging:*** US is commonly used to detect hepatic steatosis, but its sensitivity decreases with liver fat less than 30% or BMI over 40 kg/m$^2$, and it does not assess MASH or fibrosis. It is important to note, however, that US also falls short in assessing the presence of MASH or fibrosis [38]. MRI-based techniques, such as MRI proton density fat fraction (MRI-PDFF), offer superior accuracy for quantifying steatosis, with a cut-off of >5% for diagnosis [39]. FibroScan® with controlled attenuation parameter (CAP) is another noninvasive imaging technology effective for steatosis estimation in children [40]. Studies by Middleton et al. and Kwon et al. demonstrated MRI-PDFF and FibroScan®-CAP's utility in accurately assessing hepatic fat content in pediatric patients [39, 41]. Despite their benefits, validation in diverse cohorts and cost-effectiveness considerations remain challenges to their widespread adoption in diagnosing pediatric MASLD. Additionally, the lack of universally available normal cut-off values and variations in cut-off values among studies emphasize the need for further validation and standardization in pediatric population.

***Assessment and detection of fibrosis on imaging:*** Given the challenges associated with liver biopsy, the exploration of noninvasive methods for assessing fibrosis, a critical determinant of liver-related outcomes, is an area of active research in pediatric MASLD. The pursuit of alternative approaches aims to enhance diagnostic accuracy while minimizing the invasiveness and limitations associated with traditional biopsy methods.

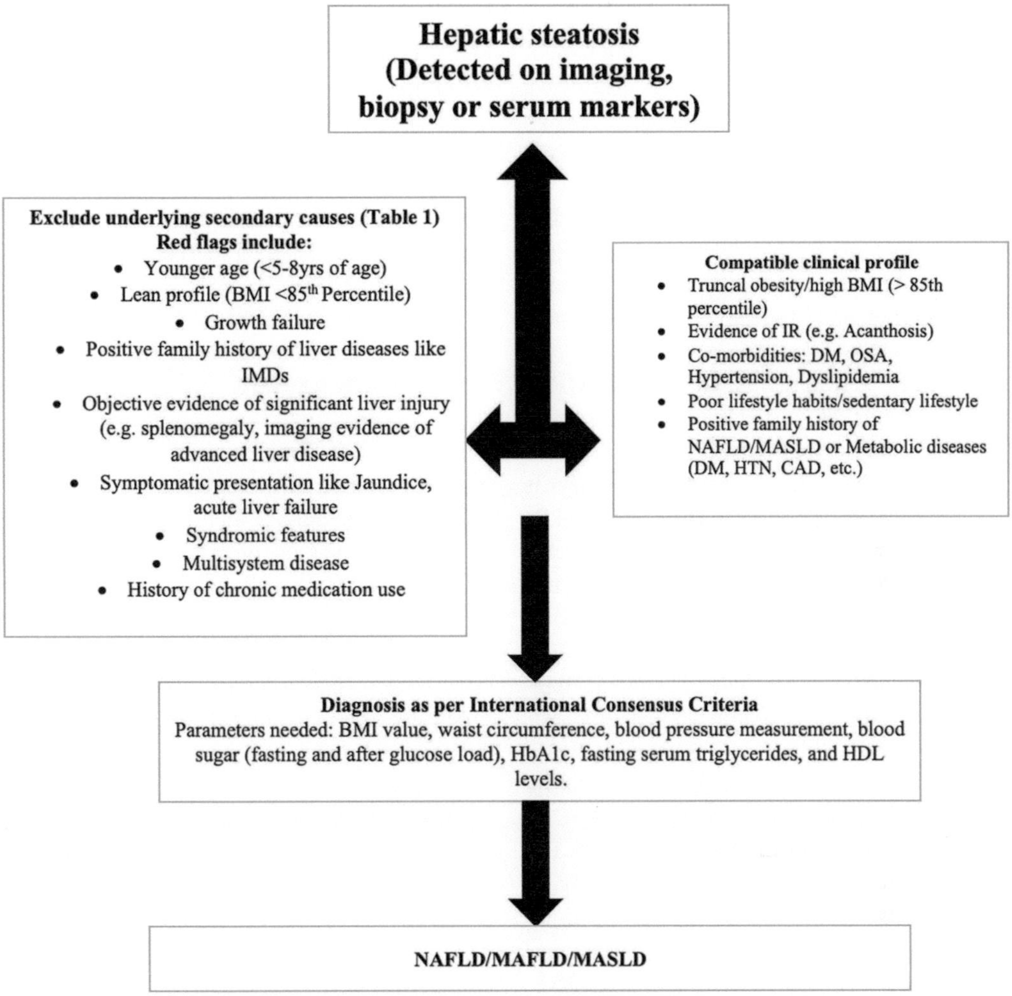


**Fig. 12.2** Suggested approach to diagnosing MASLD. *BMI* body mass index, *IMD* inherited metabolic diseases, *CLD* chronic/cirrhotic liver disease, *ALF* acute liver failure, *NAFLD* nonalcoholic fatty liver disease, *MAFLD* metabolic-associated fatty liver disease, *MASLD* metabolic dysfunction-associated steatotic liver disease, *IR* insulin resistance, *DM* diabetes mellitus, *OSA* obstructive sleep apnea, *CAD* coronary artery disease

(a) **Vibration-controlled transient elastography (VCTE)**, also known as transient elastography (TE) using FibroScan®, has shown high efficacy in assessing fibrosis severity in pediatric MASLD. In a study by Nobili et al., involving 52 children with biopsy-proven NASH, TE accurately predicted any fibrosis (F1–F4) with an AUROC of 0.977 [42]. Similarly, Alkhouri et al. further confirmed TE's proficiency, reporting an AUROC of 1.00 in predicting clinically significant (≥F2) fibrosis in a cohort of 67 children with biopsy-proven MASLD [43]. These studies demonstrate the precision of TE in identifying different fibrosis stages, supporting its potential as a valuable noninvasive tool for fibrosis assessment in pediatric MASLD.

(b) **Acoustic radiation force impulse (ARFI)** provides a dynamic assessment of liver stiffness, acting as a surrogate marker for fibrosis severity in various liver diseases, including pediatric MASLD. Its advantages include simultaneous visualization of grayscale or color Doppler images alongside ARFI images, using the same equipment through software imaging control and detection algorithms. Additionally, its versatile shear wave velocity (SWV) measurements allow assessment through different approaches, enhancing flexibility and applicability in evaluating liver stiffness. While limited data exists on ARFI's performance in children with MASLD, ongoing research in this area is evolving and showing promising results [44, 45].

(c) **Magnetic resonance elastography (MRE)** surpasses VCTE in sensitivity for detecting fibrosis stages ≥2, ≥3, and ≥4 in MASLD in adults [46]. An LSM by MRE ≥3.63 kPA is suggestive for advanced fibrosis, and ≥5 kPa is suggestive of cirrhosis in adult patients with MASLD [47]. While MRE data in children are limited, ongoing research is evolving. In a multicenter study of 90 pediatric patients, Schwimmer et al. assessed the diagnostic utility of two-dimensional gradient-recalled echo MRE (2D GRE MRE) in conjunction with liver biopsy in pediatric MASLD. The study reported an AUROC of 0.77–0.79 for detecting any fibrosis (≥ F1) and a cut-off of 3.03–3.05 for identifying advanced fibrosis (≥F3), with sensitivity ranging from 33.3% to 50%, specificity between 91.7% and 94%, PPV of 28.6–30%, and NPV of 95.2–96.2% [48].

### 12.1.7 Biomarkers

Identifying and validating novel noninvasive biomarkers for pediatric MASLD is a key research focus. While several noninvasive fibrosis scores used in adults, such as AST to ALT ratio, APRI, NAFLD fibrosis score, and Fib-4 index, have been explored, their applicability in children remains unvalidated. The pediatric NAFLD fibrosis index (PNFI), designed specifically for pediatric use, demonstrated predictive capability for advanced fibrosis [49], but lacks external validation. CK18, a hepatocyte apoptosis marker, shows promise in pediatric MASLD diagnosis and prognosis. Elevated CK18 levels correlate with MASH and outperform traditional liver enzyme markers [50–52]. In biopsy-proven MASLD, CK18 levels decrease in tandem with histologic improvements [53]. While full-length CK-18 (M65) also shows promise in diagnosing MASH [54, 55], large validation studies are necessary to confirm their clinical utility in pediatric MASLD. Despite ongoing research, there are currently no validated biomarkers for clinical use in pediatric MASLD.

### 12.1.8 Management

Pediatric MASLD management requires a multifaceted approach involving lifestyle adjustments, dietary modifications, and careful monitoring. Key aspects include dietary changes, physical activity promotion, and addressing risk factors. Effective management entails regular follow-ups, specialist collaboration, and tailored interventions while considering age-appropriate growth. Emerging pharmacological therapies and ongoing research add complexity, necessitating a comprehensive strategy. Personalized care, ongoing research, and a holistic approach are essential, emphasizing adaptability to integrate new therapies and address the unique needs of young patients.

### 12.1.9 Lifestyle Management

While Resmetirom is approved for adults with MASLD, no pharmacological treatments exist for children, making lifestyle changes critical [56]. Lifestyle management remains paramount in addressing pediatric MASLD, emphasizing dietary modifications and increased physical activity as key pillars of treatment [1]. While weight loss is a crucial target in adult populations, defining specific weight loss goals for pediatric patients is less straightforward. Nonetheless, even modest reductions in weight have demonstrated improvements in clinical biomarkers of MASLD in children, highlighting the significance of weight management [57, 58]. Various dietary interventions have been explored in pediatric MASLD, including portion control, reduced glycemic load, low carbohydrate diets,

Mediterranean diet, meal replacement, time-restricted eating, very low-calorie diets, and protein-sparing modified fasting [60–63]. The effectiveness of these dietary approaches often hinges on long-term adherence, with studies indicating varying levels of compliance across different dietary strategies. While adherence tends to be lower with low carbohydrate diets, approaches like portion control and reduced glycemic load have shown better adherence rates [60]. To enhance sustainability, involving other family members in dietary and lifestyle changes can be beneficial. In addition to dietary modifications, the importance of regular physical activity cannot be overstated in pediatric MASLD management. Engaging in physical activity is vital for proper growth and development, as well as for addressing the underlying issues of overweight and obesity associated with MASLD. While specific studies directly comparing different exercise interventions in pediatric MASLD are limited, evidence from studies focused on pediatric obesity suggests significant benefits of exercise in reducing intrahepatic triglycerides and liver enzyme levels [63]. General recommendations advocate for at least 60 min of daily moderate to vigorous physical activity, incorporating a variety of activities and including resistance training to enhance muscular strength and bone health [64]. Structured and unstructured daily activities should be enjoyable and sustainable, aligning with broader health recommendations for children. Importantly, physical activity has been shown to improve several serum biomarkers related to MASLD, even independent of significant weight loss, highlighting its multifaceted role in managing pediatric MASLD [65].

**Bariatric Surgery**

Bariatric surgery, including laparoscopic sleeve gastrectomy, is effective in reducing weight, with both adults and children experiencing approximately 20% total body weight loss [66, 67]. While less common in pediatrics, it's considered for those over 12 years old with a BMI over 35 kg/m$^2$ and comorbid MASH or type 2 diabetes [1]. However, bariatric surgery may worsen MASLD in some cases, with around 12% of adults experiencing exacerbated MASLD postoperatively [68]. The impact of bariatric surgery on pediatric MASLD warrants careful consideration on an individual basis.

**Pharmacology**

Trials in the pediatric field have not achieved desired goals and are not approved for pediatric MASLD management. The TONIC trial investigated vitamin E (800 units daily) and metformin (500 mg twice daily) in pediatric MASLD, with neither treatment meeting the primary outcome of substantial and persistent ALT reduction [69]. However, vitamin E demonstrated greater NASH resolution (58% vs. 28%; $P = 0.006$), with significant histological improvements compared to placebo. Losartan, considered for its antifibrotic effects in pediatric MASLD treatment, did not significantly reduce ALT levels in children compared to a placebo [70]. Elafibranor, a dual PPAR $\alpha/\delta$ agonist, showed well-tolerated once-daily dosing in children with a 37.4% relative reduction in ALT, suggesting potential for further exploration [71]. Omega-3 fatty acids (DHA and eicosapentaenoic acid) have shown positive outcomes in pediatric fatty liver disease trials, improving transaminases, hepatic steatosis, and BMI [72]. Ongoing trials, like NCT03867487, investigate SGLT2 inhibitors as a novel pediatric MASLD treatment, with results anticipated in the future. Given the limited effective treatments and substantial disease burden, urgent need exists for new options in managing this condition, with MASLD lacking approved therapy, relying on lifestyle changes and weight loss, yet facing challenges in implementation and long-term efficacy due to various factors. GLP1-RAs, such as liraglutide and semaglutide, show promise in managing MASLD, initial adult data do not demonstrate significant fibrosis improvements compared to placebo [73]. However, recent updates from the ESSENCE trial indicate that the trial achieved its primary endpoints, showing a statistically significant and superior improvement in liver fibrosis with no worsening of steatohepatitis, as well as resolution of steatohepatitis with no worsening of liver fibrosis, with semaglutide 2.4 mg compared to placebo. Enthusiasm persists, and AASLD suggests considering these agents in patients with obesity and diabetes due to potential MASLD benefits [74]. While adult trials for MASLD persist, historical trends show pediatric trials lagging. Optimism surrounds the prospect of future pediatric-specific trials, holding promise for advanced cases resistant to lifestyle management.

**Summary**
The surge in childhood obesity globally has led to a corresponding increase in MASLD cases, posing significant challenges for healthcare systems. These conditions not only affect the liver but also jeopardize overall health, potentially leading to long-term complications like cirrhosis. Continual research is needed to understand these conditions better and improve outcomes for affected children. As ongoing trials progress, addressing pediatric MASLD with tailored, effective approaches remains a priority in pediatric gastroenterology and hepatology. Urgent action is needed to adopt impactful management strategies, navigate lifestyle changes, and explore innovative interventions to mitigate the increasing burden and enhance outcomes for affected children.

**Key Points**

- MASLD is the most common cause of chronic liver disease in children.
- Spectrum of the MASLD may be different from that seen in the adult population; a proportion of pediatric subjects may have an underlying secondary cause of steatosis which needs to be excluded.
- Pediatric MASH presents distinct histologic patterns, suggesting potentially diverse disease pathophysiological processes influenced by age. Obtaining pediatric-specific data is essential to address knowledge gaps, providing insights into the unique progression of MASLD in the pediatric population and guiding tailored interventions and management approaches.
- The diagnostic landscape for pediatric MASLD involves a multifaceted approach, combining clinical evaluation, imaging studies, and laboratory assessments. Routine blood tests and imaging, such as ultrasound, serve as initial indicators, but advanced diagnostic modalities, including liver biopsy and emerging noninvasive tools, are crucial for comprehensive disease understanding.
- Multipronged approach should be undertaken for holistic care including strengthening of peer group/school/family support system along with standard medical management.
- In pediatric population, improved physical activity (as sports-related activities) and dietary interventions are the keystones for the management; till further evidence is available, pharmacotherapy and bariatric surgery has role in selected patients.

## 12.2 MASLD and Alcohol Consumption

Alexandre Louvet

Since alcohol and the metabolic syndrome represent the first two more prevalent causes of chronic liver disease, they coexist in a very high proportion of patients. Significant effort has been made over the last decades to understand the synergistic effects of both conditions on liver function.

Liver damage related to alcohol or to metabolic syndrome share some common pathways and it can be difficult to pathologists to distinguish histological lesions caused by alcohol-related liver disease (ARLD) or by metabolic dysfunction-associated steatotic liver disease (MASLD). Indeed, in terms of pathophysiology, both conditions are characterized by a certain degree of Kupffer cell activation, bacterial translocation, dysbiosis and leaky gut, adipose tissue inflammation, etc. [83]. For both conditions, a certain degree of systemic inflammation is observed which seems to contribute to liver inflammation and liver injury [84]. Genetics also play a major role in promoting steatosis and fibrosis progression both for ARLD and MASLD, especially polymorphisms for PNPLA3, TM6SF2, MBOAT7, and HSD17B13 [83].

While some similar pathways are activated during ARLD and MASLD, leading to steatosis, steatohepatitis, fibrosis and ultimately cirrhosis, little is known about end-stage liver disease in the two conditions, especially liver regeneration, fibrosis perpetuation and drivers of decompensation [85], mostly because animal models are at present unable to recapitulate clinical and histological damage observed in patients with decompensated cirrhosis.

As a result of some shared pathways between ARLD and MASLD, liver biopsy shows in the two conditions a certain degree of steatosis, hepatocyte ballooning, Mallory-Denk bodies and subsequently fibrosis and cirrhosis [83]. Some lesions are more specific of ARLD such as infiltration by polymorphonuclear neutrophils or cholestasis in decompensated forms (especially alcohol-related hepatitis). The composition of extracellular matrix seems also different between the two conditions while some specific comparison studies are still lacking.

Data coming from animal models have underlined the synergism between alcohol and the metabolic syndrome toward more pronounced liver injury. As an example, rodents overfed and fed alcohol show much more important steatosis and elevated transaminases compared to overfeeding or alcohol regimen alone [86]. In this study, the two regimens combined seemed more susceptible to increase fibrogenesis while one treatment alone had very limited effects. It must be kept in mind that animal models mostly cause early stages of ARLD and MASLD, especially steatosis, with very mild inflammation and almost not fibrosis [83]. From a histological point of view, it must be stressed that metabolic factors do not seem to play the same role when different elementary lesions are considered. Indeed, a recent study performed in 325 patients with a history of excessive alcohol use (defined by the authors as >24/36 g/day for women/men for at least 1 year) has demonstrated that drivers of fibrosis, steatosis and inflammation are different [87]. As an example, body mass index was associated with steatosis but not with inflammation or fibrosis, while insulin resistance correlated with inflammation and fibrosis, but not with steatosis. Active drinking was a strong predictor of steatosis and inflammation but had no impact on fibrosis. These findings underline that some metabolic factors influence ARLD at a different degree when early vs. late events are chosen as endpoints.

In individuals, the relationship between alcohol and the metabolic syndrome is difficult to analyze because the number of metabolic factors and the amount of alcohol consumed markedly change the outcome. Nevertheless, this relationship seems more synergistic and multiplicative than simply additive. As an example, a large prospective study on close to 10,000 men with a median follow-up of 29 years [88] has demonstrated that the relative risk of dying from liver cause was much higher in obese patients consuming more than 15 units of alcohol a week (relative risk of roughly 18) compared to lean patients with no alcohol consumption (set as reference). When assessing the contributions of body mass index and of alcohol to liver mortality, the authors found that body mass index alone did not significantly increase the risk, while alcohol alone was associated with a 3.66 risk and the interaction between body mass index and alcohol had a risk of liver-related death of 9.53. In women, a very large population-based study performed in more than 1 million patients screened for breast cancer has confirmed that the risk of cirrhosis was highest in case of weekly alcohol consumption greater than 15 units and obesity [89]. Again, the relationship between alcohol and body mass index was multiplicative and not only additive. Like in the previous study performed in men [88], alcohol was the most important driver of fatal outcome, accounting for 42% of deaths while body mass index was responsible for 17% of liver fatality.

Studies taking liver biochemistry as an endpoint also underline the relationship between alcohol consumption and the metabolic syndrome. For instance, a cross-sectional study on more than 2000 patients attending a research visit has demonstrated that obese people consuming more than 3 drinks/day had much higher transaminases (both AST and ALT) than individuals having only one condition after adjustment on age, sex, cholesterol, triglycerides, diabetes, and blood pressure [90].

The clinical outcome between MASLD and ARLD is largely different. Population studies have indeed shown that patients with ARLD have a much higher risk of dying or of developing liver events vs. their comparators than patients with MASLD vs. their own comparators [91, 92]. When comparing patients with steatosis related to alcohol and related to metabolic syndrome, age at death is lower in patients with ARLD than in patients with MASLD, regardless of sex [93]. Interestingly, the large Dionysos cohort has also shown that alcohol was an independent factor of steatosis persistence and of death in patients with steatosis, while body mass index played a minor role [94].

Metabolic factors play an important role in the natural history of ARLD. Indeed, in heavy drinkers, cirrhosis is more frequently observed in overweight than in non-overweight patients [95]. The same study has also found that liver inflammation (i.e., histological lesions of alcohol-related hepatitis) was more prevalent in case of excess weight for at least 10 years. The same group has also demonstrated that body mass index and serum glucose were independently associated with a higher fibrosis score in a cohort of more than 250 patients with a daily alcohol consumption higher than 50 g/day [96].

Looking more precisely at the drivers of morbidity and mortality in ARLD and MASLD help understand how the two conditions interact. The role of diabetes must be underlined because it very significantly impacts the risk of extensive fibrosis/cirrhosis. As an example, a Swedish cohort study has shown that diabetes is observed in roughly 25% of patients with cirrhosis compared to 11.2% in MASLD regardless of fibrosis stage [92]. Conversely, a large biobank from the genetic study GenomAlc [97] has observed a much more important prevalence of diabetes in patients with ARLD compared to controls. Lastly, a French study [98] has observed that most of the disease burden in patients with diabetes was related to alcohol. Indeed, this retrospective cohort of more than 50,000 patients with type 2 diabetes has calculated that alcohol use disorders carried an attributable risk of disease progression to liver-related complications of more than 50% while obesity only accounted for 7%.

While large evidence shows that obesity/diabetes/metabolic syndrome impact negatively the natural history of patients with excessive daily alcohol consumption (i.e., more than 20 g/day in women and more than 30 g/day in men), a controversy exists as to whether moderate amounts of alcohol (that is daily consumption of 10–20 g) may be beneficial by limiting the histological damage related to MASLD. As an example, a cohort of approx. 600 patients with livre biopsies has shown that modest drinkers had less steatosis, fibrosis and ballooning than lifetime nondrinkers [99]. One of the explanations could be that modest alcohol drinking is associated with improved insulin resistance and also underlines the fact that consumptions of 10–20 g/day reduce the risk of myocardial infarction. However, this is to be taken with much caution because the positive impact of modest daily alcohol consumption—if it exists—does not seem to exist in patients with MASLD who have a high fibrosis risk [100]. Indeed, it is very difficult to draw a firm conclusion about this putative effect of moderate alcohol consumption because most data come from cross-sectional studies with no intervention, without taking into account other confounders [101]. It must also be underlined that body mass index and alcohol consumption vary a lot along lifetime and for example abstainers at time of inclusion may have been former alcohol abusers. In addition, insulin resistance and drinking patterns are generally not well measured in cohort studies.

Lastly, a recent nomenclature has been proposed after a Delphi consensus [102]. Though bringing some desirable changes, the complex relationship between alcohol and the metabolic syndrome will have to be clarified. Among the major criticisms made to this new nomenclature, the fact that only one factor of the metabolic syndrome is now required to qualify the patient for a diagnosis of MASLD is very questionable. Indeed, three criteria are usually needed for a clinical diagnosis of the metabolic syndrome [103] among the following: elevated waist circumference, elevated triglyceride, reduced HDL-cholesterol, elevated blood pressure, and elevated fasting glucose. Some of these factors can be influenced by other conditions than the metabolic syndrome (e.g., diabetes caused by pancreatic disorders, elevated blood pressure related to suprarenal diseases, etc.). Thus, requiring three factors out of five is very relevant because it makes the clinician very confident about the fact that the patient has indeed a metabolic syndrome rather than an external cause of these factors. Since patients with daily alcohol consumption have frequently changes in lipid metabolism, elevated blood pressure and diabetes, the definition of the metabolic syndrome in them should not rely on a single metabolic criterion.

The choice of thresholds is also questionable in the new nomenclature [102]. Indeed, two cut-off values have been proposed to differentiate MASLD from MASLD with increased alcohol intake (termed MetALD) and ARLD. The first cut-off is set at 20 (women) and 30 (men) grams/day. This cut-off is well-established and was formerly used to define nonalcoholic fatty liver disease. The main reason for using this threshold is that meta-analyses have shown that the risk of liver damage related to daily alcohol drinking starts to increase beyond a daily alcohol consumption of 20–30 g [104, 105]. Conversely, the second cut-off to define "heavy drinking" was set at 60 g/day without firm consensus in the literature. It must be underlined that excessive drinking is poorly defined by scientific societies. The National Institute on Alcohol Abuse and Alcoholism (NIAAA) defines heavy drinking as more than 3 drinks/day in women or 4 drinks/day in men, with one drink corresponding to 14 g. The World Health Organization (WHO) defines 4 risk levels of alcohol consumption: low (1–20 grams/day in women, 1–40 g/day in men), moderate (20–40 g/day in women, 40–60 g/day in men), high (40–60 g/day in women, 60–100 g/day in men), and very high (>60 g/day in women, >100 g/day in men). The European Association for the Study of the Liver (EASL) does not define heavy drinking. These discrepancies certainly underline the need for a consensus. Caution is thus needed regarding the existence of a "second cut-off", especially when considering that the curve linking daily alcohol consumption with the risk of cirrhosis does not seem to change markedly beyond 60 g/day [104].

There is thus large evidence that alcohol and the metabolic syndrome interact and are responsible for a synergistic impact on liver damage in patients with both conditions. As mentioned above, clinical data show that daily alcohol consumption carries the more important weight in the interaction. However, more data are needed to understand more clearly which amount of alcohol can be tolerated in patients with features of the metabolic syndrome. When considering the shared pathways between the two conditions, it is tempting to imagine that an ideal drug could be efficient for both ARLD and MASLD. Special attention should thus be paid in terms of therapeutic development to design trials that will stratify patients according to their alcohol consumption and the importance of the metabolic syndrome.

## 12.3 MASLD in HIV Patients

Mariana M. Ramírez-Mejía and
Nahum Méndez-Sánchez

### 12.3.1 Introduction

Human immunodeficiency virus (HIV) remains as a major public health problem, affecting more than 39 million people living with HIV (PLWH) worldwide [106]. HIV has been converted from a fatal disease to a manageable chronic condition with the introduction of antiretroviral therapy (ART) [107, 108]. Nevertheless, the success of ART is accompanied by a number of complications, including metabolic disturbances that contribute to the development of diseases such as MASLD [109].

MASLD has emerged as a significant and growing health problem among PLWH, reflecting a complex interplay between the metabolic impacts of HIV infection, the side effects of ART and the presence of traditional metabolic risk factors such as obesity, diabetes and dyslipidemia [110, 111]. Additionally, coinfection with hepatitis C virus (HCV) or hepatitis B virus (HBV), common in PLWH, may accelerate the progression of liver fibrosis in the setting of MAFLD/MASLD [112]. Given the increased risk and potential complications associated with MASLD in PLWH, there is a critical need for early detection, risk stratification, and treatment strategies tailored to this population [113]. In this chapter we will discuss the epidemiology, pathogenesis, clinical implications, and treatment considerations of MASLD in the context of HIV infection. By elucidating the complex interplay of factors contributing to the occurrence of MASLD in PLWH, we can better inform clinical practice and optimize outcomes in this vulnerable population.

### 12.3.2 Epidemiology

The estimated worldwide prevalence of MASLD in PLWH is 33.9%, higher than in the general population [114]. Nevertheless, prevalence varies depending on the geographic region, with the highest reported in Europe (42.7%), followed by South America (35.8%) [114, 115]. The incidence rates of MASLD among PLWH also reflect significant variability across different regions and populations (Fig. 12.3) [116]. This variability is largely attributed to differences in diagnostic methods, the prevalence of risk factors, and the accessibility and quality of healthcare systems [115, 117]. Additionally, metabolic steatohepatitis (MASH) and fibrosis are increasingly recognized as significant health concerns among PLWH with estimated prevalence of 48.7% and 23.3% respectively (Figs. 12.4 and 12.5) [114, 118].

The risk factors for MASLD in PLWH are multifactorial, combining those associated with MASLD in the broader population and specific factors related to HIV infection and its treatment [110, 119]. General risk factors include obesity, type 2 diabetes mellitus (T2DM), dyslipidemia, hypertension and genetic predispositions, which contribute significantly to the development and

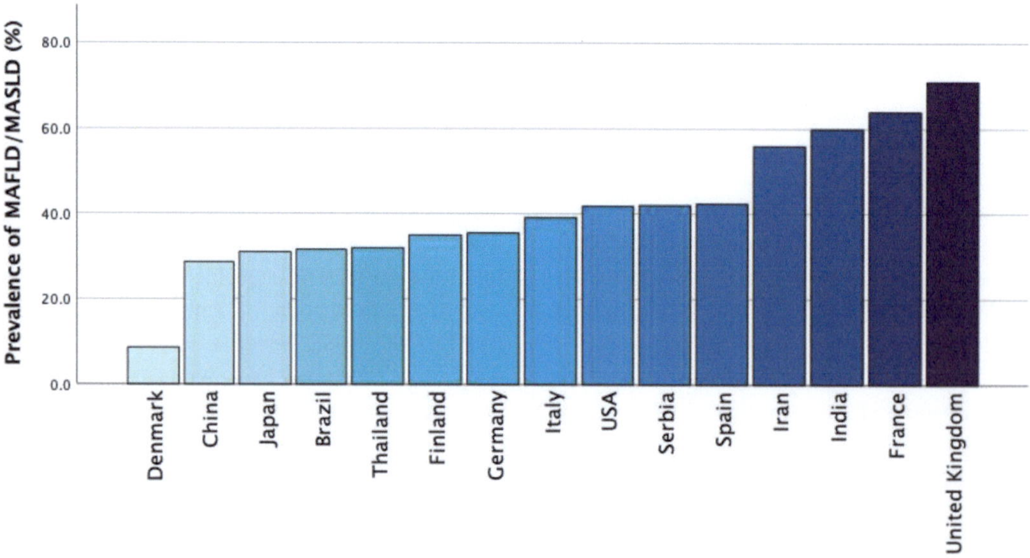


**Fig. 12.3** Prevalence of MASLD in PLWH. This chart illustrates the prevalence of metabolic dysfunction-associated fatty liver disease (MAFLD) and metabolic dysfunction-associated steatotic liver disease (MASLD) in people living with HIV (PLWH) across different geographic regions

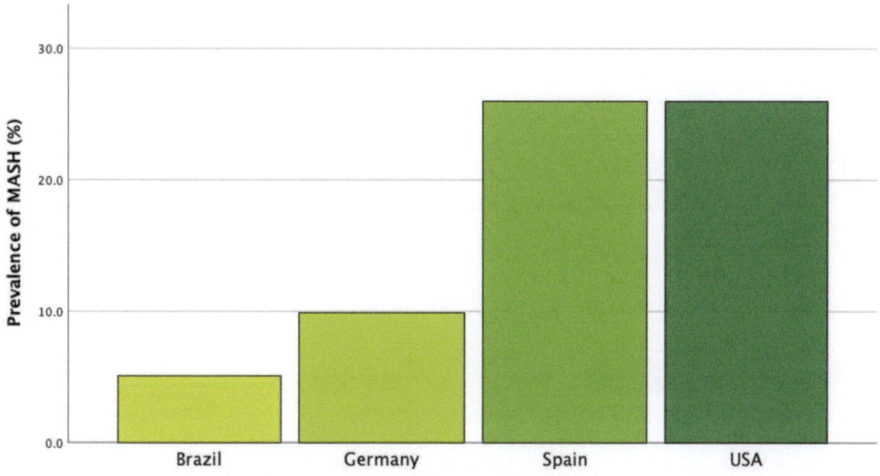


**Fig. 12.4** Prevalence of MASH in PLWH. This chart illustrates the prevalence of metabolic-associated steatohepatitis (MASH) in people living with HIV (PLWH) across different geographic regions

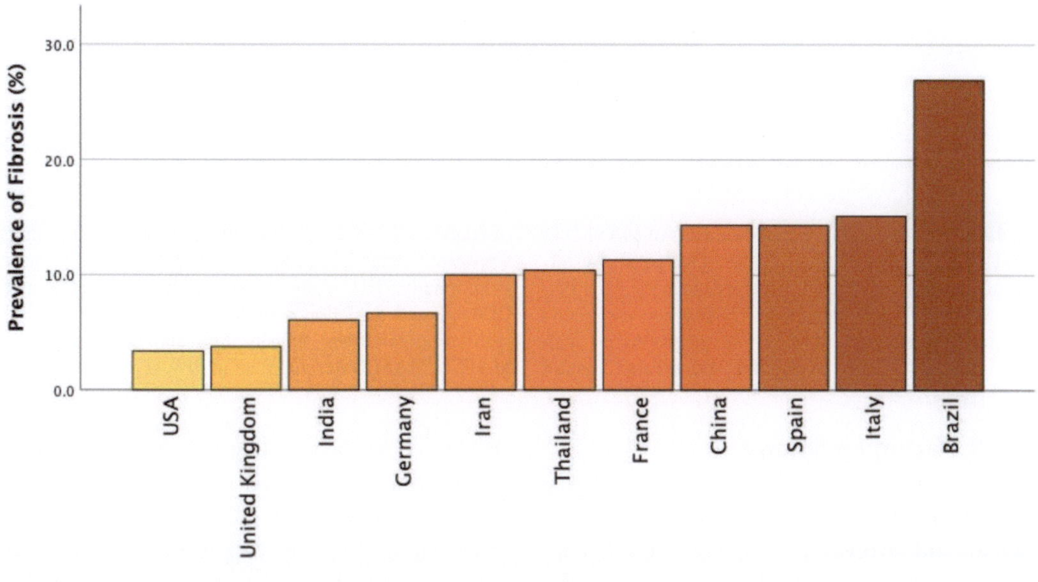


**Fig. 12.5** Prevalence of fibrosis in PLWH. This chart illustrates the prevalence of liver fibrosis in people living with HIV (PLWH) across different geographic regions

progression of MASLD [114]. PLWH face unique challenges that elevate their risk of developing MASLD. The use of certain antiretroviral therapies has been linked to metabolic alterations, such as lipodystrophy, insulin resistance (IR), and dyslipidemia [121–123]. Furthermore, HIV-associated factors such as chronic inflammation and immune dysregulation, even in the setting of virologic suppression with ART, can exacerbate liver damage [113]. Coinfections with hepatitis B virus (HBV) and hepatitis C virus (HCV) are also more prevalent in PLWH and can lead to more rapid progression of MASLD [123].

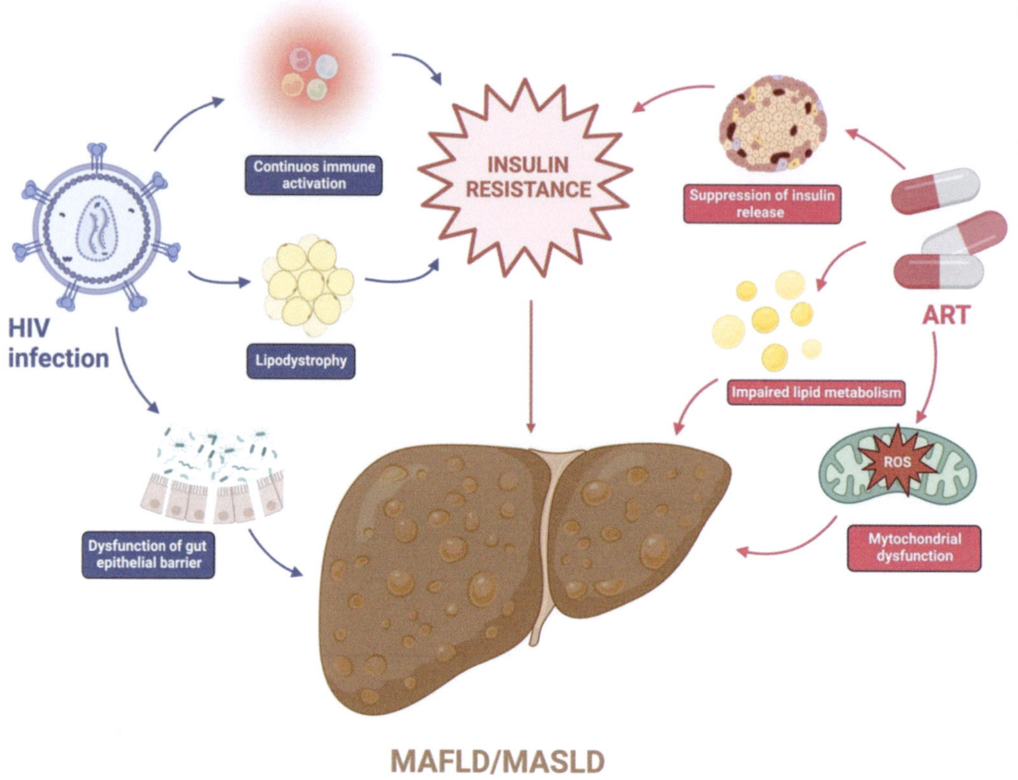


**Fig. 12.6** Pathophysiological mechanisms of MASLD in PLWH. This figure illustrates the complex pathophysiology of metabolic dysfunction-associated fatty liver disease (MAFLD) and metabolic dysfunction-associated steatotic liver disease (MASLD) in people living with HIV (PLWH). PLWH experience exacerbated insulin resistance (IR) due to HIV infection-induced immune activation and antiretroviral therapy (ART) use. Additionally, HIV-related gastrointestinal damage and CD4+ T cell depletion compromise mucosal immunity, facilitating microbial translocation and contributing to MAFLD/MASLD development in PLWH

### 12.3.3 Pathophysiology

The pathophysiology of MASLD in PLWH is complex and involves multiple pathways that are similar and distinct from those observed in the general population (Fig. 12.6) [124]. In PLWHA, IR can be exacerbated by HIV infection itself by continuous immune activation with elevated levels of pro-inflammatory markers or expansion of CD8+/HLA-DR subtype T cells [125, 126], and by the use of ART, particularly regimens that include protease inhibitors (PIs) and some nucleoside reverse transcriptase inhibitors (NRTIs) [127]. PIs can trigger IR and alter lipid metabolism, through different pathways, such as direct suppression of insulin release from pancreatic beta-cells and elevation of apolipoprotein B levels [112, 128]. On the other side, NRTIs can lead to alterations in the lipid profile and IR due to mitochondrial toxicity [127, 129]. This mitochondrial dysfunction can result in decreased fatty acid oxidation and a consequent accumulation of lipids in hepatocytes [130]. In addition to these mechanisms, the gut microbiota also plays an important role in the development of MASLD in PLWH. HIV infection is closely associated with damage to the gastrointestinal (GI) tract and depletion of intestinal CD4+ T cells, which are crucial for the maintenance of mucosal immunity. This loss of CD4+ T cells in the GI tract leads to dysfunction of the epithelial barrier, compromising its integrity. A compromised intestinal barrier allows translocation of microbial products into the systemic circulation, a phenomenon that has far-reaching consequences for the development of MASLD in PLWH [131].

### 12.3.4 Clinical Manifestations

The clinical manifestations of MASLD in PLWH are diverse and can range from asymptomatic elevations of liver enzymes to advanced liver disease [132]. Over time, if the disease progresses uncontrolled, it can lead to more serious complications, such as metabolic steatohepatitis (MASH), fibrosis, cirrhosis, and even hepatocellular carcinoma (HCC) [113]. Progression to these advanced stages of liver disease may be accelerated in PLWH due to immune dysfunction and chronic inflammation [112, 133]. In addition, the presence of comorbidities such as coinfections with HBV or HCV may synergistically increase the risk of liver-related morbidity and mortality [134].

### 12.3.5 Diagnosis and Monitoring

The approach to diagnosis and monitoring of MASLD in PLWH is complicated by the relative paucity of data specific to this population. Consequently, clinicians often adapt diagnostic guidelines and recommendations developed for MASLD in the general population to the context of PLWH [127]. Although liver biopsy is considered the definitive method for diagnosing and staging MASLD [74], its application in PLWH is limited by several factors. Liver biopsy is invasive, carries potential risks, and is associated with significant costs. In addition, the possibility of sampling error can affect diagnostic accuracy [135]. These limitations are especially relevant in PLWH, where the need for continuous follow-up to assess disease progression or response to treatment makes repeated liver biopsies impractical and undesirable [118, 127]. Therefore, noninvasive methods assume a pivotal role in the diagnosis and risk stratification of MASLD in PLWH. These methods, including biochemical markers, fibrosis scores (such as the FIB-4 index, noninvasive liver disease assessment (NILDA), and NAFLD fibrosis score) and imaging techniques (such as ultrasound, transient elastography, and MRI-based assessments) [109, 136]. Noninvasive methods not only facilitate the detection and evaluation of liver fibrosis and steatosis, but also allow monitoring of disease progression and the efficacy of therapeutic interventions over time [137]. These approaches are particularly advantageous in the management of PLWH, which may require more dynamic and less invasive monitoring strategies due to their unique clinical considerations.

### 12.3.6 Treatment

Treatment of MASLD in PLWH requires a multifaceted approach that addresses underlying metabolic risk factors, optimizes ART, and considers lifestyle modifications as key elements [110].

#### 12.3.6.1 Lifestyle Modifications

Lifestyle changes are fundamental in the treatment of MASLD, focusing on diet, exercise and weight control [138]. PLWH with MASLD should avoid a diets rich in saturated fatty acids, refined carbohydrates and processed red meat [139]. For overweight or obese individuals, a weight loss goal of 7–10% of body weight is recommended [74]. In lean individuals, who may also suffer from MASLD due to metabolic dysregulation rather than excess weight, a more modest weight loss goal of 3–5% is advised [139].

#### 12.3.6.2 Pharmacological Interventions

Although there are currently no drugs specifically approved for MASLD, treatment may include medications that address underlying metabolic conditions such as IR, dyslipidemia, and hypertension [74, 138]. In PLWH, carefully selecting and managing ART is essential, given the potential for certain ART regimens to exacerbate liver fat accumulation and metabolic disturbances [127, 140]. Modification of ART to regimens with less metabolic impact may be advantageous in some cases [141].

### 12.3.7 Conclusion

The emergence and management of MASLD in PLWH represent a major and evolving challenge in the broader context of chronic HIV care. Despite the transformative impact of ART in converting HIV from a life-threatening disease to a manageable chronic condition, this success is accompanied by new health complications, most notably MASLD due to its complex interaction with metabolic disturbances, the effects of HIV itself, ART-related side effects, and traditional metabolic risk factors such as obesity, diabetes, and dyslipidemia. As we move forward, it is clear that a comprehensive approach encompassing early detection, risk stratification, lifestyle modifications, optimized ART selection, and management of comorbidities is essential to address MASLD in PLW. Continued research and interdisciplinary management are vital to advance our understanding and improve outcomes for this growing disease in PLWH.

## References


1. Vos MB, et al. NASPGHAN clinical practice guideline for the diagnosis and treatment of nonalcoholic fatty liver disease in children: recommendations from the expert committee on NAFLD (ECON) and the north American Society of Pediatric Gastroenterology, hepatology and nutrition (NASPGHAN). J Pediatr Gastroenterol Nutr. 2017;64(2):319–34.
2. Younossi Z, et al. Global burden of NAFLD and NASH: trends, predictions, risk factors and prevention. Nat Rev Gastroenterol Hepatol. 2018;15(1):11–20.
3. Younossi ZM, et al. Nonalcoholic steatohepatitis is the Most rapidly increasing indication for liver transplantation in the United States. Clin Gastroenterol Hepatol. 2021;19(3):580–589 e5.
4. Eslam M, et al. Defining paediatric metabolic (dysfunction)-associated fatty liver disease: an international expert consensus statement. Lancet Gastroenterol Hepatol. 2021;6(10):864–73.
5. Rinella ME, et al. A multi-society Delphi consensus statement on new fatty liver disease nomenclature. J Hepatol. 2023;78(6):1966–86.
6. Lister NB, et al. Child and adolescent obesity. Nat Rev Dis Primers. 2023;9(1):24.
7. Paik JM, et al. Global burden of NAFLD and chronic liver disease among adolescents and young adults. Hepatology. 2022;75(5):1204–17.
8. Mann JP, et al. Nonalcoholic fatty liver disease in children. Semin Liver Dis. 2018;38(1):1–13.
9. Anderson EL, et al. The prevalence of non-alcoholic fatty liver disease in children and adolescents: a systematic review and meta-analysis. PLoS One. 2015;10(10):e0140908.
10. Li J, et al. The changing epidemiology of liver disease among US children and adolescents from 1999 to 2016. Am J Gastroenterol. 2021;116(10):2068–78.
11. Schwimmer JB, et al. Prevalence of fatty liver in children and adolescents. Pediatrics. 2006;118(4):1388–93.
12. Xanthakos SA, et al. High prevalence of nonalcoholic fatty liver disease in adolescents undergoing bariatric surgery. Gastroenterology. 2015;149(3):623–34 e8.
13. Shalimar, et al. Prevalence of non-alcoholic fatty liver disease in India: a systematic review and meta-analysis. J Clin Exp Hepatol. 2022;12(3):818–29.
14. Tominaga K, et al. Prevalence of fatty liver in Japanese children and relationship to obesity. An epidemiological ultrasonographic survey. Dig Dis Sci. 1995;40(9):2002–9.
15. Park HS, et al. Relation between elevated serum alanine aminotransferase and metabolic syndrome in Korean adolescents. Am J Clin Nutr. 2005;82(5):1046–51.
16. Song P, et al. Prevalence and correlates of suspected nonalcoholic fatty liver disease in Chinese children. Int J Environ Res Public Health. 2017;14(5):465.
17. Lin G, et al. Epidemiology and lifestyle survey of non-alcoholic fatty liver disease in school-age children and adolescents in Shenyang, Liaoning. BMC Pediatr. 2022;22(1):286.
18. Sahota AK, et al. Incidence of nonalcoholic fatty liver disease in children: 2009-2018. Pediatrics. 2020;146(6):e20200771.
19. Saab S, et al. Nonalcoholic fatty liver disease in latinos. Clin Gastroenterol Hepatol. 2016;14(1):5–12.
20. Patil R, et al. Screening and referral practices for nonalcoholic fatty liver disease by race and ethnicity in a primary care clinic. J Racial Ethn Health Disparities. 2023;10(3):1392–7.
21. Schwimmer JB, et al. Influence of gender, race, and ethnicity on suspected fatty liver in obese adolescents. Pediatrics. 2005;115(5):e561–5.
22. Fraser A, Longnecker MP, Lawlor DA. Prevalence of elevated alanine aminotransferase among US adolescents and associated factors: NHANES 1999-2004. Gastroenterology. 2007;133(6):1814–20.
23. Draijer L, et al. A natural history study of paediatric non-alcoholic fatty liver disease over 10 years. JHEP Rep. 2023;5(5):100685.
24. Goyal NP, Schwimmer JB. The progression and natural history of pediatric nonalcoholic fatty liver disease. Clin Liver Dis. 2016;20(2):325–38.
25. Simon TG, et al. Non-alcoholic fatty liver disease in children and young adults is associated with increased long-term mortality. J Hepatol. 2021;75(5):1034–41.

26. Xanthakos SA, et al. Progression of fatty liver disease in children receiving standard of care lifestyle advice. Gastroenterology. 2020;159(5):1731–1751 e10.
27. Carter-Kent C, et al. Relations of steatosis type, grade, and zonality to histological features in pediatric nonalcoholic fatty liver disease. J Pediatr Gastroenterol Nutr. 2011;52(2):190–7.
28. Mansoor S, et al. The evaluation of hepatic fibrosis scores in children with nonalcoholic fatty liver disease. Dig Dis Sci. 2015;60(5):1440–7.
29. Schwimmer JB, et al. Longitudinal assessment of high blood pressure in children with nonalcoholic fatty liver disease. PLoS One. 2014;9(11):e112569.
30. Furthner D, et al. Nonalcoholic fatty liver disease in children with obesity: narrative review and research gaps. Horm Res Paediatr. 2022;95(2):167–76.
31. Nobili V, et al. NAFLD in children: new genes, new diagnostic modalities and new drugs. Nat Rev Gastroenterol Hepatol. 2019;16(9):517–30.
32. Schwimmer JB, et al. Histopathology of pediatric nonalcoholic fatty liver disease. Hepatology. 2005;42(3):641–9.
33. Shah J, Okubote T, Alkhouri N. Overview of updated practice guidelines for pediatric nonalcoholic fatty liver disease. Gastroenterol Hepatol (N Y). 2018;14(7):407–14.
34. Al-Harthy F, et al. Evaluation of hepatitis in pediatric patients with presumed nonalcoholic fatty liver disease. JPGN Rep. 2022;3(2):e181.
35. Chalasani N, et al. The diagnosis and management of nonalcoholic fatty liver disease: practice guidance from the American Association for the Study of Liver Diseases. Hepatology. 2018;67(1):328–57.
36. Younossi ZM, et al. Nonalcoholic fatty liver disease: assessment of variability in pathologic interpretations. Mod Pathol. 1998;11(6):560–5.
37. Alkhouri N, et al. Development and validation of a new histological score for pediatric non-alcoholic fatty liver disease. J Hepatol. 2012;57(6):1312–8.
38. Shannon A, et al. Ultrasonographic quantitative estimation of hepatic steatosis in children with NAFLD. J Pediatr Gastroenterol Nutr. 2011;53(2):190–5.
39. Middleton MS, et al. Diagnostic accuracy of magnetic resonance imaging hepatic proton density fat fraction in pediatric nonalcoholic fatty liver disease. Hepatology. 2018;67(3):858–72.
40. Chaidez A, et al. The discriminatory ability of FibroScan liver stiffness measurement, controlled attenuation parameter, and FibroScan-aspartate aminotransferase to predict severity of liver disease in children. Hepatol Commun. 2022;6(11):3015–23.
41. Kwon YD, et al. Usefulness of transient Elastography for non-invasive diagnosis of liver fibrosis in pediatric non-alcoholic steatohepatitis. J Korean Med Sci. 2019;34(23):e165.
42. Nobili V, et al. Accuracy and reproducibility of transient elastography for the diagnosis of fibrosis in pediatric nonalcoholic steatohepatitis. Hepatology. 2008;48(2):442–8.
43. Alkhouri N, et al. Combined paediatric NAFLD fibrosis index and transient elastography to predict clinically significant fibrosis in children with fatty liver disease. Liver Int. 2013;33(1):79–85.
44. Liu H, et al. Acoustic radiation force impulse Elastography for the non-invasive evaluation of hepatic fibrosis in non-alcoholic fatty liver disease patients: a Systematic Review & Meta-Analysis. PLoS One. 2015;10(7):e0127782.
45. Kamble R, et al. Liver acoustic radiation force impulse (ARFI) in childhood obesity: comparison and correlation with biochemical markers. J Ultrasound. 2017;20(1):33–42.
46. Tamaki N, et al. Magnetic resonance elastography plus Fibrosis-4 versus FibroScan-aspartate aminotransferase in detection of candidates for pharmacological treatment of NASH-related fibrosis. Hepatology. 2022;75(3):661–72.
47. Loomba R, et al. Magnetic resonance elastography predicts advanced fibrosis in patients with nonalcoholic fatty liver disease: a prospective study. Hepatology. 2014;60(6):1920–8.
48. Schwimmer JB, et al. Magnetic resonance elastography measured shear stiffness as a biomarker of fibrosis in pediatric nonalcoholic fatty liver disease. Hepatology. 2017;66(5):1474–85.
49. Nobili V, et al. The pediatric NAFLD fibrosis index: a predictor of liver fibrosis in children with non-alcoholic fatty liver disease. BMC Med. 2009;7:21.
50. Vos MB, et al. Cytokeratin 18, a marker of cell death, is increased in children with suspected nonalcoholic fatty liver disease. J Pediatr Gastroenterol Nutr. 2008;47(4):481–5.
51. Feldstein AE, et al. Serum cytokeratin-18 fragment levels are useful biomarkers for nonalcoholic steatohepatitis in children. Am J Gastroenterol. 2013;108(9):1526–31.
52. Fitzpatrick E, et al. Serum levels of CK18 M30 and leptin are useful predictors of steatohepatitis and fibrosis in paediatric NAFLD. J Pediatr Gastroenterol Nutr. 2010;51(4):500–6.
53. Vuppalanchi R, et al. Relationship between changes in serum levels of keratin 18 and changes in liver histology in children and adults with nonalcoholic fatty liver disease. Clin Gastroenterol Hepatol. 2014;12(12):2121–30 e1–2.
54. Pagano S, et al. Serum level of cytokeratin 18 (M65) as a prognostic marker of high cardiovascular disease risk in individuals with non-alcoholic fatty liver disease. Biomol Ther. 2023;13(7):1128.
55. Lee J, et al. Accuracy of cytokeratin 18 (M30 and M65) in detecting non-alcoholic steatohepatitis and fibrosis: a systematic review and meta-analysis. PLoS One. 2020;15(9):e0238717.
56. Harrison SA, et al. A phase 3, randomized, controlled trial of resmetirom in nash with liver fibrosis. N Engl J Med, 2024;390(6): p. 497–509.
57. Nobili V, et al. Effect of vitamin E on aminotransferase levels and insulin resistance in children with

non-alcoholic fatty liver disease. Aliment Pharmacol Ther. 2006;24(11–12):1553–61.
58. Nobili V, et al. Lifestyle intervention and antioxidant therapy in children with nonalcoholic fatty liver disease: a randomized, controlled trial. Hepatology. 2008;48(1):119–28.
59. Berkowitz RI, et al. Meal replacements in the treatment of adolescent obesity: a randomized controlled trial. Obesity (Silver Spring). 2011;19(6):1193–9.
60. Kirk S, et al. Role of carbohydrate modification in weight management among obese children: a randomized clinical trial. J Pediatr. 2012;161(2):320–7 e1.
61. Schwimmer JB, et al. Effect of a low free sugar diet vs usual diet on nonalcoholic fatty liver disease in adolescent boys: a randomized clinical trial. JAMA. 2019;321(3):256–65.
62. Akbulut UE, et al. The effect of a Mediterranean diet vs. a low-fat diet on non-alcoholic fatty liver disease in children: a randomized trial. Int J Food Sci Nutr. 2022;73(3):357–66.
63. Gonzalez-Ruiz K, et al. The effects of exercise on abdominal fat and liver enzymes in pediatric obesity: a systematic review and meta-analysis. Child Obes. 2017;13(4):272–82.
64. Bull FC, et al. World Health Organization 2020 guidelines on physical activity and sedentary behaviour. Br J Sports Med. 2020;54(24):1451–62.
65. Harris SJ, et al. Exercise training improves serum biomarkers of liver fibroinflammation in patients with metabolic dysfunction-associated steatohepatitis. Liver Int. 2023;44:532.
66. Manco M, et al. The benefit of sleeve gastrectomy in obese adolescents on nonalcoholic steatohepatitis and hepatic fibrosis. J Pediatr. 2017;180:31–37 e2.
67. Inge TH, et al. Perioperative outcomes of adolescents undergoing bariatric surgery: the teen-longitudinal assessment of bariatric surgery (teen-LABS) study. JAMA Pediatr. 2014;168(1):47–53.
68. Lee Y, et al. Complete resolution of nonalcoholic fatty liver disease after bariatric surgery: a systematic review and meta-analysis. Clin Gastroenterol Hepatol. 2019;17(6):1040–1060 e11.
69. Lavine JE, et al. Effect of vitamin E or metformin for treatment of nonalcoholic fatty liver disease in children and adolescents: the TONIC randomized controlled trial. JAMA. 2011;305(16):1659–68.
70. Vos MB, et al. Randomized placebo-controlled trial of losartan for pediatric NAFLD. Hepatology. 2022;76(2):429–44.
71. Goyal NP, et al. An open label, randomized, multicenter study of Elafibranor in children with nonalcoholic steatohepatitis. J Pediatr Gastroenterol Nutr. 2023;77(2):160–5.
72. Dionysopoulos G, et al. Can omega-3 fatty acids be beneficial in pediatric NAFLD? A systematic review and meta-analysis. Crit Rev Food Sci Nutr. 2023;63(27):8545–53.
73. Newsome PN, et al. A placebo-controlled trial of subcutaneous Semaglutide in nonalcoholic steatohepatitis. N Engl J Med. 2021;384(12):1113–24.
74. Rinella ME, et al. AASLD practice guidance on the clinical assessment and management of nonalcoholic fatty liver disease. Hepatology. 2023;77(5):1797–835.
75. Manco M, et al. Metabolic syndrome and liver histology in paediatric non-alcoholic steatohepatitis. Int J Obes. 2008;32(2):381–7.
76. Benedict M, Zhang X. Non-alcoholic fatty liver disease: an expanded review. World J Hepatol. 2017;9(16):715–32.
77. Bonsembiante L, Targher G, Maffeis C. Nonalcoholic fatty liver disease in obese children and adolescents: a role for nutrition? Eur J Clin Nutr. 2022;76(1):28–39.
78. He S, et al. A sequence variation (I148M) in PNPLA3 associated with nonalcoholic fatty liver disease disrupts triglyceride hydrolysis. J Biol Chem. 2010;285(9):6706–15.
79. Carlsson B, et al. Review article: the emerging role of genetics in precision medicine for patients with non-alcoholic steatohepatitis. Aliment Pharmacol Ther. 2020;51(12):1305–20.
80. Santoro N, et al. Variant in the glucokinase regulatory protein (GCKR) gene is associated with fatty liver in obese children and adolescents. Hepatology. 2012;55(3):781–9.
81. Newton KP, et al. Low and high birth weights are risk factors for nonalcoholic fatty liver disease in children. J Pediatr. 2017;187:141–146 e1.
82. Nobili V, et al. Obstructive sleep apnea syndrome affects liver histology and inflammatory cell activation in pediatric nonalcoholic fatty liver disease, regardless of obesity/insulin resistance. Am J Respir Crit Care Med. 2014;189(1):66–76.
83. Ntandja Wandji LC, et al. Combined alcoholic and non-alcoholic steatohepatitis. JHEP Rep. 2020;2(3):100101.
84. Gao B, et al. Inflammatory pathways in alcoholic steatohepatitis. J Hepatol. 2019;70(2):249–59.
85. Boyle M, Masson S, Anstee QM. The bidirectional impacts of alcohol consumption and the metabolic syndrome: cofactors for progressive fatty liver disease. J Hepatol. 2018;68(2):251–67.
86. Xu J, et al. Synergistic steatohepatitis by moderate obesity and alcohol in mice despite increased adiponectin and p-AMPK. J Hepatol. 2011;55(3):673–82.
87. Israelsen M, et al. Metabolic and genetic risk factors are the strongest predictors of severity of alcohol-related liver fibrosis. Clin Gastroenterol Hepatol. 2022;20(8):1784–1794 e9.
88. Hart CL, et al. Effect of body mass index and alcohol consumption on liver disease: analysis of data from two prospective cohort studies. BMJ. 2010;340:c1240.
89. Liu B, et al. Body mass index and risk of liver cirrhosis in middle aged UK women: prospective study. BMJ. 2010;340:c912.

90. Loomba R, Bettencourt R, Barrett-Connor E. Synergistic association between alcohol intake and body mass index with serum alanine and aspartate aminotransferase levels in older adults: the rancho Bernardo study. Aliment Pharmacol Ther. 2009;30(11–12):1137–49.
91. Hagstrom H, et al. Mortality in biopsy-proven alcohol-related liver disease: a population-based nationwide cohort study of 3453 patients. Gut. 2021;70(1):170–9.
92. Simon TG, et al. Mortality in biopsy-confirmed nonalcoholic fatty liver disease: results from a nationwide cohort. Gut. 2021;70(7):1375–82.
93. Dam-Larsen S, et al. Long term prognosis of fatty liver: risk of chronic liver disease and death. Gut. 2004;53(5):750–5.
94. Bedogni G, et al. Incidence and natural course of fatty liver in the general population: the Dionysos study. Hepatology. 2007;46(5):1387–91.
95. Naveau S, et al. Excess weight risk factor for alcoholic liver disease. Hepatology. 1997;25(1):108–11.
96. Raynard B, et al. Risk factors of fibrosis in alcohol-induced liver disease. Hepatology. 2002;35(3):635–8.
97. Whitfield JB, et al. Obesity, diabetes, coffee, tea, and cannabis use Alter risk for alcohol-related cirrhosis in 2 large cohorts of high-risk drinkers. Am J Gastroenterol. 2021;116(1):106–15.
98. Mallet V, et al. Burden of liver disease progression in hospitalized patients with type 2 diabetes mellitus. J Hepatol. 2022;76(2):265–74.
99. Dunn W, et al. Modest alcohol consumption is associated with decreased prevalence of steatohepatitis in patients with non-alcoholic fatty liver disease (NAFLD). J Hepatol. 2012;57(2):384–91.
100. Hajifathalian K, Torabi Sagvand B, McCullough AJ. Effect of alcohol consumption on survival in nonalcoholic fatty liver disease: a National Prospective Cohort Study. Hepatology. 2019;70(2):511–21.
101. Aberg F, et al. Alcohol consumption and metabolic syndrome: clinical and epidemiological impact on liver disease. J Hepatol. 2023;78(1):191–206.
102. Rinella ME, et al. A multisociety Delphi consensus statement on new fatty liver disease nomenclature. J Hepatol. 2023;79(6):1542–56.
103. Alberti KG, et al. Harmonizing the metabolic syndrome: a joint interim statement of the international diabetes federation task force on epidemiology and prevention; National Heart, Lung, and Blood Institute; American Heart Association; world heart federation; international atherosclerosis society; and International Association for the Study of obesity. Circulation. 2009;120(16):1640–5.
104. Rehm J, et al. Alcohol as a risk factor for liver cirrhosis: a systematic review and meta-analysis. Drug Alcohol Rev. 2010;29(4):437–45.
105. Roerecke M, et al. Alcohol consumption and risk of liver cirrhosis: a systematic review and meta-analysis. Am J Gastroenterol. 2019;114(10):1574–86.
106. Mody A, et al. HIV epidemiology, prevention, treatment, and implementation strategies for public health. Lancet. 2024;403(10425):471–92.
107. Arts EJ, Hazuda DJ. HIV-1 antiretroviral drug therapy. Cold Spring Harb Perspect Med. 2012;2(4):a007161.
108. Broder S. The development of antiretroviral therapy and its impact on the HIV-1/AIDS pandemic. Antivir Res. 2010;85(1):1–18.
109. van Welzen BJ, et al. A review of non-alcoholic fatty liver disease in HIV-infected patients: the next big thing? Infect Dis Ther. 2019;8(1):33–50.
110. Michel M, et al. Metabolic dysfunction-associated fatty liver disease in people living with HIV. Sci Rep. 2023;13(1):9158.
111. Crum-Cianflone N, et al. Nonalcoholic fatty liver disease among HIV-infected persons. J Acquir Immune Defic Syndr. 2009;50(5):464–73.
112. Coronel-Castillo CE, et al. Nonalcoholic fatty liver disease and nonalcoholic steatohepatitis in HIV infection: a metabolic approach of an infectious disease. Expert Rev Gastroenterol Hepatol. 2019;13(6):531–40.
113. Seth A, Sherman KE. Fatty liver disease in persons with HIV infection. Top Antivir Med. 2019;27(2):75–82.
114. Kalligeros M, et al. Prevalence and characteristics of nonalcoholic fatty liver disease and fibrosis in people living with HIV Monoinfection: a systematic review and meta-analysis. Clin Gastroenterol Hepatol. 2023;21(7):1708–22.
115. Jin D, et al. Regional variation in NAFLD prevalence and risk factors among people living with HIV in Europe: a meta-analysis. Front Public Health. 2023;11:1295165.
116. Manzano-Nunez R, et al. Uncovering the NAFLD burden in people living with HIV from high- and middle-income nations: a meta-analysis with a data gap from Subsaharan Africa. J Int AIDS Soc. 2023;26(3):e26072.
117. Lemoine M, et al. Diagnostic accuracy of noninvasive markers of steatosis, NASH, and liver fibrosis in HIV-Monoinfected individuals at risk of nonalcoholic fatty liver disease (NAFLD): results from the ECHAM study. J Acquir Immune Defic Syndr. 2019;80(4):e86–94.
118. Squillace N, et al. Nonalcoholic fatty liver disease and steatohepatitis in people living with HIV. Expert Rev Gastroenterol Hepatol. 2019;13(7):643–50.
119. Biały M, Czarnecki M, Inglot M. Impact of combination antiretroviral treatment on liver metabolic health in HIV-infected persons. Viruses. 2023;15(12):2432.
120. Willig AL, Overton ET. Metabolic complications and glucose metabolism in HIV infection: a review of the evidence. Curr HIV/AIDS Rep. 2016;13(5):289–96.
121. Soti S, et al. NAFLD and HIV: do sex, race, and ethnicity explain HIV-related risk? Curr HIV/AIDS Rep. 2018;15(3):212–22.

122. Thet D, Siritientong T. Antiretroviral therapy-associated metabolic complications: review of the recent studies. HIV AIDS (Auckl). 2020;12:507–24.
123. Lacombe K, Rockstroh J. HIV and viral hepatitis coinfections: advances and challenges. Gut. 2012;61(Suppl 1):i47–58.
124. Papagianni M, Tziomalos K. Non-alcoholic fatty liver disease in patients with HIV infection. AIDS Rev. 2018;20(3):171–3.
125. Pedro MN, et al. Insulin resistance in HIV-patients: causes and consequences. Front Endocrinol (Lausanne). 2018;9:514.
126. Gutierrez AD, Balasubramanyam A. Dysregulation of glucose metabolism in HIV patients: epidemiology, mechanisms, and management. Endocrine. 2012;41(1):1–10.
127. Kaplan A, Price JC. HIV-associated NAFLD: disease burden and management. Curr Hepatol Rep. 2019;18(4):482–91.
128. Behrens G, et al. Impaired glucose tolerance, beta cell function and lipid metabolism in HIV patients under treatment with protease inhibitors. AIDS. 1999;13(10):F63–70.
129. Kakuda TN, et al. Nucleoside reverse transcriptase inhibitor-induced mitochondrial toxicity as an etiology for lipodystrophy. AIDS. 1999;13(16):2311–2.
130. Gardner K, et al. HIV treatment and associated mitochondrial pathology: review of 25 years of in vitro, animal, and human studies. Toxicol Pathol. 2014;42(5):811–22.
131. Duarte MJ, et al. The human microbiome and gut-liver axis in people living with HIV. Curr HIV/AIDS Rep. 2023;20(3):170–80.
132. Vodkin I, et al. Clinical, biochemical and histological differences between HIV-associated NAFLD and primary NAFLD: a case-control study. Aliment Pharmacol Ther. 2015;41(4):368–78.
133. Fourman LT, et al. Clinical predictors of liver fibrosis presence and progression in human immunodeficiency virus–associated nonalcoholic fatty liver disease. Clin Infect Dis. 2020;72(12):2087–94.
134. Shahriar S, et al. Insights into the coinfections of human immunodeficiency virus-hepatitis B virus, human immunodeficiency virus-hepatitis C virus, and hepatitis B virus-hepatitis C virus: prevalence, risk factors, pathogenesis, diagnosis, and treatment. Front Microbiol. 2021;12:780887.
135. Sumida Y, Nakajima A, Itoh Y. Limitations of liver biopsy and non-invasive diagnostic tests for the diagnosis of nonalcoholic fatty liver disease/nonalcoholic steatohepatitis. World J Gastroenterol. 2014;20(2):475–85.
136. Sterling RK, et al. Diagnostic ability of simple noninvasive blood tests to predict increased liver stiffness in people living with HIV and Steatotic liver disease. Am J Gastroenterol. 2024;119:1483.
137. Karanjia RN, et al. Hepatic steatosis and fibrosis: non-invasive assessment. World J Gastroenterol. 2016;22(45):9880–97.
138. Rong L, et al. Advancements in the treatment of non-alcoholic fatty liver disease (NAFLD). Front Endocrinol (Lausanne). 2022;13:1087260.
139. Cinque F, et al. Nutritional and lifestyle therapy for NAFLD in people with HIV. Nutrients. 2023;15(8):1990.
140. Bischoff J, et al. Stratifying the risk of NAFLD in patients with HIV under combination antiretroviral therapy (cART). EClinMed. 2021;40:101116.
141. Shengir M, et al. Switch to a raltegravir-based antiretroviral regimen in people with HIV and non-alcoholic fatty liver disease: a randomized controlled trial. HIV Med. 2024;25(1):135–42.

# 13 MASLD: Looking Ahead

Ziyan Pan and Mohammed Eslam

The rates of metabolic dysfunction is increasing due to the large increase in caloric consumption and lack of physical activity. As a result, there has been an increase in the prevalence of metabolic dysfunction-associated steatotic liver disease (MASLD), which poses a substantial challenge to global health by leading to significant morbidity and mortality, especially in cases where fibrosis is evident [1].

MASLD is a complex condition affecting multiple systems, exhibiting heterogeneity in terms of its underlying causes, modifiers, range of disease severity, and natural progression. Additionally, there is significant variability among patients across the spectrum of MASLD. MASLD is linked to a greater likelihood of experiencing both liver-related complications and non-hepatic diseases, including cardiovascular disease, type 2 diabetes mellitus, chronic kidney disease, and some extrahepatic tumours [2, 3]. The increasing frequency of MASLD and the subsequent associated hepatic and extrahepatic consequences pose significant health, economic, and societal challenges. How do we move forwards? Advancement can only be achieved by addressing issues at the societal, population, and individual levels. In the subsequent section, we elucidate several prominent obstacles and prospective avenues within the domain of MASLD.

In 2020, an international expert consensus panel proposed a new definition of fatty liver disease to address the various limitations of the previous definition of non-alcoholic fatty liver disease (NAFLD), which reflects our increasing knowledge of the significant influence of metabolic dysfunction on this condition [4, 5]. The redefinition process involves the modification of the disease nomenclature from NAFLD to metabolic dysfunction-associated fatty liver disease (MAFLD) and the introduction of a simple and inclusive set of diagnostic criteria for the disease, thereby replacing the prior set of diagnostic criteria that relied on exclusion [4, 5]. The proposal has received support from various national and pan-national regional liver societies, patient advocacy groups, and professionals in the nursing and allied health fields [1, 6–13]. A multitude of studies have provided evidence supporting the efficacy of these criteria in the identification of patients exhibiting metabolic dysfunction, advanced hepatic fibrosis, and extrahepatic outcomes, including cardiovascular disease and chronic kidney disease [14–16]. Moreover, MAFLD effectively circumvents the stigmatization and trivialization that often accompany NAFLD. Additionally, due to the intricate and varied character of metabolic disorders, MAFLD is positioned alongside other metabolic diseases, thereby diverging from the limited and

Z. Pan · M. Eslam (✉)
Storr Liver Centre, Westmead Institute for Medical Research, Westmead Hospital and University of Sydney, Westmead, NSW, Australia
e-mail: mohammed.eslam@sydney.edu.au


N. Méndez-Sánchez, X. Qi (eds.), *Metabolic Dysfunction-Associated Steatotic Liver Disease*, https://doi.org/10.1007/978-981-97-9519-2_13

narrow perspective centred solely on hepatology. This makes MAFLD a disease that is of interest to medical and health policy-making teams from other fields. It also has the potential to promote the establishment of MAFLD clinics led by teams of experts from several fields. These clinics would allow for proactive evaluation and timely intervention of metabolic comorbidities [2]. A new term, metabolic dysfunction-associated steatotic liver disease (MASLD), along with its accompanying diagnostic criteria, was suggested in the year 2023. Currently, there is challenge in achieving a unified nomenclature and definition and there is great anticipation for future efforts to align the definitions of MASLD and MAFLD. However, it is important that these efforts also involve a thorough reassessment of the diagnostic criteria, taking into account strong clinical and epidemiological evidence rather than relying solely on expert opinion.

The identification of high-risk patients is of utmost importance and poses an additional hurdle, given that only a minority of patients with MASLD will experience complications associated with the condition. The primary determinant for both hepatic and extrahepatic symptoms of MASLD is the presence of severe fibrosis [17]. While liver biopsy continues to be the gold standard method for assessing histological severity in these individuals, its limitations and unsuitability for large-scale applications have prompted extensive research efforts to identify reliable non-invasive biomarkers for MASLD. This finding is particularly relevant to the recent release of resmetirom as the first approved drug for treating MASLD. The identification and widespread utilization of a diverse range of proprietary and non-proprietary biomarkers and scores have been achieved [17]. The progress made in understanding the pathophysiology of MASLD and elucidating the involvement of genetics, epigenetics, the microbiome, and metabolomics in disease pathogenesis presents a promising opportunity for the identification of innovative biomarkers facilitating enhanced patient classification and tailored management strategies. Additional research, such as cost-effectiveness studies, will be necessary prior to endorsing the integration of these innovative biomarkers or multiomics techniques into clinical practice.

Although lean individuals with MASLD have greater morbidity and mortality, they may be mistakenly labelled as healthy and disregarded by healthcare personnel. They are significantly underrepresented in clinical trials compared to their obese counterpart [18, 19]. There are numerous uncertainties in our understanding of disease progression in persons with a normal body weight. Addressing these questions will serve as the foundation for developing efficient preventative and therapeutic strategies for MASLD in nonobese individuals and perhaps for nonobese individuals with a normal weight who have additional metabolic comorbidities. There is a need for a deeper characterization of the genetic and environmental elements that influence the variations in individuals' responses to various forms of management.

Furthermore, MASLD is a heritable polygenic condition that is highly likely to have a common genetic foundation with other metabolic diseases. Genome-wide association studies and candidate gene investigations have revealed several genetic variants that are associated with illness susceptibility and progression, as well as the regulation of crucial pathways in disease pathogenesis. Additional research is necessary to further advance our knowledge of the genetic underpinnings of MASLD. The emergence of genomics has also sparked high expectations as an approach for drug exploration and the creation of a non-invasive marker for disease detection [3, 20–22].

Although there has been significant progress in the development and exploration of drug targets for MASLD, driven by advancements in pathophysiology understanding, the outcomes have fallen short of initial expectations. We are now witnessing excitement about the first drug approved for MAFLD treatment. Multiple open questions are emerging. For example, can non-invasive tests (NITs) be used as tools for identifying patients to be treated with resmetirom and identifying the follow-up and stopping rules? This is especially important for expensive drugs, such as resmetirom, for which only 16% of patients on the highest dose achieved both co-primary histological outcomes [23]. Additionally, identifying baseline and dynamic predictors of treatment response is crucial. Finally, the role of combination and 'add-on' or 'switch-to' strategies has yet to be clarified.

Ultimately, due to the primary influence of metabolic dysfunction on the pathogenesis of MASLD and the multisystemic nature of the disease, a multidisciplinary management approach involving the engagement of various stakeholders is crucial to offer tailored, prompt, fair, and cost-effective health interventions for individuals with MASLD. Enhanced patient involvement in all facets of research and implementation pertaining to the prevention and care of MASLD will contribute to improved adherence to clinical recommendations [2]. It is imperative to enhance societal understanding regarding the ramifications of metabolic dysfunction and incorporate public health interventions for MASLD into policies about non-communicable diseases [2, 24].

**Acknowledgements** ME is supported by a National Health and Medical Research Council of Australia (NHMRC) Program Grant (APP1053206) and Project and ideas grants (APP2001692, APP1107178 and APP1108422).

**Competing Financial Interests** The authors declare no competing financial interests.

## References

1. Eslam M, et al. The Asian Pacific Association for the Study of the Liver clinical practice guidelines for the diagnosis and management of metabolic associated fatty liver disease. Hepatol Int. 2020;14(6):889–919.
2. Eslam M, et al. Incorporating fatty liver disease in multidisciplinary care and novel clinical trial designs for patients with metabolic diseases. Lancet Gastroenterol Hepatol. 2021;6:743–53.
3. Bayoumi A, et al. The epigenetic drug discovery landscape for metabolic-associated fatty liver disease. Trends Genet. 2020;36(6):429–41.
4. Eslam M, et al. MAFLD: a consensus-driven proposed nomenclature for metabolic associated fatty liver disease. Gastroenterology. 2020;158(7):1999–2014 e1.
5. Eslam M, et al. A new definition for metabolic dysfunction-associated fatty liver disease: an international expert consensus statement. J Hepatol. 2020;73(1):202–9.
6. Gómez MR, Ampuero J. Looking for a new name for Non-alcoholic fatty liver disease in Spanish: Esteatosis Hepática Metabólica (EHmet). Rev Esp Enferm Dig. 2021;113(3):161–3.
7. Tan SS, et al. Endorsing the redefinition of fatty liver disease. Lancet Gastroenterol Hepatol. 2021;6(3):163.
8. Mendez-Sanchez N, et al. The Latin American Association for the Study of the Liver (ALEH) position statement on the redefinition of fatty liver disease. Lancet Gastroenterol Hepatol. 2021;6(1):65–72.
9. Shiha G, et al. Nomenclature and definition of metabolic-associated fatty liver disease: a consensus from the Middle East and North Africa. Lancet Gastroenterol Hepatol. 2021;6(1):57–64.
10. Shiha G, et al. Redefining fatty liver disease: an international patient perspective. Lancet Gastroenterol Hepatol. 2021;6(1):73–9.
11. Fouad Y, et al. What's in a name? Renaming 'NAFLD' to 'MAFLD'. Liver Int. 2020;40(6):1254–61.
12. Spearman CW, et al. The sub-Saharan Africa position statement on the redefinition of fatty liver disease: from NAFLD to MAFLD. J Hepatol. 2021;74(5):1256–8.
13. Clayton M, et al. From NAFLD to MAFLD: nurse and allied health perspective. Liver Int. 2021;41(4):683–91.
14. Lee H, et al. Metabolic dysfunction-associated fatty liver disease and incident cardiovascular disease risk: a Nationwide cohort study. Clin Gastroenterol Hepatol. 2021;19(10):2138–2147.e10.
15. Sun DQ, et al. MAFLD and risk of CKD. Metabolism. 2021;115:154433.
16. Yamamura S, et al. MAFLD identifies patients with significant hepatic fibrosis better than NAFLD. Liver Int. 2020;40(12):3018–30.
17. Alharthi J, Eslam M. Biomarkers of metabolic (dysfunction)-associated fatty liver disease: an update. J Clin Transl Hepatol. 2022;10(1):134.
18. Eslam M, et al. Metabolic (dysfunction)-associated fatty liver disease in individuals of normal weight. Nat Rev Gastroenterol Hepatol. 2022;19(10):638–51.
19. Eslam M, Fan J-G, Mendez-Sanchez N. Non-alcoholic fatty liver disease in non-obese individuals: the impact of metabolic health. Lancet Gastroenterol Hepatol. 2020;5(8):713–5.
20. Plenge RM, Scolnick EM, Altshuler D. Validating therapeutic targets through human genetics. Nat Rev Drug Discov. 2013;12(8):581–94.
21. Eslam M, George J. Genetic contributions to NAFLD: leveraging shared genetics to uncover systems biology. Nat Rev Gastroenterol Hepatol. 2020;17(1):40–52.
22. Eslam M, Valenti L, Romeo S. Genetics and epigenetics of NAFLD and NASH: clinical impact. J Hepatol. 2018;68(2):268–79.
23. Harrison SA, et al. A phase 3, randomized, controlled trial of resmetirom in NASH with liver fibrosis. N Engl J Med. 2024;390(6):497–509.
24. Sarin SK, et al. Integration of public health measures for NAFLD into India's national programme for NCDs. Lancet Gastroenterol Hepatol. 2021;6(10):777–8.

# Metabolic Steatohepatitis After Liver Transplantation

# 14

Alberto Ferrarese, Sara Battistella,
Francesco Paolo Russo, and Patrizia Burra

## Abbreviation

| | |
|---|---|
| MASLD | Metabolic dysfunction-associated steatotic liver disease |
| MASH | Metabolic dysfunction-associated steatohepatitis |
| PNPLA3 | Patatin-like phospholipase domain-containing 3 |
| T2DM | Type 2 diabetes mellitus |

## 14.1 Introduction

### 14.1.1 Definition, Epidemiology, Outcome

In the last decades, metabolic liver disease has emerged as a leading indication for liver transplantation in Western countries [1, 2]. Furthermore, many studies have demonstrated the high prevalence of metabolic syndrome following surgery. Consequently, the issue of recurrent or de novo metabolic dysfunction-associated steatotic liver disease (MASLD) has become crucial in many transplant centers.

Recently, international consensus has been achieved to change the nomenclature, in order to reduce the stigma associated with previous definitions such as nonalcoholic fatty liver disease and nonalcoholic steatohepatitis [3–5]. Therefore, new terms have been introduced, and will be applied in this chapter. By definition, MASLD is characterized by hepatic steatosis, confirmed by histological or radiological evidence, in conjunction with at least one cardiometabolic risk factor and the absence of any other cause. Copresence at histology of MASLD and steatohepatitis (hepatocellular ballooning and inflammation), is defined as metabolic dysfunction-associated steatohepatitis (MASH) [3]. Allograft steatohepatitis is further classified as "recurrent", in patients who have been transplanted for metabolic disease, or "de novo", in patients transplanted for other etiologies (Table 14.1) [6].

The epidemiological landscape of MASLD after transplantation is still heterogeneous. This is primarily because, since histology remains crucial for diagnosis (particularly of MASH) the actual prevalence may be biased due to the absence of per-protocol biopsies in many centers. Additionally, several confounding factors, such as chronic alcohol use (which is not uncommon among patients transplanted for nonalcoholic indications [7]) or immunological issues, may

Alberto Ferrarese and Sara Battistella contributed equally with all other contributors.

A. Ferrarese · S. Battistella · F. P. Russo · P. Burra (✉)
Multivisceral Transplant Unit, Department of Surgery, Oncology and Gastroenterology, Padua University Hospital, Padua, Italy
e-mail: burra@unipd.it



N. Méndez-Sánchez, X. Qi (eds.), *Metabolic Dysfunction-Associated Steatotic Liver Disease*, https://doi.org/10.1007/978-981-97-9519-2_14

**Table 14.1** Definitions of MASLD and MASH and their application in the transplant setting

| | Definition |
|---|---|
| MASLD | Macrovesicular steatosis (fat in >5% of hepatocytes) |
| MASH | Macrovesicular steatosis (fat in >5% of hepatocytes)<br>And<br>Hepatocellular ballooning (enlarged round cells with clear, vacuolar cytoplasm)<br>And<br>Inflammation (predominantly lobular, composed mainly of clusters of mononuclear cells, Kupffer cells possibly present, microgranulomas with or without lipid droplets, e.g., lipogranulomas) |
| Recurrent MASH | Histological evidence of MASH in patients who underwent LT for MASLD |
| De novo MASH | Histological evidence of MASH in patients who underwent LT for other etiologies |

add further diagnostic bias. A meta-analysis of 17 retrospective studies revealed that the mean incidence rates of recurrent and de novo MASLD at 1, 3, and 5 years are 59%, 57%, and 82%, and 67%, 40%, and 78%, respectively. Additionally, the incidence of recurrent MASH (53%, 57.4%, and 38% at 1, 3, and 5 years after transplantation, respectively) was higher compared to de novo disease (13%, 16%, and 17%, respectively) [8]. A recent multicenter study from France reported even higher rates of biopsy-proven recurrent steatohepatitis at 5 years (60.3%) [9].

These findings have significant epidemiological implications. Firstly, there is a notable difference in incidence between MASLD and MASH, especially in long-term follow-up, indicating that less than half of patients with MASLD would progress to MASH. Secondly, recurrent MASH is high at 1 year after liver transplantation, underscoring the need for strategies to prevent its recurrence early after surgery.

The gold standard for diagnosing recurrent and de novo MASH remains liver biopsy. Noninvasive, tests based on biochemical parameters, or ultrasound/transient elastography are useful screening tools but lack accuracy. Magnetic resonance has emerged as an accurate noninvasive technique for diagnosing both steatosis and fibrosis, but it is constrained as a first-line approach due to high costs and limited availability.

Data on the prognostic role of MASH on graft and patient survival are still scarce. Reported rates of significant histologically proven fibrosis at long-term follow-up in patients with recurrent or de novo MASLD are around 20% and 48% at 5- and 10 years posttransplantation, respectively [8]. It is currently unknown if advanced fibrosis due to de novo or recurrent MASH significantly affect patient and graft survival. According to available data, there is a low rate of late re-transplantation for such condition, perhaps for disease underdiagnosis and late occurrence (perhaps in elderly patients who are considered too old for re-LT) [10].

## 14.2 Risk Factors

Risk factors for recurrence and de novo MASLD after liver transplantation can be distinguished as modifiable and non-modifiable (Fig. 14.1). Among **modifiable risk factors**, obesity, type 2 diabetes mellitus (T2DM), and metabolic syndrome are well-established factors associated with the onset and progression of MASLD before transplantation. Obesity is diagnosed in more than one-third of liver transplant recipients, with the majority of weight gain occurring within the first 3 years after surgery [11]. T2DM prevalence ranges from 31% to 38% posttransplant, with de novo T2DM occurring in 13–28% of cases [12]. The prevalence of dyslipidemia posttransplant is estimated at approximately 70% [13]. Although the net effect of hypercholesterolemia after transplant is still not fully understood, recent studies have indicated that it may affect graft function during long-term follow-up [14]. Lifestyle factors such as cigarette smoking and sedentary habits may significantly contribute to the development of MASH after transplant, too. Cigarette smoking is not only clearly associated with cardiovascular disease, cancer, and T2DM, but has also been directly linked to MASH in the non-

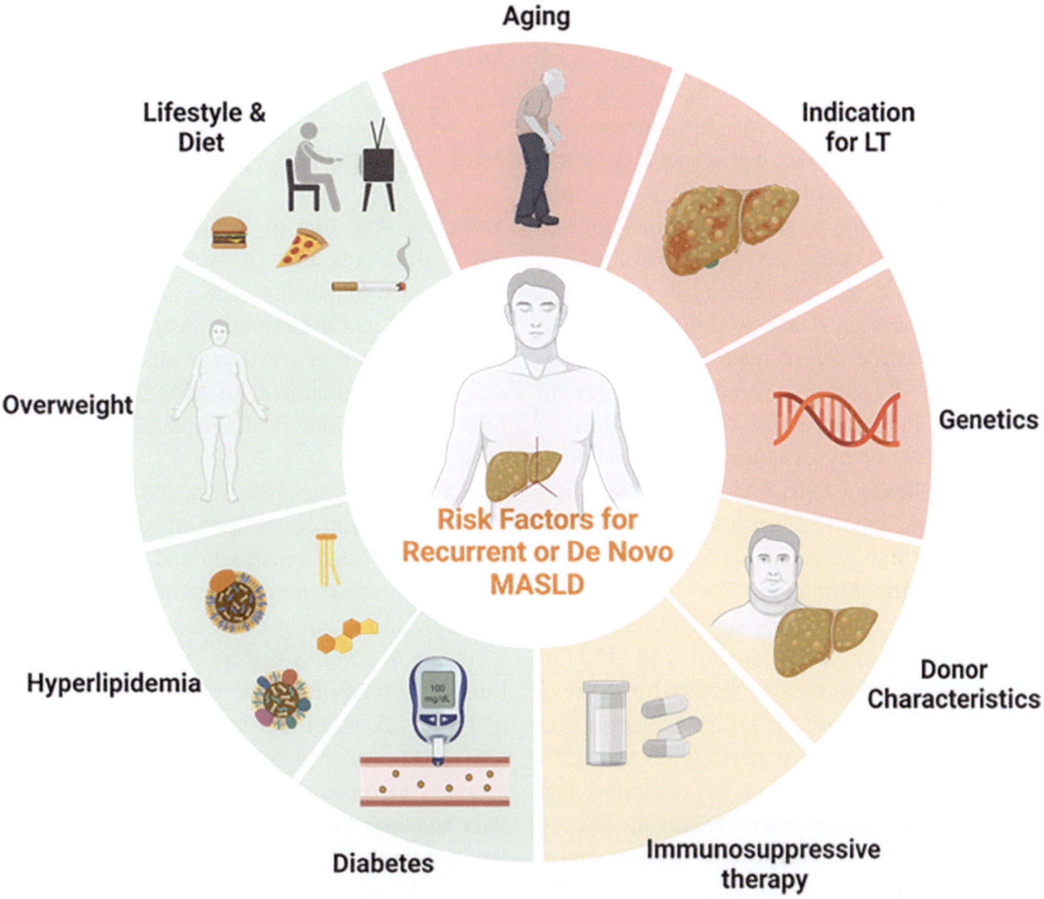


**Fig. 14.1** Risk factors for recurrent and de novo MASH after liver transplantation

transplant setting, with a strong linear association between the duration of smoking and the number of cigarettes smoked per day [15].

While these considerations primarily pertain to the pretransplant setting, it is conceivable that the same mechanisms apply to the posttransplant scenario as well. Therefore, it is likely that the set of pathologies causing metabolic syndrome may contribute to the development of steatosis and/or steatohepatitis in the graft. This can occur both in patients who had these factors before transplantation and in those who develop them after surgery. It is also probable that the presence of multiple metabolic factors may have a synergistic effect on the development of steatosis and/or steatohepatitis post-liver transplantation. Indeed, we have recently demonstrated, in a single-center prospective cohort, a significant association between renal function (assessed by estimation of glomerular filtration rate) and the development of de novo metabolic syndrome after liver transplantation, opening new perspectives about the impact on renal function on de novo MASLD [16].

Immunosuppressive therapy may play an additional role in the development of recurrent or de novo MASH after transplant. Glucocorticoids not only exacerbate hyperglycemia in transplant recipients with known T2DM, but can also induce T2DM in patients without preoperative hyperglycemia. Steroids are also associated with hyperlipidemia as they stimulate fatty acid synthesis, leading to elevated concentrations of total cholesterol and triglycerides [17]. However, steroids are usually tapered early after liver transplantation, minimizing their long-term influence. Cyclosporine induces hypercholesterolemia by inhibiting sterol 27-hydroxylase: a dose-dependent increase in low-density lipoproteins and decrease in high-density lipoproteins has been observed with serum concentration of cyclosporine. Tacrolimus has a more favorable impact than cyclosporine in terms of lipidemic effect, but presents a greater pro-diabetogenic action [18]. The use of mycophenolate mofetil, combined with reduced doses of calcineurin inhibitors, has been shown to reduce cardiovascular risk and the risk of renal function impairment [19]. Regarding mammalian target of rapamycin inhibitors, some studies suggest an increased risk of hyperlipidemia by promoting lipoprotein-lipase activity and insulin resistance, while others report a cardioprotective effect attributed to improved endothelial function and reduced plaque formation [20]. In summary, immunosuppressive therapy needs careful management in patients transplanted for MAFLD or in those who had many risk factors for de novo steatosis/steatohepatitis, tailoring protocols and preferring CNI-sparing or steroid-free regimens. On the other hand, it is crucial to remember that a stable immunosuppressive regimen, able to avoid fluctuations and patient nonadherence, appears important to ensuring good graft function and preventing rejection.

Among **non-modifiable risk factors**, ageing is characterized by the redistribution of adipose tissue, with accumulation in visceral areas. This visceral fat accumulation is associated with heightened systemic inflammation, metabolic syndrome, T2DM, all of which are risk factors for MASH. Women of reproductive age typically have a lower risk of metabolic dysfunction due to the protective effects of estrogen, but this advantage diminishes after menopause [21]. Whether these gender differences persist after transplant, it remains to be established. Genetic polymorphism, particularly for the patatin-like phospholipase domain-containing 3 (PNPLA3) rs738409 variant, is a widely recognized risk factor for MASLD development. The risk of steatosis significantly increases when both the donor and recipient share this polymorphism [22]. Other genetic variants potentially linked to hepatic steatosis development after liver transplantation include PCSK9 and PCSK7 [23], although these findings require validation in larger studies.

## 14.3 Diagnosis

The early detection of hepatic **steatosis** in the liver graft remains a subject of debate. Noninvasive diagnostic tools, such as the Fatty Liver Index and the Hepatic Steatosis Index, can be helpful, even in a validated algorithm for the diagnosis and treatment of MASLD and metabolic complications posttransplant does not yet exist [24, 25].

A recent meta-analysis revealed that transient elastography with continuous attenuation parameter exhibits good sensitivity and specificity for detecting steatosis compared to histology, though its diagnostic accuracy decreases in patients with moderate to severe steatosis. Additionally, it has limited accuracy in obese patients, who constitute a significant proportion of MASLD patients [26]. Studies investigating the accuracy of continuous attenuation parameter for diagnosing liver steatosis after transplant, showed a prevalence of up to 70% of steatosis and up to 40% of advanced steatosis. However, neither of them compared the results with histology [27–29]. However, a consensus on the optimal cut-off value of this parameter for diagnosing steatosis after transplant has not yet been reached. Among radiological techniques, magnetic resonance imaging demonstrates higher sensitivity and specificity for detecting liver fat (90% and 91%, respectively) compared to computed tomography scan (sensitivity 74%, specificity 70%) and ultrasound (sensitivity 65%, specificity 77%) [30]. However, as previously said, costs and limited availability may reduce its implementation as first-line diagnostic tool in clinical practice. Liver biopsy remains the gold standard for diagnosing recurrent or de novo MASLD and MASH, using the abovementioned histological definition. Currently, no histological features differentiate recurrent from de novo MASLD, necessitating a clinical-based differential diagnosis [6].

Liver biopsy is recommended as the reference test for the assessment of **fibrosis**, too.

Noninvasive tests may be useful for ruling out advanced fibrosis in MASLD patients in clinical practice [31]. Among noninvasive tests, NAFLD fibrosis score (NFS) and FIB-4 are the most commonly used in clinical practice and in the non-transplant setting. NAFLD fibrosis score incorporates 6 variables (age, BMI, AST/ALT ratio, platelet count, hyperglycemia, and albumin), while FIB-4 relies solely on age, AST, ALT, and platelet count. The accuracy of such noninvasive tests in the context of liver transplantation appears suboptimal in many cases, as some parameters such as thrombocytopenia and increased transaminases are not always predictive of potential fibrosis.

Other patented serum fibrosis biomarkers (such as FibroMeter™ and Enhanced Liver Fibrosis test™), which have demonstrated comparable accuracy to aforementioned non patented test in general population, require further validation in the transplant setting. Transient elastography currently represents the most widely available tool for liver stiffness measurement. In a metanalysis, it shows the best performance to diagnose recurrent fibrosis in transplant recipients compared with other noninvasive tests, however, the only a minority of patients has MASLD/MASH [32]. Promising data on Magnetic Resonance elastography in general population with metabolic liver disease warrants further clarification in the transplant setting [33].

## 14.4 Pharmacological Treatment of MASH After Liver Transplantation

There currently are few data on pharmacological management of posttransplant MASH. Evidence could therefore be extrapolated from the non-transplant setting. Among the most significant clinical trials, a study by Sanyal et al. demonstrated so far the superiority of vitamin E over placebo in terms of histological improvement in non-transplanted, nondiabetic MASH patients in a cohort of approximately 250 patients [34]. The same study, however, showed the lack of efficacy of pioglitazone compared to placebo, not confirming the previously demonstrated data from a smaller randomized controlled trial [35]. It is worth noting, however, that there were no significant improvements in fibrosis, which is an important driver in the natural history of the MASH disease [36]. Furthermore, both of these agents have adverse risk profiles including weight gain, CVD, and malignancies, which can be encountered after liver transplantation. In the last 10 years, many other randomized controlled trials demonstrated improvement of steatosis with novel molecules, as liraglutide, semaglutide, tirzepatide, and SGLT2 inhibitors, significantly increasing the number of therapeutic options available, especially in patients with diabetes [37–40]. No significant steps have been made on fibrosis, however, as occurred in two recently published studies. The first, a phase 3 randomized study (including patients with F4 fibrosis), showed that resmetirom, a thyroid hormone receptor beta–selective agonist, was able to determine fibrosis improvement in 24.2–25.9% (according to drug dosage), compared with 14.2% of those in the placebo group [41]. This drug has been recently approved for MASH patients by European and US Medicine Agency. A further phase 2b study has shown promising evidence regarding pegozafermin, a long-acting glycol-pegylated fibroblast growth factor 21 (FGF21) analogue, capable of significantly improving fibrosis compared to placebo after 24 weeks of therapy, in a cohort of patients with moderate-severe fibrosis (F2-F3) [42].

Putting together all these data, it appears the number of effective therapeutic options before transplant is significantly growing in the field of MASH, mainly in patients with moderate fibrosis. Therefore, new guidelines are awaited to address therapeutic algorithms. This process will find subsequent application in the field of liver transplantation, where there are only few data. Siddiqui et al. recently showed promising data on saroglitazar, a dual peroxisome proliferator-associated receptor $\alpha/\gamma$ agonist, in a phase 2A, single-center, open-label, single-arm study involving transplant patients, who experienced an improvement of some biochemical and radiological parameters [43].

However, there are still several uncertainties: it remains to be understood which endpoints should be used in clinical trials (resolution/improvement of fibrosis at histology vs. composite endpoints comprising or not histology); the role of liver biopsy in the management of therapy and/or the space for liquid biopsy; the possibility of extracting more accurate prognostic information from histological sampling, with the new technologies available; the correct timing for starting therapy, in post-liver transplant setting [44–46]. Finally, special patient subgroups should not be forgotten, such as patients who develop MASH in pediatric age after liver transplantation, or those who present significant comorbidities (e.g., recurrence of underlying disease posttransplant with de-novo MASH superimposed), whose management will need to be based on specific research.

## 14.5 Management of Metabolic Complications Associated with MASH

### 14.5.1 Principles of Management

The management of MASH posttransplantation requires a proper treatment of the associated complications. Overweight and/or obesity, dyslipidemia, hypertension, and diabetes are the main therapeutic targets. Two preliminary aspects require attention before any treatment. First, the need for a network that allows, on the one hand, interaction with the General Practitioner, and on the other hand, a close collaboration with Dieticians, experts of metabolic complications within the Hospital. This allows for identification of those patients, who can be managed by the Transplant Hepatology together with the General Practitioner (both therapeutically and in terms of follow-up), or who may need to be referred to dedicated outpatient clinic (for example, following the failure of first- or second-line therapy) [6, 47, 48]. The second aspect concerns the peculiarity of the solid organ transplant patient, especially regarding immunosuppressive therapy. This involves not only the presence of drug-drug interactions, which are nowadays well known and easy to recognize, but also the potential combined effects on hepatic and/or extrahepatic (e.g., kidney) function between immunosuppressive therapy and novel drugs. For this reason, the management involving Transplant Hepatologists still finds justification.

### 14.5.2 Old and Novel Strategies for Weight Loss

The management of metabolic comorbidities after transplantation should always begin with **prevention**. Intervention to prevent weight gain may be more successful than weight loss attempts after weight gain has occurred. For this reason, such interventions should be planned even before transplantation and implemented in the posttransplant phase, based on the patient's outcome and characteristics. It is known that physical performance after transplantation cannot be similar for all patients, therefore a personalized recovery plan capable of identifying achievable goals should be tailored [49]. Physical activity appears to be effective to prevent weight gain, especially if supervised and performed for a sufficiently long period of time to improve physical performance parameters [50].

Once overweight/obesity has been developed, the combination of lifestyle, diet for weight loss are the first therapeutic options. A meta-analysis of intervention studies in non-transplanted patients showed that, for every 1 kg of weight loss by an individual with MASLD, there was a 0.8% reduction in hepatic steatosis, whereas a 5-kg weight loss was associated with a 5% reduction in steatosis. However, although the extent of weight loss was also associated with corresponding histological improvements in hepatic inflammation, ballooning and resolution of MASH, there was limited evidence of a dose-dependent benefit of weight loss on hepatic fibrosis [51]. These findings support the notion that there is a dose-dependent association between the amount of weight loss and the extent of improvements in MASLD [52].

The current guidelines recommend the Mediterranean diet as the cornerstone of dietary management for MASLD patients [53]. Additionally, energy restriction and the exclusion of processed foods, fructose-enriched foods, and beverages are also advised. A Dietitian can provide further guidance in implementing these dietary recommendations.

Regarding pharmacological interventions, orlistat (a reversible inhibitor of gastric and pancreatic lipase) has been used in the postoperative setting in a small cohort of patients, without providing significant improvement in body weight [54]. Phentermine (a hypothalamic adrenergic agonist which stimulates decreased appetite and increased resting energy expenditure) in combination with topiramate (an anti-epileptic medication that increases satiety), or naltrexone-bupropion are two combinations of drugs approved for weight loss. However, no data are currently published in the liver transplant setting. Conversely, warnings about potential liver-related injuries have been raised, therefore their use should be carefully weighed [55].

Interesting data have been published on liraglutide, a glucagon-like peptide 1 analogue which increases glucose-dependent insulin secretion and decreases inappropriate glucagon secretion. A preliminary study on 17 kidney transplant patients found no significant weight loss in diabetic recipients with 1 year of liraglutide use, although there was a reduction in insulin requirement [56]. This molecule provided, in a small cohort of liver transplant recipients, with a higher weight loss than patients who received other anti-obesity medications [57]. A similar amount of weight loss (8.4% weight reduction at 12 months) has been achieved in a small cohort of transplanted patients who received semaglutide, without significant side effects [58]. However, multiple aspects need clarification, including the correct patient target and timing of initiation of such therapy after-transplant; the possible protective effect of such drugs on renal function and on the development of cardiovascular events; the possibility in the future of extending their use beyond diabetes; the best combination between such therapies and non-pharmacological therapies.

The role of bariatric surgery in weight loss is well established, as are the strong indications for surgery in non-transplanted obese patients. In the liver transplant setting, however, the field appears to be more heterogeneous. The study by Heimbach et al., in 2013 highlighted the effectiveness in terms of weight loss and the safety of simultaneous bariatric surgery with liver transplantation [59]. Many other centers then started a bariatric program associated with liver transplantation, especially in countries like the USA where the prevalence of MASLD is high. A recent international survey has shown significant heterogeneity among centers regarding the timing of bariatric surgery (pre- vs. during- vs. post-transplant), the interval between transplantation and bariatric surgery, and the type of surgical intervention [60]. In general, data on simultaneous bariatric surgery with liver transplantation (or in close proximity to it, as proposed by Tariq et al. [61]) confirm the safety of such procedures, which should be proposed only at high-level Expert Centers.

Bariatric surgery in individuals who develop morbid obesity long after transplantation should be considered too, especially if there are no significant improvements after medical therapy. A retrospective series from France described the outcome of 14 patients who underwent bariatric surgery 5 years after transplantation, with significant weight loss in a large percentage of patients [62]. A recent systematic review collected case reports that described bariatric surgery after transplantation: no significant information can be drawn given the heterogeneity among studies and the low sample size [63]. In this context, careful preoperative anesthesiologic evaluation is warranted, as these patients are getting old and typically develop cardiovascular comorbidities. Studies capable of demonstrating the efficacy of bariatric surgery as a treatment for recurrent or de novo MASLD after liver transplantation are still awaited.

## 14.6 Treatment of Metabolic Complications After Liver Transplantation: What's New?

Metabolic complications are the cornerstone of the development of posttransplant MAFLD, alongside weight gain. There are two main pathways in the management of these comorbidities in the liver transplant setting. The first is a wise minimization over time of immunosuppressive therapy, through a judicious use of therapeutic protocols tailored to the patient's characteristics. Recent studies have, for example, demonstrated the usefulness and effectiveness of therapy with everolimus in the early posttransplant phase, successfully mitigating the risk of side effects associated with high doses of tacrolimus [64]. Similarly, a steroid-free immunosuppressive strategy appears effective in selected patients without immunological issues nor previous autoimmune hepatitis in preventing metabolic complications.

The second approach is the need to aggressively prevent and manage at the earliest these metabolic complications, through new and potent pharmacological strategies. This can be carried out in selected cases and in collaboration with Expert Physicians. Two interesting examples concern diabetes and hypercholesterolemia.

Progress in the treatment of diabetes has been achieved in recent years with novel, effective, and safe drugs. A recently published review proposed a step-up approach, where insulin was considered exclusively as the last step, preferring the new glucose-lowering drugs such as dipeptidyl peptidase-4 inhibitors and glucagon-like peptide-1 receptor agonists [65]. This is also in relation to the cardioprotective effect of these novel molecules, now extensively reported both in the non-transplanted population and in solid organ transplant recipients as well, where the incidence of major adverse cardiovascular events was reduced [66].

Regarding hypercholesterolemia, although the pleiotropic properties of statins are recognized in both pre- and posttransplant settings [67], they can cause hypertransaminasemia and/or other side effects. In this regard, the possibility of using the new Proprotein Convertase Subtilisin Kexin Type 9 inhibitors will be a strategy to explore in selected cases, as already done in patients undergoing other solid organ transplants [68].

In conclusion, the treatment of metabolic complications post-liver transplantation appears standardized and well-defined. Increasing therapeutic advancements will lead to further updates, with the potential for increasingly tailored therapy, as evidence in liver transplantation becomes available.

## References


1. Younossi ZM, Stepanova M, Ong J, et al. Nonalcoholic steatohepatitis is the Most rapidly increasing indication for liver transplantation in the United States. Clin Gastroenterol Hepatol. 2021;19:580–589.e5.
2. Ferrarese A, Battistella S, Germani G, et al. Nash up, virus down: how the waiting list is changing for liver transplantation: a single center experience from Italy. Medicina (Kaunas). 2022;58:290.
3. Rinella ME, Lazarus JV, Ratziu V, et al. A multisociety Delphi consensus statement on new fatty liver disease nomenclature. Hepatology. 2023;78:1966–86.
4. Mendez-Sanchez N, Arrese M, Gadano A, et al. The Latin American Association for the Study of the Liver (ALEH) position statement on the redefinition of fatty liver disease. Lancet Gastroenterol Hepatol. 2021;6:65–72.
5. Eslam M, Newsome PN, Sarin SK, et al. A new definition for metabolic dysfunction-associated fatty liver disease: an international expert consensus statement. J Hepatol. 2020;73:202–9.
6. Germani G, Laryea M, Rubbia-Brandt L, et al. Management of recurrent and de novo NAFLD/NASH after liver transplantation. Transplantation. 2019;103:57–67.
7. Russ KB, Chen NW, Kamath PS, et al. Alcohol use after liver transplantation is independent of liver disease etiology. Alcohol Alcohol. 2016;51:698–701.
8. Saeed N, Glass L, Sharma P, et al. Incidence and risks for nonalcoholic fatty liver disease and steatohepatitis post-liver transplant: systematic review and meta-analysis. Transplantation. 2019;103:e345–54.
9. Villeret F, Dharancy S, Erard D, et al. Inevitability of disease recurrence after liver transplantation for NAFLD cirrhosis. JHEP Rep. 2023;5:100668.
10. Bhati C, Idowu MO, Sanyal AJ, et al. Long-term outcomes in patients undergoing liver transplantation for nonalcoholic steatohepatitis-related cirrhosis. Transplantation. 2017;101:1867–74.
11. Fussner LA, Heimbach JK, Fan C, et al. Cardiovascular disease after liver transplantation: when, what, and who is at risk. Liver Transpl. 2015;21:889–96.
12. Watt KD. Metabolic syndrome: is immunosuppression to blame? Liver Transpl. 2011;17(Suppl 3):S38–42.
13. Hüsing A, Kabar I, Schmidt HH. Lipids in liver transplant recipients. World J Gastroenterol. 2016;22:3315–24.
14. Park J, Lee SH, Han S, et al. An observational study on the effect of hypercholesterolemia developed after living donor liver transplantation on cardiac event and graft failure. Sci Rep. 2021;11:959.

15. Jang YS, Joo HJ, Park YS, et al. Association between smoking cessation and non-alcoholic fatty liver disease using NAFLD liver fat score. Front Public Health. 2023;11:1015919.
16. Becchetti C, Ferrarese A, Zeni N, et al. A prospective longitudinal assessment of de novo metabolic syndrome after liver transplantation. Clin Transpl. 2022;36:e14532.
17. Laish I, Braun M, Mor E, et al. Metabolic syndrome in liver transplant recipients: prevalence, risk factors, and association with cardiovascular events. Liver Transpl. 2011;17:15–22.
18. Galvin Z, Rajakumar R, Chen E, et al. Predictors of de novo nonalcoholic fatty liver disease after liver transplantation and associated fibrosis. Liver Transpl. 2019;25:56–67.
19. Neuberger JM, Mamelok RD, Neuhaus P, et al. Delayed introduction of reduced-dose tacrolimus, and renal function in liver transplantation: the 'ReSpECT' study. Am J Transplant. 2009;9:327–36.
20. Kurdi A, Martinet W, De Meyer GRY. mTOR inhibition and cardiovascular diseases: dyslipidemia and atherosclerosis. Transplantation. 2018;102:S44–6.
21. DiStefano JK. NAFLD and NASH in postmenopausal women: implications for diagnosis and treatment. Endocrinology. 2020;161:bqaa134.
22. Míková I, Neřoldová M, Hubáček JA, et al. Donor PNPLA3 and TM6SF2 variant alleles confer additive risks for graft steatosis after liver transplantation. Transplantation. 2020;104:526–34.
23. Eshraghian A, Moasser E, Azarpira N, et al. Variations in TM6SF2, PCSK9 and PCSK7 genes and risk of hepatic steatosis after liver transplantation: a cross-sectional study. BMC Gastroenterol. 2021;21:458.
24. Lee JH, Kim D, Kim HJ, et al. Hepatic steatosis index: a simple screening tool reflecting nonalcoholic fatty liver disease. Dig Liver Dis. 2010;42:503–8.
25. Bedogni G, Bellentani S, Miglioli L, et al. The Fatty Liver Index: a simple and accurate predictor of hepatic steatosis in the general population. BMC Gastroenterol. 2006;6:33.
26. Pu K, Wang Y, Bai S, et al. Diagnostic accuracy of controlled attenuation parameter (CAP) as a non-invasive test for steatosis in suspected non-alcoholic fatty liver disease: a systematic review and meta-analysis. BMC Gastroenterol. 2019;19:51.
27. Chayanupatkul M, Dasani DB, Sogaard K, et al. The utility of assessing liver allograft fibrosis and steatosis post-liver transplantation using transient elastography with controlled attenuation parameter. Transplant Proc. 2021;53:159–65.
28. Karlas T, Kollmeier J, Böhm S, et al. Noninvasive characterization of graft steatosis after liver transplantation. Scand J Gastroenterol. 2015;50:224–32.
29. Mak LY, Chan AC, Wong TC, et al. High prevalence of de novo metabolic dysfunction-associated fatty liver disease after liver transplantation and the role of controlled attenuation parameter. BMC Gastroenterol. 2023;23:307.
30. van Werven JR, Marsman HA, Nederveen AJ, et al. Assessment of hepatic steatosis in patients undergoing liver resection: comparison of US, CT, T1-weighted dual-echo MR imaging, and point-resolved 1H MR spectroscopy. Radiology. 2010;256:159–68.
31. EAftSotLEa easloffice@easloffice.eu, Panel CPG, Chair, et al. EASL Clinical Practice Guidelines on non-invasive tests for evaluation of liver disease severity and prognosis - 2021 update. J Hepatol. 2021;75:659–89.
32. Bhat M, Tazari M, Sebastiani G. Performance of transient elastography and serum fibrosis biomarkers for non-invasive evaluation of recurrent fibrosis after liver transplantation: a meta-analysis. PLoS One. 2017;12:e0185192.
33. Liang JX, Ampuero J, Niu H, et al. An individual patient data meta-analysis to determine cut-offs for and confounders of NAFLD-fibrosis staging with magnetic resonance elastography. J Hepatol. 2023;79:592–604.
34. Sanyal AJ, Chalasani N, Kowdley KV, et al. Pioglitazone, vitamin E, or placebo for nonalcoholic steatohepatitis. N Engl J Med. 2010;362:1675–85.
35. Belfort R, Harrison SA, Brown K, et al. A placebo-controlled trial of pioglitazone in subjects with nonalcoholic steatohepatitis. N Engl J Med. 2006;355:2297–307.
36. Friedman SL, Neuschwander-Tetri BA, Rinella M, et al. Mechanisms of NAFLD development and therapeutic strategies. Nat Med. 2018;24:908–22.
37. Latva-Rasku A, Honka MJ, Kullberg J, et al. The SGLT2 inhibitor dapagliflozin reduces liver fat but does not affect tissue insulin sensitivity: a randomized, double-blind, placebo-controlled study with 8-week treatment in type 2 diabetes patients. Diabetes Care. 2019;42:931–7.
38. Newsome PN, Buchholtz K, Cusi K, et al. A placebo-controlled trial of subcutaneous semaglutide in nonalcoholic steatohepatitis. N Engl J Med. 2021;384:1113–24.
39. Armstrong MJ, Gaunt P, Aithal GP, et al. Liraglutide safety and efficacy in patients with non-alcoholic steatohepatitis (LEAN): a multicentre, double-blind, randomised, placebo-controlled phase 2 study. Lancet. 2016;387:679–90.
40. Jastreboff AM, Aronne LJ, Ahmad NN, et al. Tirzepatide once weekly for the treatment of obesity. N Engl J Med. 2022;387:205–16.
41. Harrison SA, Bedossa P, Guy CD, et al. A phase 3, randomized, controlled trial of resmetirom in NASH with liver fibrosis. N Engl J Med. 2024;390:497–509.
42. Loomba R, Sanyal AJ, Kowdley KV, et al. Randomized, controlled trial of the FGF21 analogue pegozafermin in NASH. N Engl J Med. 2023;389:998–1008.
43. Siddiqui MS, Parmar D, Shaikh F, et al. Saroglitazar improves nonalcoholic fatty liver disease and metabolic health in liver transplant recipients. Liver Transpl. 2023;29:979–86.
44. Angelini G, Panunzi S, Castagneto-Gissey L, et al. Accurate liquid biopsy for the diagnosis of non-

alcoholic steatohepatitis and liver fibrosis. Gut. 2023;72:392–403.
45. Wood-Trageser MA, Lesniak AJ, Demetris AJ. Enhancing the value of histopathological assessment of allograft biopsy monitoring. Transplantation. 2019;103:1306–22.
46. Siddiqui MS, Muthiah M, Satapathy SK, et al. Defining an approach for therapeutic strategies in metabolic dysfunction-associated steatotic liver disease after liver transplantation. Hepatology. 2023;
47. Burra P, Becchetti C, Germani G. NAFLD and liver transplantation: disease burden, current management and future challenges. JHEP Rep. 2020;2:100192.
48. Toniutto P, Germani G, Ferrarese A, et al. An essential guide for managing post-liver transplant patients: what primary care physicians should know. Am J Med. 2022;135:157–66.
49. Dunn MA, Rogal SS, Duarte-Rojo A, et al. Physical function, physical activity, and quality of life after liver transplantation. Liver Transpl. 2020;26:702–8.
50. Totti V, Tamè M, Burra P, et al. Physical condition, glycemia, liver function, and quality of life in liver transplant recipients after a 12-month supervised exercise program. Transplant Proc. 2019;51:2952–7.
51. Koutoukidis DA, Koshiaris C, Henry JA, et al. The effect of the magnitude of weight loss on non-alcoholic fatty liver disease: a systematic review and meta-analysis. Metabolism. 2021;115:154455.
52. Lonardo A, Mantovani A, Petta S, et al. Metabolic mechanisms for and treatment of NAFLD or NASH occurring after liver transplantation. Nat Rev Endocrinol. 2022;18:638–50.
53. (EASL) EAftSotL, (EASD) EAftSoD, (EASO) EAftSoO. EASL-EASD-EASO clinical practice guidelines for the management of non-alcoholic fatty liver disease. J Hepatol. 2016;64:1388–402.
54. Cassiman D, Roelants M, Vandenplas G, et al. Orlistat treatment is safe in overweight and obese liver transplant recipients: a prospective, open label trial. Transpl Int. 2006;19:1000–5.
55. Brown SA, Izzy M, Watt KD. Pharmacotherapy for weight loss in cirrhosis and liver transplantation: translating the data and underused potential. Hepatology. 2021;73:2051–62.
56. Kukla A, Hill J, Merzkani M, et al. The use of GLP1R agonists for the treatment of type 2 diabetes in kidney transplant recipients. Transplant Direct. 2020;6:e524.
57. Richardson SH, Wong G, Garner E, et al. Utility of glucagon-like peptide 1 receptor agonists as anti-obesity medications in liver transplant recipients. Liver Transpl. 2024;30:226–8.
58. Chow KW, Ibrahim B, Rahal K, et al. Semaglutide is effective in achieving weight loss in liver transplant recipients. Liver Transpl. 2024;30:223–5.
59. Heimbach JK, Watt KD, Poterucha JJ, et al. Combined liver transplantation and gastric sleeve resection for patients with medically complicated obesity and end-stage liver disease. Am J Transplant. 2013;13:363–8.
60. Widmer J, Eden J, Abbassi F, et al. How best to combine liver transplantation and bariatric surgery?-results from a global, web-based survey. Liver Int. 2024;44:566–76.
61. Tariq N, Saharia A, Nwokedi U, et al. Combined liver transplantation and sleeve gastrectomy: report of a brief-interval staged approach. Liver Transpl. 2023;29:422–30.
62. Dumortier J, Erard D, Villeret F, et al. Bariatric surgery and liver transplantation, here we are now: a French nationwide retrospective study. Clin Res Hepatol Gastroenterol. 2023;47:102164.
63. de Barros F, Uba CF, PH. Liver transplantation and bariatric surgery: a new surgical reality: a systematic review of the best time for bariatric surgery. Updat Surg. 2021;73:1615–22.
64. Cholongitas E, Burra P, Vourli G, et al. Safety and efficacy of everolimus initiation from the first month after liver transplantation: a systematic review and meta-analysis. Clin Transpl. 2023;37:e14957.
65. Brodosi L, Petta S, Petroni ML, et al. Management of Diabetes in candidates for liver transplantation and in transplant recipients. Transplantation. 2022;106:462–78.
66. Dotan I, Rudman Y, Turjeman A, et al. Glucagon-like peptide 1 receptor agonists and cardiovascular outcomes in solid organ transplant recipients with diabetes mellitus. Transplantation. 2024;108:e121.
67. Becchetti C, Dirchwolf M, Schropp J, et al. Use of statins after liver transplantation is associated with improved survival: results of a nationwide study. Aliment Pharmacol Ther. 2022;56:1194–204.
68. Jennings DL, Sultan L, Mingov J, et al. PCSK9 inhibitors safely and effectively lower LDL after heart transplantation: a systematic review and meta-analysis. Heart Fail Rev. 2023;28:149–56.

MIX
Papier aus verantwortungsvollen Quellen
Paper from responsible sources
FSC® C105338

If you have any concerns about our products, you can contact us on
**ProductSafety@springernature.com**

In case Publisher is established outside the EU, the EU authorized representative is:
**Springer Nature Customer Service Center GmbH**
**Europaplatz 3, 69115 Heidelberg, Germany**

Printed by Libri Plureos GmbH
in Hamburg, Germany